SOURCEBOOK OF
MEDICAL COMMUNICATION

ROBERT C. REEDER, M.D., F.A.C.S.

Clinical Associate Professor of Plastic Surgery, University of Tennessee
Center for the Health Sciences; Chief, Plastic Surgery Service,
Baptist Memorial Hospital, Memphis, Tennessee

with 421 illustrations

The C. V. Mosby Company

ST. LOUIS • TORONTO • LONDON   1981

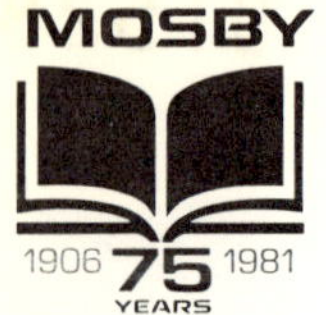

MOSBY
1906 **75** 1981
YEARS

A TRADITION OF PUBLISHING EXCELLENCE

Editor: Karen Berger
Manuscript editor: Nelle Garrecht
Design: Susan Trail
Production: Jeanne Gulledge

Copyright © 1981 by The C.V. Mosby Company

All rights reserved. No part of this book may be reproduced in any manner without written permission of the publisher.

Printed in the United States of America

The C.V. Mosby Company
11830 Westline Industrial Drive, St. Louis, Missouri 63141

Library of Congress Cataloging in Publication Data

Main entry under title:

Sourcebook of medical communication.

   "Result of a symposium . . . sponsored by the Educational Foundation of the American Society of Plastic and Reconstructive Surgeons"—Pref.
   Bibliography: p.
   Includes index.
   1.   Communication in medicine.   I.   Reeder, Robert C.
II.   American Society of Plastic and Reconstructive Surgeons.   Educational Foundation.
R118.S63   610'.141   81-2089
ISBN 0-8016-4177-2   AACR2

AC/M/M   9 8 7 6 5 4 3 2 1   03/A/299

Contributors

EARL BAUER

President, Bauer Audio-Video, Inc., Dallas, Texas

KAREN BERGER

Editor, Medical/Dental Division, The C.V. Mosby Company, St. Louis, Missouri

LINDA CAMPBELL

Director, Department of Meetings Management and Communications, American Society of Plastic and Reconstructive Surgeons, Inc., Chicago, Illinois

JOEL W. COLE

Account Executive AGS&R Studios, Incorporated, Chicago, Illinois

ROBERT M. GOLDWYN, M.D.

Clinical Professor of Surgery, Harvard Medical School; Editor, *Plastic and Reconstructive Surgery*

RICHARD A. HEIMBURGER, M.D., F.A.C.S.

Consulting Plastic Surgeon, Department of Corrections, Jefferson City, Missouri; Active Staff, Columbia Midwest Regional Hospital and Boone County Hospital; formerly Associate Professor, Chief of Plastic Surgery, University of Missouri Medical Center, Columbia, Missouri

NORMAN E. HUGO, M.D.

Associate Professor, Surgery, Northwestern University–McGaw Medical Center, Chicago, Illinois

JEROME KLINGBEIL, M.D.

Associate Clinical Professor of Surgery (Plastic), University of California School of Medicine, Irvine, California

THOMAS J. KRIZEK, M.D.

Professor of Surgery, College of Physicians and Surgeons of Columbia University, and Chief, Division of Plastic and Reconstructive Surgery, Columbia–Presbyterian Medical Center, New York, New York

DENIS C. LEE, M.D.

Associate Professor of Art and Postgraduate Medicine; Assistant Professor of Plastic Surgery; Director of Services, Medical and Biological Illustration Unit; Director of Medical Sculpture, Department of Medical Illustration and Sculpture, University of Michigan, Ann Arbor, Michigan

JOEL MATTISON, M.D., F.A.C.S.

Clinical Professor of Surgery (Plastic Surgery), Department of Surgery, University of South Florida, Tampa, Florida

MARY MENDELOWITZ

Formerly Assistant Executive Vice-President, American Society of Plastic and Reconstructive Surgeons, Inc., Chicago, Illinois

STEPHEN H. MILLER, M.D.

Professor of Surgery, Chief of Plastic and Reconstructive Surgery, Department of Surgery, University of Oregon Health Sciences Center, Portland, Oregon

RICHARD MLADICK, M.D.

Professor, Department of Plastic Surgery, Eastern Virginia Medical School, Norfolk, Virginia

ROSS MUSGRAVE, M.D., Sc.D., F.A.C.S.

Clinical Professor of Surgery (Plastic), University of Pittsburgh School of Medicine, Pittsburgh, Pennsylvania; Past President, American Society of Plastic and Reconstructive Surgeons, Inc.

ROBERT W. PARSONS, M.D.

Associate Professor of Surgery and Pediatrics, Section of Plastic Surgery, The University of Chicago, Chicago, Illinois

SHELDON PHILLIPS

Coordinator, Scientific and Technical Photography, Customer Technical Service, Professional and Finishing Markets Division, Eastman Kodak Company, Rochester, New York

LINDA PORTERFIELD

Managing Editor, *Plastic Surgery News*, American Society
of Plastic and Reconstructive Surgeons, Inc.;
formerly Executive Editor and Executive Business Manager,
The Ohio State Medical Journal, Ohio State
Medical Association, Columbus, Ohio

ROBERT C. REEDER, M.D., F.A.C.S.

Clinical Associate Professor of Plastic Surgery,
University of Tennessee Center for the Health Sciences;
Chief, Plastic Surgery Service, Baptist Memorial Hospital,
Memphis, Tennessee

MARTIN C. ROBSON, M.D.

Professor of Surgery and Chief of Plastic and
Reconstructive Surgery, Department of Surgery,
University of Chicago, Chicago, Illinois

MELVIN SPIRA, M.D., D.D.S.

Professor and Head, Division of Plastic Surgery,
Cora and Webb Mading Department of Surgery,
Baylor College of Medicine, Houston, Texas

KATHRYN L. STEPHENSON, M.D.

Former Editor, *Plastic and Reconstructive Surgery*

HALE TOLLETH, M.D., F.A.C.S.

Assistant Clinical Professor of Plastic Surgery,
Stanford University School of Medicine; Instructor in
Plastic Surgery, University of California at Davis,
California; Clinical Adjunct, Plastic and Reconstructive
Surgery Center, St. Francis Memorial Hospital,
San Francisco, California

CHARLES R. VAN WINKLE

Vice-President, General Manager, Med-Video,
New York, New York

RICHARD WARREN, M.D.

Professor of Surgery Emeritus, Harvard Medical School,
Boston, Massachusetts; former Editor, *Archives of Surgery*

PEGGY WILLIAMSON

Medical Illustrator, Carefree, Arizona

Preface

Sidney Bailey drives a taxicab in Memphis. Often he entertains his passengers with quotes, limericks, and one-liners. The response to this has been so good that he decided to write a book of taxicab humor. He soon found, however, that his ninth grade education did not prepare him for such a venture, so he went to night school and completed his high school education. More importantly, he obtained a number of books about basic grammar, composition, and word usage which he keeps in his cab and studies between fares. He explains his philosophy thus: "Just talking to people everyday is okay. But when you try to write English you have to be exact about it. So I try to write intelligently and to learn the things you need to know to do that."

All of us can take a lesson from Mr. Bailey. Too often when we have something important to say we do not take the time or effort to learn how to say it properly. Just as none of us has the innate ability to repair a cleft lip, remove an appendix, or recognize the murmur of aortic stenosis, neither are we born with the ability to write or speak intelligibly. These skills, like the medical ones, are learned by study and repeated practice.

Sourcebook of Medical Communication is not intended to be the all-knowing beginning and end of scientific communication. It is, rather, a collection of basic communicative skills and ideas that will, hopefully, pique your interest and provide a starting point for study and honing of your communications skills.

This book is the result of a symposium on medical communications sponsored by the Educational Foundation of the American Society of Plastic and Reconstructive Surgeons. When the collected papers were gathered for publication, it was apparent that not all aspects of this important subject had been covered in the symposium, so additional manuscripts were solicited to fill the gaps. The authors of these are due a special thanks, since it was often necessary to impose short deadlines for the submission of the manuscripts.

Profound gratitude is due my long-suffering secretary, Bonnie Seitz, who uncomplainingly typed and retyped the many manuscripts; to my partners, Allen Hughes and Thad Ferrell, who made it possible for her to do so; and to the quintessence of medical editors, Karen Berger, of The C. V. Mosby Company, who not only shepherded this project through its inception and growth but who also contributed a most important chapter. Finally, I wish to thank my devoted wife, Billie Dean, who endured days, weekends, and nights of preparation of this volume. Her counsel and patience have made it all possible.

I leave you with this advice which, if not original, is apropos: "If you would be a writer, write; if you would be a speaker, speak." Use every opportunity to communicate more effectively, whether it be dictating an operative report, writing a progress note, or making a presentation on teaching rounds. Learn the basics and hone your skills. Then when you have something of value to say you will know how to say it properly and you can say it in a way that will never be dull and with the assurance that it will be welcomed by your colleagues.

Robert C. Reeder

Contents

SECTION I

Writing

CHAPTER 1

Getting started

Kathryn L. Stephenson, M.D.

BEFORE A WORD IS WRITTEN
Determine your purpose

Journals purport to disseminate what is new, true, and important. For which of these reasons do you want to write? (1) Do you want to report an original investigation? (2) Do you want to confirm or criticize a new technique? (3) Have you rediscovered something that has new importance when combined with new information in the field? (4) Do you want to enhance your professional economic status? (5) When asked to write an article or paper are you unable to say "No" firmly?

Search the literature

After you have determined your purpose, the next step is to review the literature to obtain the information relative to the status of your proposed experiment or observations. To obtain the material most quickly and with the least trauma, see "Searching the Literature Comes before Writing the Literature" by William K. Beatty (see also Appendix A-1).

The main bibliography of medical literature after 1960 is the *Index Medicus*. Works published between 1952 and 1959 are listed in the *Current List of Medical Literature*. Recent information is more easily acquired with Medlars (Medical Literature Analysis and Retrieval System) based at the National Library of Medicine in Bethesda, Md. Medline provides direct access to the articles within a few minutes but is not available everywhere. However, when it can be used, it facilitates obtaining the essential information for beginning a study. There are other indices as well, and it is well worth reading the seven-page article by Beatty to determine which ones will best serve your purpose. Although the literature search may take weeks, it can save you months of experimentation or work on a problem previously investigated—and years of embarrassment if your publica-

tion would contain some gross oversight. You would be wise to ferret out the references yourself and not rely completely on a system or librarian.

OUTLINE THE INVESTIGATION

A logical outline does much to clarify thinking and is essential if you wish to convince an editor of the validity of your work. After outlining a proposed study, it might be well at this time to discuss it with a biostatistician to determine that all bases are covered with regard to procuring adequate data to be significant.

Select an audience

After the data are acquired and the results are known, the next step is to determine who will be interested in the study. At this time you can select the specific journal in which you aspire to publish and get its guidelines for authors.

The reader's degree of sophistication in the field will determine both what material should be included and how much explanation is appropriate. One physician tells of spending months working on a paper on the parotid gland and presenting it to a colleague for approval. After reading the article his colleague said, "Earl, this may be all right for your friends but my friends know all this." What may seem fundamental for understanding for one audience may be insulting to another.

Determine the format of the article

The form a paper will take depends, of course, on the results of the study to be reported. Negative results warrant only a short paper and a summary of the findings. Perhaps a case report, a case report with a review of the literature, or even a preliminary report is appropriate. Regardless, it is necessary to check the material and put it into a comprehensive form. This is not easy, and you will go through many drafts of the paper. If possible, ask someone to read the draft to delete unnecessary words or phrases and to clarify ambiguities. DeBakey's book, *The Scientific Journal: Editorial Policies and Practices*, will be invaluable.

COMMON PITFALLS

A paper that lacks organization, adequate data to support the thesis, or verification to support the authors point of view will be rejected for publication. Likewise, if the discussion is not relevant, if the author fails to follow publication guidelines, or if the bibliography is inaccurate, the manuscript may well be rejected. If the manuscript is carelessly presented, the editor will suspect that the work reported was performed with equal carelessness.

The fact that a manuscript is accepted for publication does not mean that the author has avoided all of the problems common to many papers. Many of these problems arise because the author was motivated by something other than the desire to publish information that would help in the care of patients.

Consequences of "publish or perish"

What is a person's motivation for publishing and what are the consequences? One motivation is obvious: Some individuals' names are associated with particular procedures by virtue of repetition, although often it is not the originator but the popularizer of the procedure who becomes well known. Publishing is a good way to become known as an authority.

If dissemination of information were the only reason for writing, the number of papers published annually would be relatively constant. Perhaps the increase in numbers in recent years is the result of the "publish or perish" dicta. Healy has proposed a one-year moratorium on listing the names of individuals and institutions on papers published and then comparing the number of papers submitted during that year with the number submitted in preceding and subsequent years.

Duplication of material, credit and title padding, and "me-tooism" may all be symptoms of the publish or perish syndrome. Other problems include incomplete bibliographies and loading the text with jargon. Each of these problems is discussed briefly below.

Duplication of material. There is much in the various medical journals that does not merit publication. However, as P. L. Wilson notes, the affluence of some physicians and the fact that professional books are tax deductible are two reasons why established medical publishers increase their lists each year and why other publishers are either acquiring or developing medical divisions.

Because of this increase in the number of publications available, there is often duplication of material. This can be direct duplication, as occurred when an editorial appeared in one journal in one year and in a similar journal the following year. More common, perhaps, is duplication of the same information without any fundamental change of thesis. The same material is often published in slightly altered form in several journals. There are three journals on plastic surgery in the United States at present in addition to the British and Scandinavian journals, which are also published in English. Duplication here is inexcusable, since the audience for all of these journals is similar. However, if the same information is published in a different language or is addressed to a different audience, as, for example, articles on the same subject appearing in both a plastic surgery and a pediatric journal, there is no criticism.

Multiple authorship. I. M. Siegel's letter to the editor of the *Lancet*, entitled "Games Authors Play," is worth quoting in entirety in this regard:

The listing of faculty publications for the past year from one of our major medical centres reveals some interesting findings. The majority of papers had more than one author, most had more than two, and it was not uncommon to find four or even five colleagues sharing authorship. Giving credit where due is all to the good, but the bibliographies of several departments (reflecting this credit explosion) numbered five times more authors than papers!

Although such publications serve the "bibliographic needs" of each contributor (four or five rather than a mere one or two), it is sometimes difficult to tell which investigator deserves the most credit. There is little doubt who did the work where a single or only several writers are listed. In the case of the multi-authored treatise, it is sometimes (not always, but sometimes) the last-listed participants who really deserve the most mention.

Credit padding, especially the noblesse-oblige practice of placing a chief's name on every publication issuing from his department, unfairly decreases credit due those who did the work, demeans the office of department head, and seriously dilutes the value of having published.

Plurality of authorship represents a horizontal parley which slices the pie of publication, so many may share. It is often the case of the whole being less than its parts, for although a senior author is usually regarded as most important, some bibliographies do not stipulate shared authorship or, at best, indicate that the paper was written "with . . .".

Crafty as credit loading may be, it only encumbers a journal with names. Its vertical counterpart, title-multiplying, is more burdensome, as it gluts the literature with superfluous publications. It works like this. A study is designed, and as soon as early data is available, a preliminary report published. This establishes precedence, and the authors can then relax, but not for long. The possibility of someone publishing with evidence of earlier work or, worse yet, disproving the theory before it has been adequately proved, poses an imminent threat. Here begins a crash course toward the printers. Once a paper is published, vertical fragmentation can begin. A preliminary report and the major work are already in print. The title can now be reworded, a bit more data added, the format and phrasing slightly revised, the illustrations changed, and lo and behold the article is ready for republication in another journal. This can be repeated p.r.n. as tolerated by the literature. A review of the Indices Medicus reveals this tolerance to be high indeed. Mutants can even metastasise to a related literature. But like cellular metastasis, though superficially distinct, the marks of their parentage are revealed upon close scrutiny.

Finally, any controversial subject may provoke correspondence and reply in a journal's letters department (more credits), and another study (follow-up review) is usually feasible a year or so after initial publication.

At least quintuplet mutations are possible from a well conceived paper: (1) preliminary report which submits limited data and reaches tentative conclusions; (2) major paper presenting bulk of data and confirming tentative conclusions; (3) similar paper(s) elsewhere in the literature (new title, different format, additional data, same conclusions); (4) article(s) in related literature applying thesis and data in different context, same conclusions; (5) review article (a rewording or summary of 1, 2, 3, and 4 above).

Well, if the base is one (paper), and the horizontal credit loading component five (authors), and the vertical fragmentation factor five (mutations), it follows that the product of this publication parley is $(1 \times 5 \times 5)$ or twenty-five credits!

It was John Ryle who, in the foreword to his *Fears May be Liars*, so aptly stated: "Although our instruction, as well as our destruction, now comes from the air, the written word still has its little part to play."*

"Me-too" papers. Another type of paper often submitted for publication is the "me-too" paper. A surgeon, for example, publishes a paper (with or without merit), but if it is a real *tour de force* it is certain to generate many papers. Other surgeons desiring to display their virtuosity publish on the same subject as soon as they can collect a few cases to justify the publication by some inconsequential modification. They ignore Gertrude Stein's statement that, "A difference to be a difference must make a difference." Again, the motivation is not to inform but to obtain professional stature—another result of "publish or perish."

In some instances the consequence of me-tooism may lead to medical disaster. With the publication of many papers on one subject a vogue is established. To recall a few: hemipelvectomy for the individual melanoma, the radical en bloc or "commando" procedure for the patient with oral malignancies, and the immediate alveolar graft for the newborn with a cleft palate defect.

Incomplete bibliography

The bibliography must be accurate. Otherwise, it leads to frustration for the reader who wishes to check material from a preceding paper. Limiting the bibliog-

raphy to previous papers by yourself, no matter how relevant, is certainly not scholarly. In college the name of the game was to *not* quote the work from which most of the material was taken for a term paper. This tactic has no place in medicine. Since many readers may well be familiar with the various sources, they should be credited at the outset. Many authors are also guilty of not reading the original work and thus perpetuating misquotation and misinterpretation for many years.

It is remarkable that many authors think they have made an adequate search of the literature if they have reviewed the past ten years. This leads to unjustified claims of originality or priority. "Priority," according to DeBakey, depends upon the date of publication. Journal editors keep a record of the date the paper was received in their office. However, for legal reasons they will not be responsible for assessing priority. Every author should keep his or her own dated record of conception and completion of the work.

Jargon: "Medispeak"

King is of the opinion that every medical journal, even specialty journals, should be intelligible to third-year medical students. Jargon often is so ambiguous as to be meaningless. Do you pull the pants up or the vest down in the "vest-over-pants" procedure? To one author the procedure is the former, to another it is the latter, and for the reader the term may be cute but confusing. Medical literature is replete with jargon and vogue words. Young and Tilney, in a letter to the editor of the *New England Journal of Medicine*, wrote about "Medispeak," making this point with regard to the spoken word. It is not limited to the spoken word but is recurrent in the medical literature:

The language of medicine was once Latin. Then, in the interests of clarity it became English. Now, a separate language has appeared: "Medispeak." Medispeak is the language of case presentations and of medical and scientific lectures. For those who have difficulty understanding it we offer the following observations on construction:

At this point in time we have learned from sequential interfacing with science-oriented personnel that there is usually a positive feasibility for using the language of computers. When the potential for this integration is inoperative, then the significant parameters of mathematic jargon can be factored into the idea track as an alternative semantic modality.

One should, wherever possible, sanctify the mundane with sociologic suffixes. It is more valuable to have a learning experience than to learn, and a positive interactive ongoing interpersonal relationship is more satisfying than friendship.

We must remember that nouns have weight and that language, like a hamburger, is to be judged by its weight. We should not, therefore, have patients but "a patient population," not time but "a time course," and not a crisis but "a crisis situation."

---

*Siegel, I. M.: Games authors play, Lancet 2(7831):733, Sept, 29, 1973. Reprinted by permission.

We must also remember never to refer to the body simply. Our patients do not breathe—they have a "respiratory status"; they are clothed not in skin but an "integumentary apparatus"; they do not feed but "aliment"; they are not confused but have a "clouded sensorium with decreased mental status"; they do not walk, they "ambulate"; they do not die but merely reach "the terminal event".

In addition to obfuscating experiential realities we can with "Medispeak" enhance the importance of our activities. Technologists are more clever than technicians. A "critical overview" is so much more "significant" than a mere opinion. "Therapeusis" works better than treatment and a "misadventure" is less reprehensible than a mistake.*

RESPONSIBILITIES OF A JOURNAL EDITOR

An editor's life is not an easy one. He or she does not simply have to keep the paper circulating to the board and compose the publication. The editor must also decide which of the board members is best suited to review a manuscript and evaluate the several reviews, which

---

*Young, A. E., and Tilney, N. L.: "Medispeak" (letter to the editor), New Engl. J. Med. 19(17):1011, 1977. Reprinted by permission.

may differ considerably. He or she must screen the material for possible legal problems, compose the budget, and cope with the publishers. Publishers are in business to make money, and wide circulation is important in acquiring advertisers who are essential for financial support. If international distribution is desirable the editor may be faced with accepting an inferior paper from a foreign contributor.

CONCLUSION

Do not be discouraged if you get a refusal from the journal, but as in all experiences in life, profit by it. Often editors will indicate why the paper was refused and perhaps with further work you can make it acceptable. After answering "What did I do, what did I find, what does it mean?" you should write the results in a comprehensible form so that we all can share them and take better care of our patients.

The notes found in Appendix A-2 are not an attempt to replace any of the accepted texts on manuscript preparation, but they should be of some help in getting started.

CHAPTER 2

The rough draft

Robert M. Goldwyn, M.D.

OBSTACLES TO BEGINNING THE DRAFT

For most writers the first draft is the most difficult because it involves thinking something different and doing something new. To overcome the inertia of habit and to break, even temporarily, with the familiar require courage and concentration, two indispensable qualities of a good writer (or any good professional). If, indeed, the author does not feel the exertion, then what he or she is writing is probably not worth reading.

Inexperience as an author is an obvious deterrent to doing the first draft. More important is lack of something worth communicating. "Another meeting, another paper" is the all-too-familiar sequence. Junior staff and residents are mustered and someone is conscripted to review a disease and treatment that have already been well reported. With remarkable parochialism the decision is to commit duplication, the rationale being that "our patients have been better managed and our study will be the best." Perhaps but not likely. Whoever is to write the paper may be only mildly interested but assumes the burden in order to further his or her career. Absence of enthusiasm and staleness of the subject are inauspicious conditions for creative work. The project would best be aborted before it gains life through a first draft—before it grows into a dull presentation and a duller paper. Uninspired at its inception, it will be spiritless at its delivery.

Other considerations that may impede the execution of a first draft concern authorship. Frequently, would-be writers are in conflict. Although they had the idea and did the work, they will be either listed as junior authors or, if lucky, the first co-author with the chief of the service or the head of the laboratory, whose presence on the paper will be due less to intellectual contributions to the project than to his or her financial support and status. The young author may justifiably resent acquiescing to the rules of academe. A sign of this institutionalized "me-tooism" is the unbridled multiple authorship of today.

Pertinent are the observations of Asher: "Six people can no more write an article than six people can drive a car. . . . Although heads of departments may provide inspiration, encouragement, and example, surely it is better to reward them with a polite acknowledgement at the end instead of a downright lie at the beginning."*

Therefore, at the outset clearly establish authorship. Will you be doing all the writing? If not, who will write what and how will the authors be listed? Settling these sticky points early prevents later acrimony and disappointment. Be certain that the paper you are planning is original and is not soon to be published. Aside from dishonesty, that strategy reflects the unwise ambition of an impoverished mind.

MECHANICS OF THE FIRST DRAFT

How does the first draft get done? Do you write it, type it yourself, or dictate it? There are almost as many ways of writing as there are writers. The important thing is not to get stalled in the first stage. As in learning a foreign language, it is better to speak with grammatical imperfections than to be so precise and careful that you become mute. My preference is to write a brief outline in longhand; then let it age a few days and to dictate what I consider a "proper" first draft (by no means the final draft). If you cannot do much on a particular day, stop and begin on another occasion. Hemingway advised writers to leave their desk when they still had something to say so they would not begin "cold" the next time. As bad as the first draft may be, it is better than blank paper.

---

*Asher, R.: Six honest serving men for medical writers, J.A.M.A. **208:** 83, 1969.

Composing the first draft is always easier if you know what you want to say and to whom. Will it be a case report, a review, or the report of an experiment? If it involved laboratory investigation, you should already know about previous work. If it is a case report, consult the *Index Medicus* before believing that you alone have witnessed this remarkable clinical event. If you have established that your case actually merits reporting (and is not the 104th case report following a review of the literature that appeared just two years ago) then it is important to scrutinize the journal to which you will submit your offering. Who and how many read it? Who are the editors? Are their standards high? How much lag time between the acceptance of an article and its publication? Since each journal has its own requirements, you will save much effort by following their guidelines for authors.

Choosing a title

Start the first draft by choosing a title that will reflect the content of your paper and entice both editor and reader. The title should not be ambiguous or cumbersome. Commenting on a title of excessive length, Dr. Morris Fishbein, late editor of the *Journal of the American Medical Association*, asked: "With that title, why write a paper?"

Parts of the article

Introduction. The introduction should be only two or three paragraphs and should contain the purpose and scope of the paper. Allude briefly to previous publications so that the reader will be aware of the importance of the article. Later, in the discussion, you will have the opportunity to expand on past relevant studies.

Remember that a busy editor may never go beyond a tedious introduction.

Material and methods. This section is usually next in a scientific paper. The advice of O'Connor and Woodford is pertinent:

Follow a logical order in describing the methods and provide enough details for an experienced investigator to repeat the experiments, or at least to assess the reliability of the methods and therefore the results. Often, the best order is chronological. . . . If you have used methods which are described elsewhere, it is pointless to give full details again; refer to a published text instead. Do, however, orientate the readers by stating the principle on which these methods are based, unless the methods are so well known that this would be naive.*

If you are reporting a clinical project, clarify for the reader whether it is prospective or retrospective, how the series of patients was obtained, and whether there is a control group (If so, what were the criteria for matching?).

Results. Helpful to the reader are results reported with some explanation of relevance and significance. Statistical analysis can be used if required but the tests employed should be stated. If tables are necessary they should be aids, not obstacles, to understanding.

Discussion. This section should recapitulate the essential findings. You may let your mind soar but if you speculate, label it such. Fit your work and observations into the greater whole to give the reader perspective. Cite the labors of others accurately, and if you criticize, be civil. Remember that you are authoring a scientific communication, not a polemic.

In the discussion, do not confuse the reader by suddenly presenting results that have not previously appeared in the paper.

Conclusion or summary. Depending upon the journal or the book, a summary and/or conclusions may be necessary. One is not the same as the other. A summary "does not pretend to general truth." It contains the gist and important findings of the article or chapter. It should be brief, not a humdrum rerun of the results. Conclusions are "statements of general truth established in the course of the work reported. . . . Conclusions are not warranted unless the work was conclusive."*

In either a summary or conclusion, never introduce concepts and data not given earlier in your article.

References. Admittedly, for the first draft, it would be best to have all references available and complete. The reality is usually different. To pause while writing the first draft in order to insert correct citations interrupts the creative tempo. Blanks can be left to be filled in later.

Abstract. Increasingly, journals are requiring abstracts for computerized storage and retrieval of information. For many journals the abstract has replaced the summary. A good abstract has features of both the summary and the conclusion. It is the marrow and soul of your paper. It is what you want others to retain when they have forgotten everything else.

Remember that the first draft is not the final version. You have just begun. To paraphrase George S. Kaufman: papers are not written, they are rewritten. The wastebasket is the writer's best friend.

---

*O'Connor, M., and Woodford, E. P.: Writing scientific papers in English. An ELSE—CIBA Foundation guide for authors, Amsterdam, 1975, Associated Scientific Publishers.

*Hewitt, R. M.: The physician-writer's book . . . tricks of the trade of medical writing, Philadelphia, 1957, W. B. Saunders Co.

CHAPTER 3

Style in medical writing

Richard Warren, M.D.

MEANINGS OF STYLE

The word "style" can have various connotations. Casey, that immortal batsman, said as he let the first pitch go by, "That ain't my style!" He was referring to the quality of the pitch that did not suit his individual preference. In that sense style indicates a characteristic that identifies a person. In writing, for instance, only a sentence or two from Hemingway, Joyce, Gertrude Stein, or Le Carré identify the author. In addition, this identity-style can indicate a discipline. Every profession or trade has its own argot. We know the medical one well. Lawyers, space scientists, even thieves, have theirs. Gibson* in his book, *Tough, Sweet, and Stuffy* divertingly proposes that there are three different styles in writing that identify their class of author. "Tough" is the hard-hitting prose of Hemingway and Churchill; "sweet" is the ad-man's style, wherein he ingratiatingly protests that his only concern is the readers' comfort and well-being; "stuffy" is the bureaucratese of government directives. In addition, because identity-styles change with time, they can also identify eras. Writers in the early nineteenth century, for example, used an ornate style filled with classical allusions to an extent that we impatient, late 20th-century readers find difficult to read and comprehend.

The style I am discussing here, however, requires a different definition, one with no implication of identity or period. I will call it "good writing-style," a matter which authors, teachers, and editors have made the subject of grammars and style manuals for centuries.

There are two or three categories of good writing-style to be considered, a division that is not new. St Augustine (AD 354-430) said, "To be eloquent is to be capable of

using a simple style for teaching, a moderate style for entertaining, and a lofty style when persuading."* And Boyle in 1661 distinguished a style where "the design is only to inform our readers, not to delight or persuade."† For our purposes, if we can recognize two styles, the scientific and rhetorical, we will find it easier to control our impulses to use high-flown language in scientific writing.

Although delighting and persuading our readers has little place in scientific writing, we must still write readably and not "stuffily." However, this is a special art, much more difficult than writing a letter, dictating an operative note, or making a case presentation at rounds. As Buffon stated, "Those who write as they talk, even though they talk well, write badly."‡ This caveat should be remembered especially when you are asked to submit for publication a paper that was previously read at a medical meeting. Although the program chairman will no doubt warn participants that the documents to be submitted to the journal must be different from the speech manuscript, we too often find it difficult to resist the temptation to hand in the spoken version.

DEVELOPING A GOOD WRITING STYLE

All our training, all the major activities of our day-to-day lives work against our writing properly. As doctors whose major interest is the well-being of our patients, we must communicate all our actions. The clinical record and the rounds presentation generate an argot, which is

---

*Gibson, W.: Tough, sweet, stuffy, Bloomington, 1966, University of Indiana Press.

*Augustinus Aurelius (St. Augustine): Oeuvres, vol. II, Le Magistère Chrétien, Paris, 1949; Desclée de Brouwer et Cie, p. 481.
†Boyle, R.: Certain physiologic essays and other tracts, ed. 2, London, 1969, printed for Henry Heningman at the Blew Anchor in the Lower Walk of the New Exchange, p. 12.
‡Buffon, G. L.: Discours sur le syle, Paris, 1875, Hachette et Cie.

necessary to save time in order to get the day's work done. For example, using the term "Fogartization" when you mean "the removal of intra-arterial clots by means of the Fogarty catheter" is an obvious timesaver. In their proper setting such words are useful, yet we should know how to convert these shortcuts into good medical terminology for purposes of publication.

Good medical writing must satisfy:

1. *Lazy persons* (all of us), who do not want to puzzle over unfamiliar construction
2. *Busy persons,* who do not want to waste their time reading superfluous or hyperbolic material
3. *Fastidious persons,* who are easily offended by grammatical mistakes and affected expressions
4. *Critical persons,* who are bored by material too rounded or polished or too familiar

Allbutt makes two pertinent statements concerning style: (1) "A writer who writes to convince must lay his mind alongside that of the reader, who must be carried along in a quick and equable current." (2) "Clear vision will make a sound style. Force, lucidity, simplicity, economy of expression are virtues which we may all attain: originality will be as God pleases."*

Four specific steps can be taken to help develop a good writing style:

1. Be brief.
2. Be forceful.
3. Be equable.
4. Be civil.

Be brief

Make your sentences as short as can be compatible with your message. If you need a subordinate clause, keep it shorter than the main one. Gibson's checklist suggests that any dependent clause containing more than 40% of the total words of the sentence labels the author as "stuffy." Of course, some sentences must be long, but follow a long one with a short one to break the monotony. Use short words where possible. In choosing among the nouns "use," "usage," and "utilization," for example, employ "use" wherever possible. Gibson uses a device he calls his "style machine." One of its suggestions is that a sentence contain a ration of $2/3$ monosyllabic words and a maximum of 20% of words with more than three syllables.

Be judicious about deciding whether to use the "ic" or "-ical" ending to words. Whenever possible, omit the "-al," but keep in mind that the omission will change the meaning of some words: politic, political; economic, economical.

---

*Allbutt, T. C.: Notes on the composition of scientific papers, ed. 3, London, 1923, MacMillan Publishers Ltd.

Many phrases intrude that should be eliminated. Phrases such as "the use of," "the effect of," "a report of" abound in titles of articles. They are redundant, since the presentation of the material in itself implies use or effect or report. Also, in the text, phrases such as "the fact that" and "I think that" can usually be eliminated.

Be forceful

Passive statements such as "Tom was hit by Bill," are weaker than active ones: "Bill hit Tom." Therefore, whenever possible, use an active verb. If you are reporting an experience with a new operation, "we operated on twenty-one patients" is better than "twenty-one patients were operated on." The agent is known and so the active voice is in order. (Most editors now consider the obsequious avoidance of the first person to be an affectation.) Each time you consider using a form of the verb "to be," particularly "there was" or "there were," reconsider. "There were 60 patients in the series who were agonadic" sounds better as "We found 60 patients in this series to have no gonadal tissue."

Eliminate most modifiers. E. B. White, in his editing of William Strunk's *The Elements of Style,* states, "Write with nouns and verbs." For example, "The results approximated our predictions" is better than "The results were nearly in agreement with (or even "nearly agreed with") our predictions." You have a strong verb, "approximate," so use it.

Use as few adverbs as possible. Nouns and verbs should be strong enough to provide the emphasis one often delegates to "very" or "really" or "exactly" or "approximately." These adverbs have their important uses, but during the revision process you should examine each of them to determine whether it is essential. Does "It is a very important experiment" add anything to "It is an important experiment"?

Using nouns as modifiers can create vexing decisions. In the first place they are here to stay. We cannot and should not expunge such phrases as "cancer operation" and "skin flap" from our daily usage or scientific writing. They have worked their way into the idiom. But we should avoid strings of nouns as modifiers, such as "off-campus residence permission application."

Often we can add a touch of force by using a verb form, a gerund or gerundive, to replace a phrase. An example would be in a prepositional construction. "By examining the results" is stronger than "by examination of the results."

To illustrate how a sentence can be made more forceful I have taken at random the following from a recent issue of a surgical journal: "However, in half of these observations a tendency of liver circulatory variables to return to baseline values was observed after 45 minutes of vasopressin fusion." A better version would be, "However, half of the values for liver circulation tended to return to normal after 45 minutes."

Be equable

"Equable" is Allbutt's term indicating that thoughts must travel evenly and the language of the text should reassure the reader that the writer is adhering to the topic at hand. There should be no surprises. The text should be polished and smooth.

Parallelism. Parallelism is an effective device that can be used to advantage. It can take many forms. Macaulay used it so freely that many books on style quote passages from his works as illustrations:

> Never, not even under the tyranny of Laud, had the condition of the Puritans been so deplorable as at that time. Never had spies been so actively employed in detecting congregations. Never had magistrates, grand jurors, rectors, or church-wardens been so much on the alert.*

> When I was a child, I spoke as a child, I understood as a child, I thought as a child; but when I became a man, I put away childish things. (I Corinth. 13:11)

> It was the best of times, it was the worst of times, it was the age of wisdom, it was the age of foolishness . . .(Dickens, A Tale of Two Cities)

> My objections are obvious: (1) it is unnecessary, (2) it costs too much, (3) it won't work.†

Scientific writing must not strive to be great literature, but parallelism can be used to good effect in a medical text:

> Should we follow the great Hugh Owen Thomas whose clear thinking has so much influenced English surgery and apply the principle of "rest, complete, absolute, and uninterrupted" until firm union has occurred? Or should we subscribe to the philosophy of his contemporary, Just Lucas-Championniere, who was convinced that "motion is life," and that splints were of secondary importance?‡

If you tell the reader that there are two reasons or two items of discussion to follow, make sure that they are pointed up clearly and that they are recognizable as the two you meant. To add a third or fourth concept unannounced and unidentified causes the reader to stumble unhappily. If you must add them you should rewrite the whole section.

---

*Macaulay, T. B.: The history of England from the accession of James the Second, ed. 4, London, 1849, vol. 1, p. 661.
†Baker, S.: The practical stylist, ed. 4, New York, Thomas Y. Crowell Co., Inc., 1977.
‡Quigley, T. B.: Fractures, dislocations, and sprains, in R. Warren (ed.), Surgery, Philadelphia, 1963, W. B. Saunders Co.

Beware also of the "dangling comparative," a frequent device of the ad-man, the "sweet" style of Gibson. If something is "better," "more effective," or "causes fewer side effects," be sure that the reader can find whatever it is that the "something" is being compared to. Better than what? More effective than what? Fewer side effects than what?

Also avoid the promissory note. The reader should not be told at the very end of a paper that this was merely an interim report. The reader will be frustrated, if not angry, at such a late discovery.

Connectives. Lead the reader logically from thought to thought. You have the conjunctions "and," "or," "but," and the adverbs "yet," "still," and "so" to serve you. Permit yourself to start an occasional sentence with the one of these connectives even though you may have been taught otherwise. Remember that there are many others also: "therefore," "thus," "nevertheless," "however," "moreover." Beware of those that interject a tone of emotional judgment, such as "surprisingly," "interestingly," and "happily." Also avoid introductory clichés such as "basically."

Subject and verb. Keep the subject and the verb together. "The adenocarcinoma, which was located in the splenic flexure and had revealed itself only by the presence of a mass, was anaplastic and invaded the bowel wall." Compare this to: "The adenocarcinoma of the splenic flexure had presented in the form of a palpable mass. Its histologic appearance was anaplastic and showed invasion of the bowel wall." This change brings the subject and the verb closer together; changing it to two sentences appropriately separates the two thoughts conveyed.

Commas. Rather than attempt to touch on this whole subject I will say just two things: First, although most accept the concept of separating clauses by commas, much individual variation exists concerning the location of commas, particularly to set off introductory phrases. Buffon, after his fourteenth and final revision of a piece, would have it read aloud to him so that he could then finally decide where to place the commas. Here, as in other aspects in writing, you must attune your ear. Allbutt's classic contains a major heading entitled "Sound and Rhythm."

Tenses. The admonition to be consistent concerning tense could have been made under the heading of parallelism. The reader is disconcerted by a change of horses in midstream. "Examination of Table 2 shows that simple rhinoplasty *is* successful in 70% of the cases and *was* without significant complications." It should have been "rhinoplasty was . . ."

Decisions about tenses can be difficult. Place most accounts of work performed in the past tense. The work was done and the results should also take the past tense, as should most statements in a summary or abstract. Reserve the present tense for conclusions and recommendations, whether they appear in the discussion, the abstract, or in a separate conclusions paragraph.

Be civil

Under this heading falls a list of cautions against expressions that are not necessarily considered incorrect grammar, but are, nevertheless, inappropriate "barbarisms."

Which vs that. A common dilemma appears to be whether to use "which" or "that" as a relative pronoun. The rule states that if the clause being introduced defines the main clause, use "that"; if it is not defining, use "which." "We selected the larger of the two doses that Smith had proposed." Here "Smith had proposed" defines the two doses and the usage is correct. If "which" were used, the meaning would have been clear, but the flow of the sentence would have been interrupted. "That" must always be the first word in its clause, and since it is a direct modifier of the main clause, a comma does *not* precede it. "That" can also be used by implication only. "We selected the larger of the two doses Smith had proposed" would be quite correct.

Similar clauses introduced by "which" are those that are not required for sense in that particular sentence, but provide additional information—which, of course, should be relevant. "Which" as a relative pronoun should be preceded by a comma. "We used the larger dose, which had the desired effect." Because many writers overuse "which," one thing that should be on your revisions list is a "which hunt."

Split infinitives. "I entreated him to further pursue that line of investigation." "I entreated him to carry that line of investigation further." Surely the latter is best, and also preferable to "further to carry." Allbutt states:

. . . as the verb is one of the most important words of the sentences, to divorce it from its attendant participle is a suspension without reward, and therefore, tiresome. Thus, besides imparting an air of jauntiness, a split infinitive is rarely or never telling; usually indeed it weakens the sense and puts an adverb in a less effective place.*

Plurals of medical terms. Fishbein† lists the accepted plurals of various medical terms; another source of information is the first alternative listed in *Webster's Unabridged Dictionary.* Generally, the English plural is preferred if it is at all possible to use it. "Fistulas" is better than "fistulae," "syndromes" than "syndromata,"

"carcinomas" than "carcinomata." "Sulcuses," "sinuses," "cerebellums," and "appendices," are preferred. For some words, however, the English is awkward: "diverticula" is better than "diverticulums." In some instances either form is permissible: "symposiums" or "symposia," "memorandums" or "memoranda." Individual publishers have slightly different preferences. These should be consulted.

"-ize.". Although "-ize" is an accepted verbal ending, availability should not indicate total freedom to change a noun to a verb. Adding "-ize" indiscriminately is the stuffiest of all stuffy techniques. Recognizing that there are hundreds of words ending in -ize that have found acceptance (categorize, systematize) and that there are illogical boundaries ("minimize" is acceptable, "maximize" is not), let us be moderate. Words such as "inferiorize" and "prioritize" probably are best forgotten.

Overshortened sentences. Sometimes, having learned that the way to Heaven is by shortening sentences, we overdo it and interfere with sense or civil language. Resist the impulse to tack on an additional thought to a sentence using a prepositional phrase. "We have used the procedure twenty times with a success rate of 60%" can be better said, "In twenty attempts we achieved twelve successes." The sentence, "Twenty-three patients died for a mortality rate of 46%" is clearer when rephrased as, "Twenty-three patients died; the mortality was 46%."

• • •

Orwell is worth reading because his gentle ridicule of our bad habits makes them memorable and therefore less likely to be repeated. Here are a few items:

1. Never use a metaphor, simile, or other figure of speech that you are used to seeing in print; "toe the line."
2. Do not replace simple conjunctions with more elaborate ones: "with respect to," "by dint of."
3. Avoid foreign words and expressions: "status quo," "deus ex machina."
4. Shun the double negative: "A not unblack dog was chasing a not unsmall rabbit across a not ungreen field."

RHYTHM

A good ear for style can be developed. Many teachers state that the best approach is to read extensively from famous authors, but when you do this you will find repeated violations of the guidelines in this chapter. A good writer may use long sentences in one instance and a sentence fragment in another; many writers abuse the which-that rule. What then, are you accomplishing? You are assimilating a sense of rhythm and, in most in-

---

*Allbutt, T.: Notes on the composition of scientific papers, ed. 3, London, 1923, MacMillan Publishers Ltd.
†Fishbein, M.: Medical writing: the technic and the art, Chicago, 1938, American Medical Association.

stances, good taste, which will serve you on the rocky and endless road toward developing your own style. All good teachers of style are humble persons. They would admonish any writer not to obey all their rules at once!

CRITICISM AND REVISION OF THE MANUSCRIPT
Criticism

Should you show your paper to others for criticism? This is a difficult thing to make oneself do. We develop a sensitivity about our own efforts born of the agonies we have undergone to produce the present version. Although a copy should be shown to others, steel yourself against an inevitable wounding of sensitivities. Remember, also, you do not have to attend to all of your critics comments. When asked whether he showed his material to anyone else before it was published, humorist Art Buchwald answered that he would take it down the hall to his friend who would read it and tear it apart, whereupon Buchwald would not change a word. However, he avowed, the exercise was helpful in improving his writing of the *next* article. In this way you can learn and still save face. You must sooner or later develop calluses on this interface between you and your reviewers, whether their comments are solicited or unsolicited and whether they are your superiors or peers. It is an acquired art, part of a medical writer's development.

Submitting a paper for criticism before sending it to the publisher is particularly important for those writers whose first language is not English. Most of these physicians have learned English in the hurly-burly of the clinic or laboratory. When it comes time to write a formal paper, they may have difficulty with the vagaries of English grammar.

For an editor to wax indignant over material received from foreign graduates is inappropriate. But on the other hand, a paper full of grammatical errors and odd sentence construction cannot be accepted. If indignation has any place it should be directed at the writer's professor or chief who did not find the time to perform the necessary instructing and editing.

Revision

Buffon put his material through 14 drafts; at least three are mandatory. As Garland said, "There is no such thing as good writing, only good rewriting."* One must remember that it is impossible to revise one's own material without putting it aside for overnight at least. The next day one can approach the process of revising, which the time has made more objective. Horace advised putting writing aside for 10 years. This, of course, would be ridiculous for anyone in a scientific discipline who is writing to communicate. But the strength of his feeling on the matter emphasizes the importance of taking time. Most of us simply do not have extra time, but like all other matters that face us each twenty-four hours, we must arrange our priorities. Without strong enough motivation to find time to do it, you cannot achieve a good finished product. The alternative is for medical "literature" to continue in its present state of banality. Medical progress would not be arrested, but the quality of life—a term plastic surgeons use often, and rightly, to justify many procedures—would be poorly served.

---

*Garland, J.: The printed word, J. Med. Ed. **38:**292, Apr. 23, 1963.

CHAPTER 4

The final draft

Jerome Klingbeil, M.D.

If a writer has completed everything that should have been done in a manuscript, the final draft is then just a neat, clean retyping of the work draft. Such is rarely the case and usually a significant amount of rewriting and editing is necessary.

An accurate record of scientific findings is an absolute necessity as is conformity to standards of good writing and grammar. All revisions must have been made and the material put in proper order. The final draft is the first exposure an editor has to your work; it represents the culmination and quality of the work. It should be neat.

PREPARING THE FINAL MANUSCRIPT

In each issue of a journal there is a page entitled "Information for Authors" or "Directions for contributors" (see Appendixes A-3 and A-4). This defines the requirements that a manuscript must meet if submitted to that journal, including the format for photographs, tables, and graphs, and the form of the bibliography. You should review this section before preparing your final draft to ensure that it will conform to the journal's standards.

Once you have decided upon the journal to which your paper is to be submitted, make certain that it conforms to the standards of that journal. Some general rules that are applicable to any journal are as follows:

1. Type the report on clean, white, nonerasable, bond paper (8½ × 11) of 16 pound content.
2. Type on only one side of the sheet.
3. Leave a one-inch margin at the top and bottom of each page, except the title page where the top margin should be two inches. The lateral margins should be 1¼ inches.
4. Make certain that all pages have uniform margins, spacing, and type style.
5. Use a typewriter with sharp clear type and a new black ribbon. Preferably use pica type (ten characters per inch).
6. Double-space all typing, including notes, references, legends, etc.
7. Properly label and place in sequence all graphs, tables, illustrations, and photographs and be sure that they conform to the specifications of the journal.
8. Number all pages consecutively in the upper right corner.
9. Indent each paragraph five spaces.
10. Include name, title, and address for each author. Some journals prefer this on the first page of the manuscript, others on a separate cover page. Consult the "information for authors" page to determine the requirements of the journal to which you are submitting the paper.
11. Do not fold or roll the manuscript.
12. Make extra copies on a copier rather than with carbon paper. This ensures that each copy will be uniform. The number of copies to be submitted to the editor will be specified by each journal.

After the manuscript has been typed and all graphs, illustrations, and photographs placed in their proper sequence, put the manuscript aside for a day or so before checking it over for revisions and corrections. I then put the manuscript at arm's length and turn the pages rapidly. The appearance should remain uniform and each page should blend into the next. I do this several times. Since a manuscript is the author's introduction to the editor, a good impression is the first step to acceptance.

SPECIAL CONSIDERATION

Few authors are able to submit a manuscript without errors. Having worked with the material for so long and having become so familiar with its content, the author may overlook minor errors in content, spelling, or punctuation. While an editor will note and correct these, every effort should be made to submit a manuscript with as few errors as possible. Remember, also, that it is not the responsibility of the editor to verify the accuracy of quotations and references.

Many authors have problems with the proper use of special words, symbols, or abbreviations. These should not be used without spelling them out in full when first used in the article. For example: acetylsalicylic acid (ASA); upper respiratory infection (URI).

The use of foreign words is also a problem. In journals published in the United States the spelling of a word used in this country is preferable to the English style. For example: labor as opposed to labour. Many physicians practicing in the United States have immigrated here from foreign countries. While most of them have a good general knowledge of spoken English, many may have a problem with sentence structure and the written language. A solution to this problem is to have an American colleague read the manuscript and make suggestions for correction.

PROFESSIONAL EDITING OF MANUSCRIPT

Once your work has been submitted to a journal, you must anticipate that it will be edited. Regardless of your skill and experience in writing, some changes will be necessary. For instance, you have probably become so familiar with your manuscript that some typographical or spelling errors may have been overlooked. These will be corrected and an editor will read for content and to assure that the manuscript conforms to the required style of the journal. You must expect and be prepared to accept editorial criticism and recommendations. Minor problems can usually be resolved by a discussion between author and editor. Major problems with the manuscript may entail a complete rewrite or at least significant revision.

Regardless of the journal, the editor will be concerned with:

1. Appropriateness of content
2. Accuracy of content
3. Practicality of publishing this manuscript in the journal
4. Conformity with the literary style of the journal

EDITORIAL CONCERNS

Editors must consider the needs of the people to whom an article is directed. In a surgical specialty journal, for example, the audience is pretty well defined. Subject matter that is too broad in scope or presented in a random, hodgepodge manner will rarely be accepted by such a journal. Journals also have a specified number of pages that will be published during the year. This

limitation is often reflected in the "advice to authors," in which the maximum length of an acceptable article is spelled out. If your manuscript exceeds the acceptable length, you may have to rewrite it and eliminate redundant material or consider submitting it to another journal.

Some organizations require that all papers presented at their annual meeting be submitted to their official journal for possible publication. The rejection of a manuscript submitted in this instance does not always reflect a negative attitude but, rather, a lack of space in the journal. The editor may indicate other journals that might accept the article. *Never* submit the same manuscript to two journals at the same time. To do so is unprofessional and may result in any further manuscripts from you being summarily rejected in the future.

REJECTION OF THE MANUSCRIPT

You should also check the final draft against the usual causes of rejection of manuscripts and make the necessary changes before submission to the journal. The most common causes for rejection of a manuscript—some of which are out of an author's control—are the following:

1. Lack of space
2. Too much material on a single subject
3. Too little fact—too much fancy
4. Length—too long, too short
5. Prior publication of the same or similar material
6. Evidence does not prove theory
7. Dull writing
8. Dogmatic ideas
9. Cluttered drawings and graphs
10. Poor photographs
11. Graphs and figures not explained or labeled
12. Nonconformity to published rules and standards of the journal
13. A questionable ethical situation in which the editor feels the study violates the rights or privacy of the patients involved

Thoroughly study all suggestions and comments made by the editor. This may help you in preparing the final draft of your next paper. You should also review all suggested corrections to ensure that with these changes the text still accurately reflects your intent and meaning. You will also receive a galley proof of your typeset manuscript. Read it carefully. There will, undoubtedly, be errors in spelling and punctuation, some of which were overlooked in the original manuscript, others resulting from typesetting errors. The accuracy of the published manuscript is *your* responsibility, so review the galley proofs thoroughly. The editor will usually ask you to sign the galley proof, attesting that you have read it carefully and have made all necessary corrections. Corrections in the galley proof should be limited to errors in spelling or punctuation. Do not attempt to revise the text at this stage, unless there is a significant error in content. Such revisions require retypesetting. Because they are expensive, major revisions are rarely permitted unless done at the author's expense.

In summary, when writing the final draft of your paper, familiarize yourself with the requirements and policies of the journal to which it will be submitted and prepare the manuscript accordingly. Ensure the accuracy of the contents and use the principles of good writing, grammar, and syntax. Even the best of authors must follow these rules and be prepared to accept editing of their manuscripts.

CHAPTER 5

Abstracts

Jerome Klingbeil, M.D.

The abstract has become an increasingly important part of medical literature. It is used as an informative summary at the beginning of a scientific article, as a capsule description of papers published in other journals, as a summary of a paper submitted to a program chairman to consider including in the program, or as part of the published proceedings of a meeting.

An abstract should convey the scope of a study and give as much information as possible in a limited space. It should outline the purpose and methods of the work and detail important findings and conclusions, but include a minimum of the theory upon which it is based.

An abstract should have a standard format, regardless of the purpose for which it is written. It should outline the following aspects of the study:

1. *Problem:* Describe the purpose of your study.
2. *Methods:* Discuss concisely how you conducted the experiment.
3. *Results:* Describe significant findings, giving supporting data.
4. *Conclusions:* State your conclusions succinctly. Do not use statements that add no further information, such as, "The implications of this study are discussed."

The order of importance, thus dictating the amount of space devoted to each, is: results, methods, conclusions, and problem. No more than one sentence should be devoted to the problem or conclusions, and either can often be omitted. The selected results should be expressed in numbers, where possible. In general, the past tense should be used, although the present can be used occasionally, especially when stating the problem and conclusions.

Most journals and program sponsors have a limit to the length of an abstract. While the maximum number varies, most agree that 150 words is appropriate. You will write a better abstract if you limit yourself to a defi-nite word count. There is no reason, however, why you cannot stay below the specified word count.

ABSTRACT AT THE BEGINNING OF AN ARTICLE

In the past, scientific articles did not begin with an abstract, but, rather, ended with a summary. This was an attempt to pull things together, but required the reader to read through the entire article or to go to the end of it to find the results. The recent proliferation of medical journals and the number of articles published has made it imperative to provide the reader with a capsule version of the work so that he or she may decide whether or not to read the entire article. The abstract fulfills the need for such an abbreviated summary by succinctly describing the contents of the paper.

Many more will read a title and abstract than will read an entire article, thus these are the keys to your work and must be the most thoughtfully written parts of your paper. Since the abstract is not an intrinsic part of your paper, it must be intelligible on its own and must be comprehensible to someone who has not read the entire paper. It should enable the reader to decide whether or not to read the article, it should be suitable for filing, and it should be able to be reproduced in an abstract journal or other scientific publication. Abstracting services strive to publish summaries of articles from the various journals promptly. Their work is made easier if they can copy an author's abstract verbatim. A good title and a good abstract help these services to publicize the work as soon as possible and also facilitate future retrieval.

There are things that must be avoided when writing an abstract. Do not place information in the abstract that is not in the paper. Do not publish a summary in addition to the abstract; the abstract should completely replace the summary. (A list of conclusions at the end of an article, however, is most helpful.) Avoid, also, merely listing or describing the contents: "ten cases are presented and the results analyzed" does not provide any information. Do not include conclusions alone without the evidence on which they were based. Nor should you present convictions (author's prejudices) without supporting evidence.

An abstract should be written with the same attention to proper word usage, grammar, and syntax as the manuscript of an article. Try to avoid the use of abbreviations and medical jargon. Be brief and succinct, but do not eliminate needed prepositions, adjectives, and conjunctions, such as "of," "the," and "a." At the same time, however, try not to use words or phrases that add nothing to the content of the abstract.

ABSTRACT OF AN ARTICLE FROM ONE PUBLICATION FOR USE IN ANOTHER

The purpose of this type of abstract is to inform the reader that the original article has sufficient merit to warrant reading it in depth. This type abstract can be provocative and stimulating, and emphasize what is new or different. While some scientific journals provide abstracts that may be reproduced and published without written permission, most editors prefer to have abstractors who prepare an independent abstract after reading the original article.

It has been stated that abstracts should be a certain length and contain information presented in a specified manner. When abstracting from one journal to another, however, such attempts to formalize abstract writing can be both good and bad. A neophyte using an outline can produce an acceptable abstract from the start; however, an innovative, interesting writer may find that overemphasis on format can be counterproductive.

A clever abstract writer can usually limit the reader's interest, thus abstracts that are highly critical of the original article are rarely necessary. This is not to say, however, that there is not a place for the negative abstract. This type abstract can, for example, point out that certain material is covered in a limited manner and that the original article has few references of real value.

A good medical writer may not be a good abstractor. The effective abstractor must have the ability to communicate the essence of the original article in few words. To cover all aspects of a paper from introduction to conclusion and to include all data are almost impossible, particularly when first attempted. The ability to condense such material into a satisfactory abstract comes with time, practice, and interest. Most abstracts have to be written several times to obtain the desired length and clarity.

A discussion of the philosophical reasons for a paper must be avoided. Likewise, emphasizing the importance of a particular paper must be backed up with sufficient information to ensure that the reader of the abstract clearly understands why this importance is stressed. The abstractor must not minimize the principal points of the original paper while emphasizing those that he or she feels are important. It is not the privilege of an abstractor to rewrite the original paper; neither should an article be glamorized or made into something it is not.

Every abstract of an article from one publication that is prepared for publication in another should:

1. Be backed up by notes containing all essential data of the original article
2. Contain data that are clear, accurate, and complete
3. Accurately represent the views of the original author
4. Minimize the personal views of the abstractor
5. Review the complete article, not just a portion
6. Have nothing in the abstract that is not in the original article
7. Not be too wordy, but shortened where possible

ABSTRACTS PRINTED IN PROCEEDINGS

Many scientific organizations are now printing in a bound volume abstracts of all papers presented at their meetings. These abstracts are usually photographed and printed exactly as submitted. Most organizations send each speaker a form on which to submit the abstract. On this there will be a space outlined into which the abstract must fit.

ABSTRACT SUBMITTED TO A PROGRAM COMMITTEE

Most program committees or program chairmen require that an abstract of a paper for presentation be submitted to determine whether it has sufficient merit to be included in their scientific program. Since this may be the only information concerning your work that the committee has, you must write the abstract very carefully if your paper is to be considered. The abstract must carefully describe your work and must be sufficiently well prepared and informative to interest those who will select the papers to be presented as a part of the program.

While the abstract submitted to a program committee should generally follow the format of an abstract appearing at the beginning of a scientific paper for publication, certain latitude is permitted. In the abstract to a program committee explanation is frequently given more room than actual data, since some data may change between the time of the submission of the abstract and the presentation of the paper. Again, however, avoid simply listing or describing the contents, but strive to make the abstract as informative and representative of your work as possible.

In summary, the abstract is an important part of scientific communication. The format is relatively simple and straightforward, but its use must be mastered if you are to have your work selected for publication or for inclusion in a scientific program.

CHAPTER 6

Submitting a paper to a journal

Linda Porterfield

You have a message to convey as a result of research, clinical findings, or merely thoughts on an issue. As a physician, your topic will likely be medical in nature and your audience comprised of others in the health care field. You elect the written word as your communications medium, placing your ideas in manuscript form. At this point, short of paying a printer to produce this manuscript or mimeographing hundreds of copies for distribution, your next step is to have the manuscript accepted for publication by a medical journal.

There are numerous journals on the market. Some are official publications of medical organizations; others are owned by publishing houses or individuals. Content varies from totally scientific to wholly socioeconomic, with a few being combinations of the two. Although a publisher may pay authors for their manuscripts, more frequently there is no fee for authors or they must bear part or all of the printing costs.

Obviously, the first step after completion of a manuscript is to determine the journal to which it will be submitted. Not so obvious is the fact that this step is best accomplished *prior* to completion of the manuscript's final draft.

SELECTION OF A JOURNAL

Even as authors and their material vary, publishers vary. The basic difference between medical publications is the area of medical specialty. A potential author should determine those journals most likely to be interested in the selected topic. Of course, prior to selection of a topic, a physician should be sure that it is not a duplicate of something already in the medical literature.

A specialty society publication is concerned with an individual medical field and often will not be interested in scientific information outside that field. A wider scope can be found in journals covering broad areas, such as surgery or internal medicine; however, limitations may be placed on the number of manuscripts published in each field. With memberships comprised of physicians in all specialties, state association publications must select material because it appeals to the greatest number of this diverse readership.

Once the physician has chosen a topic, a letter to the editor of a particular publication may elicit information on whether a manuscript on that subject would even be considered. Such information should not be construed as acceptance, but merely as interest or lack thereof. In most instances, no editor will accept a manuscript without reading it first.

An author must decide on submission priority: to which journal the paper will be submitted first; if rejected, to which second; and so on. Do not be afraid to "shoot for the top" when selecting a possible publisher, but do attempt to appraise realistically the chances for acceptance. Since the acceptance or rejection procedure may be lengthy, time can become a factor as the manuscript moves from publication to publication. Choosing the most appropriate journal first can mean earlier acceptance and publication. As a point of information, the smaller or less prestigious journals often will offer more assistance to an author because they are not inundated with manuscripts. First-time authors may find this help a stepping-stone to publication in more prestigious journals at a later date.

Beware of dual submission. Editors ask that manuscripts be considered by *one* publisher at a time (Fig. 6-1).

MANUSCRIPT FORMAT

After determining the submission priority, you should obtain a copy of the manuscript guidelines of the publication to which the paper will be submitted. (See Figs.

```
Date:


To whom it may concern:

This is to certify that the manuscript entitled ____________________

____________________________________________________________

has been contributed to The Ohio State Medical Journal only and has not been

submitted to or published in any other media.


Signed:


____________________________
(Author)
```

Fig. 6-1.

6-2 through 6-5 and Appendixes A-3 and A-4.) Most editors place these guidelines in each issue of the journal. Publications containing the guidelines of selected medical journals also are available.

As the final draft is compiled, significant attention should be paid to the manuscript guidelines since many publications will not even consider papers that do not appear in the correct form. Format for such items as abstract, bibliography, and illustrative material as well as overall appearance of the paper varies from publication to publication. Although requirements for specific margins and double- or triple-spacing may seem superfluous, remember that the paper will be evaluated and that easy readability will assist in this evaluation.

Illustrations should be submitted exactly as specified in the guidelines. With today's offset printing, four-color photographs can be reproduced as black and white, often without losing clarity. Some publications will request that the author submit only black-and-white photographs; others will handle the conversion from four colors themselves.

Beware of requesting that four-color photographs appear as such. Because of the high cost of four-color printing, many editors require authors to pay part, if not all, of the reproduction costs. If you do not wish to incur this cost and want your photographs to be as explanatory as possible, be sure to select prints that will not lose effectiveness when printed in black and white.

However, if your topic requires four-color photographs, pay. Although the saying may be trite, a picture *is* worth a thousand words. If cost is a problem, shop around. Ask editors for estimates on reproduction before submitting the manuscript and then choose a journal for its appropriateness and four-color cost.

Other illustrative material, such as graphs, charts, and tables, usually must be submitted in a form suitable for reproduction; however, a few publications will assist authors by typesetting tables or completing art work. The costs involved will often be billed to the author. Again, thought should be given to use of color; a second color (in addition to black) is much less expensive than four-color work.

No matter what the illustrative material, it should be clear in both visual appearance and in its ability to be comprehended. In addition, the amount of illustrative material should be in proportion to the length of the text. A manuscript should not be overwhelmed by visuals. (Such limitations should also be placed on the number of references and the amount of quoted material in the manuscript.) In addition, identify on the back of each photograph your name, title of the paper, illustration number, and the top of the illustration. Write with a grease pencil or attach a typed label. Do not mark on the face of the illustration.

When the manuscript is ready for submission, prepare a cover letter to the editor of the journal introducing the manuscript and indicating the person and address to whom the editor should respond. Mail the cover letter and the original manuscript, a number of copies (as noted in the manuscript guidelines), and the originals of

Text continued on p. 28.

The American Journal of Surgery

Information for Authors

The Editors and Publisher of *The American Journal of Surgery* invite concise original articles in the field of *clinical* and *experimental* surgery. Historical reviews and descriptions of new instruments and modern operative technics are also welcomed. Statements in articles are the responsibility of the authors. Articles must be contributed solely to *The American Journal of Surgery* and become the property of the Publisher. The Publisher reserves copyright and renewal on all published material and such material may not be reproduced in any form without the written permission of the Publisher.

MANUSCRIPTS

Manuscripts should be typed double space with one inch margins. The authors should retain a carbon copy and send the original to the Editor. Please include the full name, address, schools, degrees, staff position and affiliation (past and present) of all authors.

Drug names: generic names must be used, with brand name in parentheses indicating whether it is registered by US Patent Office.

References must follow the style of the Index Medicus. They should be listed on a separate sheet in numeric order as referred to in the article, *not alphabetically*. Only references mentioned in the text should be listed.

Periodicals:

Katz S, Wahab A, Murray W, Williams LF: New parameters of viability in ischemic bowel disease. *Am J Surg* 127: 136, 1974.

Books:

Prosser CL, Bortoff A: Electrical activity of intestinal muscle under in vitro conditions, p 2025. Handbook of Physiology, sect 6, vol 4. Baltimore, Williams & Wilkins, 1968.

Summary of approximately fifty words must be supplied for inclusion in the Table of Contents when the article is published.

Address for reprint requests must be included.

ILLUSTRATIONS AND TABLES

A minimum of illustrations, professionally prepared, is encouraged and will receive favorable consideration. Color reproduction is not recommended. If color illustrations are accepted, the cost will be borne by the author.

Illustrations must be glossy prints in sharp focus. Original artwork is not acceptable. Do not mount on cardboard. All printing on illustrations must be done by a professional artist. Illustrations must be mentioned in the text in consecutive order. Please write author's name and the figure number on the back of each illustration and indicate the top. Only those illustrations that increase the understanding of the text should be included. Please note that illustrations of published articles will not be returned.

Legends for the illustrations must be typed on a separate sheet and not attached to the picture.

Permission to reproduce photographs of patients without a disguise should be sent with the manuscript. If not, eyes will be blocked out.

The Publisher allows a limited sum toward the reproduction of illustrations. Any charges in excess of this sum must be assumed by the author. The Editor reserves the right to limit the number of illustrations.

Tables should supplement rather than duplicate the text. They should be numbered consecutively as mentioned in the text and each must have a heading.

BOOK REVIEWS, BOOK LISTINGS, AND ABSTRACTS

Books for review or listing may be sent directly to *The American Journal of Surgery.* 666 Fifth Avenue. New York, New York 10019.

REPRINTS

Price schedules and order cards for reprints are mailed to each contributor on publication. Individual reprints of an article must be obtained through the author.

Fig. 6-2.

Instructions for Authors and Correspondents

Send manuscripts by first-class mail to the Chief Editor, Arthur E. Baue, MD, PO Box 7614, Kilby Station, New Haven, CT 06519. Manuscripts are received with the understanding that they are not under simultaneous consideration by another publication. Accepted manuscripts become the permanent property of the ARCHIVES and may not be published elsewhere without permission from the publisher (AMA).

In view of the provisions of *The Copyright Revision Act of 1976*, effective Jan 1, 1978, the author(s) of manuscripts, including correspondence and brief communications, will be required to sign and date the following statement: "In consideration of the American Medical Association's taking action in reviewing and editing my submission, the author(s) undersigned hereby transfers, assigns, or otherwise conveys all copyright ownership to the AMA in the event that such work is published by the AMA." We regret that transmittal letters not containing the foregoing language signed by all authors of the submission will necessitate delay in review of the manuscript.

Author Responsibility.—All accepted manuscripts are subject to copy editing. The author will receive an edited typescript rather than galley proofs for approval. The author is responsible for all statements in his work, including changes made by the copy editor.

Designate one author as correspondent and provide his address and telephone number. Order reprints at the time the typescript is returned after editorial processing. Specify address to which requests for reprints should be sent.

Manuscript Preparation.—Submit an original typescript and two high-quality copies of the entire manuscript. All copy (including references, legends, and tables) must be typed double-spaced on 22 × 28 cm (8½ × 11-inch), heavy-duty white bond paper. Ample margins should be provided.

Refer to patients by number (or, in anecdotal reports, by fictitious given names). Real names or initials should not be used in the text, tables, or illustrations.

Titles.—Titles should be short, specific, and clear. They should not exceed 42 characters per line, including punctuation and spaces, and be limited to two lines, if possible. The title page should include the full names and academic affiliations of all authors, the address to which requests for reprints should be sent, and, if the manuscript was presented at a meeting, the name of the organization, place, and date on which it was read.

Style of Writing.—The style of writing should conform to acceptable English usage and syntax. Slang, medical jargon, obscure abbreviations, and abbreviated phrasing are to be avoided.

Informed Consent.—Manuscripts reporting the results of experimental investigations on human subjects must include a statement to the effect that informed consent was obtained after the nature of the procedure(s) had been fully explained.

Abstract.—Provide an abstract (135-word maximum) of the article, including statements of the problem, method of study, results, and conclusions. The abstract replaces the summary.

References.—List references in consecutive numerical order (not alphabetically). Once a reference is cited, all subsequent citations should be to the original number. All references must be cited in the text or tables. Unpublished data and personal communications should not be listed as references. References to journal articles should include (1) author(s), (2) title, (3) journal name (as abbreviated in *Index Medicus*), (4) volume number, (5) inclusive page numbers, and (6) year, in that order. References to books should include (1) author(s), (2) chapter title (if any), (3) editor (if any), (4) title of book, (5) city of publication, (6) publisher, and (7) year. Volume and edition numbers, specific pages, and name of translator should be included when appropriate. The author is responsible for the accuracy and completeness of the references and for their correct text citation.

Metrication.—All measurements must be in metric units. English units may also be given parenthetically if the measurements were originally done in English units.

Illustrations.—Use only those illustrations that clarify and augment the text. Submit illustrations in duplicate, unmounted and untrimmed. Do not send original artwork. Send high-contrast glossy prints (not photocopies). Figure number, name of senior author, and arrow indicating "top" should be typed on a gummed label and affixed to the back of each illustration. All lettering must be legible after reduction to column size. Artwork submitted for publication may be relettered to achieve uniformity of lettering style throughout the journal. Magnification and stain should be provided when pertinent. Illustrations should preferably be in a proportion of 12.5 × 18 cm (5 × 7 inches).

An experienced medical illustrator should be employed whenever possible for the preparation of all artwork. Template lettering or preset type is preferred to hand-lettered labels. If halftone artwork with labels is submitted, affix type and leaders to a clear acetate overlay registered to the base drawing. Labels and leaders should be applied directly to the drawing board surface if the artwork consists only of line ink technique.

Illustrations in full color are accepted for publication if the editors believe that color will add significantly to the published manuscript. The ARCHIVES will pay part of the expense of reproduction and printing color illustrations, the remainder to be borne by the author or his sponsor. After deducting the ARCHIVES contribution, the author's share is $275.00 for up to six square-finished illustrations that can be arranged on a one-page layout. Any additional illustrations or special effects will be billed to the author at cost. Positive color transparencies (35 mm preferred) must be submitted for an evaluation. Do not send color prints unless accompanied by original transparencies. All transparencies should be carefully packed and sent with the manuscript.

Legends.—Legends should be typed double-spaced, beginning on a separate sheet of paper. Length should be limited to a maximum of 40 words.

Photographic Consents.—A letter of consent must accompany all photographs of patients in which a possibility of identification exists. It is not sufficient to cover the eyes to mask identity.

Acknowledgments.—Illustrations from other publications must be acknowledged. Include the following when applicable: author(s), title of article, title of journal or book, volume number, page(s), month, and year. The publisher's permission to reprint should be submitted to the ARCHIVES after the manuscript has been formally accepted.

Statistical Review.—Manuscripts containing statistical evaluations should include the name and affiliation of the statistical reviewer.

Tables.—Each table should be typed double-spaced, including all headings, on a separate sheet of 22 × 28 cm (8½ × 11-inch) paper. Do not use larger size paper. If a table must be continued, use a second sheet and repeat all heads and stubs. Each table must have a title.

Correspondence and Brief Communications.—The editor will be pleased to receive letters that pertain to material published in the ARCHIVES and brief communications concerning other matters of interest to its readers. Such contributions should be 250 words or less, typewritten, double-spaced, and clearly marked "For Publication." No more than two references are permitted and illustrations or tables are acceptable only when essential to the message.

News and Announcements.—Brief notices may be submitted of meetings, seminars, or symposia that are of interest to the readers of the ARCHIVES. News items of appointments, promotions, and developments in the field of surgery and related disciplines are invited.

Brief Clinical Notes.—The ARCHIVES welcomes the submission for review of Brief Clinical Notes. These are to consist of no more than 400 words, two references, and one illustration. The Synopsis-Abstract should not exceed 80 words.

Fig. 6-3.

INFORMATION TO CONTRIBUTORS

All manuscripts, editorial correspondence, and galley proofs should be addressed to Betty Jane McWilliams, Ph.D., Editor, <u>Cleft Palate Journal</u>, Cleft Palate Center, University of Pittsburgh, Pittsburgh, Pennsylvania 15261.

MANUSCRIPTS

An original and three complete copies should be submitted. The author should retain a fifth copy in his own files.

<u>The format</u> for manuscript preparation should be <u>strictly</u> adhered to. Manuscripts should be typed, double-spaced, with one-inch margins on $8\frac{1}{2}$" x 11" white, bond paper. Pages should be numbered consecutively in the upper right-hand corner of each page, and the authors' last names should appear in the upper left-hand corner of each page or illustration. An abbreviated title should appear opposite the names on each page or illustration.

Page one should include the full title and the authors' names and degrees, along with information about the institutional affiliations.

Page two should list the authors' names and institutional affiliations, along with the name, address, and telephone number of the author to whom editorial correspondence should be addressed. If the paper is based upon an oral presentation at a professional meeting, the name, place, and dates should be included on page two. If the project reported was supported by any agency, credit should be given and appropriate grant numbers included.

Page three should contain the shortened title along with the authors' last names as they appear at the top of each page.

Page four should contain a carefully prepared abstract which will appear at the beginning of each article. The abstract, not to exceed 150 words, should include a brief description of subjects, methods, findings, and conclusions. Key words, up to ten, should be underscored in the summary. These will be printed in italics so that they may be used for reference purposes.

Continued.

Fig. 6-4.

The actual manuscript, not to exceed 5,000 words, should begin on page five. Headings must be used to designate the major divisions of the paper, and up to three levels of sub-headings may be incorporated where appropriate.

Tables and Figures are encouraged where they will clarify the manuscript. They should be typed using double spacing on pages separate from the main text. Each should carry an appropriate and complete title and be numbered consecutively using Arabic numerals. All tables and figures should be complete in themselves and should be referred to in the manuscript. For figures or other illustrative material, original art work is required. All photographs should be critically sharp, glossy prints. Mark the "Top" on the back of each illustration along with appropriate identification. Figure numbers and titles or legends should be listed on a separate page. Each copy of the manuscript should contain a complete set of tables, figures, and illustrations.

References are listed in double-spaced typing at the end of the manuscript in alphabetical order (unnumbered) according to the last name of the first-named author. References are noted in the text by author(s) surname(s) followed by the year of publication. Examples include: Smith (1975); as previously noted (Smith, 1975). Two or more works by the same author in the same year should carry suffixes a, b, c in both the list of references and in the text as in: Smith (1975a); Smith (1975b). The abbreviation et al is not acceptable in the list of references but may be used in the text where there are three or more authors. It is never used if there are two authors. Every reference in the text should be included in the list of references, and no reference that is not cited should appear in the list. Reference style for journal articles should be consistent and should conform to the following fictitious example: Smith, J. H., and Smith, John H., Hearing problems in adults with cleft palate, J. Speech Hear. Res., 1, 439-442, 1964. References to books should give Author, Title (with the first letter in each word capitalized), Publisher's City: Publisher, pages, year. Each author must accept responsibility for the accuracy of his references since they cannot be routinely checked by the Editor or the Section Editors.

Fig. 6-4, cont'd.

Footnotes should be avoided where possible. If they must be used for a purpose such as identifying brand names, the content of the footnote should be identified and typed on a separate page.

Original Material only should be submitted for publication. It must not have been published elsewhere in whole or in part or be in the process of such publication unless the author(s) so acknowledge. Each manuscript should be accompanied by a letter of transmittal in which the status of the work is clarified.

COST TO AUTHORS

Per page costs to the author(s) will be assessed at $40 per printed page for any pages in excess of eight except for unusual contributions where the extra-page charge may be waived. Authors are not charged for any other manufacturing costs. The Journal will pay the cost of minor changes made on the galley. The author will be assessed for any expense incurred because of major alterations.

GALLEY PROOFS

Galley proofs are sent by the printer directly to the author(s) for proof-reading within 48 hours after receipt. Authors are to note in red any errors made by the printer. Minor changes may be indicated in black. Authors should be aware that major alterations in a manuscript cannot be made on the galley unless the author is willing to bear the expense personally. Galleys must then be returned to the Editor who reserves the right to publish any manuscript as it appears on the galley if the author(s) have not responded within 14 days.

This policy does not apply to galleys of articles submitted from abroad since the time involved is usually too great to meet publication deadlines. Such galleys are proof-read in the Editor's office. However, all authors are informed of proposed changes prior to the printing of the Journal. Waverly Press will provide authors with the necessary instructions for ordering reprints.

Fig. 6-4, cont'd.

PLASTIC AND RECONSTRUCTIVE SURGERY

Information for Authors

The goal of *Plastic and Reconstructive Surgery* is to inform its readers of advancements in clinical medicine, significant research, and new developments in areas related to plastic and reconstructive surgery. This Journal provides a forum for responsible discussion among identified individuals. Unless otherwise clearly specified, the views expressed in articles, editorials, book reviews, and letters published by *Plastic and Reconstructive Surgery* represent the opinion of the author and do not reflect the official policy of the institution with which the author is affiliated, or the American Society of Plastic and Reconstructive Surgeons, Inc., the American Association of Plastic Surgeons, or the American Society for Aesthetic Plastic Surgery. Acceptance by this Journal of advertisements for products or services does not imply endorsement or preference over other similar products or services.

Papers on any aspect of plastic surgery—operative procedures, clinical or laboratory research, and case reports—are invited for publication if they contribute significantly to the literature.

The prose used in manuscripts must conform to acceptable English usage and syntax; and the contents must be clear, accurate, coherent, and logical. In accepting or rejecting a manuscript, the editors will also consider its originality, teaching value, and validity.

Manuscripts should not exceed approximately 4,000 words, with a maximum of ten diagrams, illustrations, or both. Occasional exceptions will be made for prize-winning essays, collective reviews, solicited material, or special works.

All manuscripts must be sent to:

Robert M. Goldwyn, M.D., Editor
Plastic and Reconstructive Surgery
1101 Beacon Street
Brookline, Massachusetts 02146, U.S.A.

The author should submit the original manuscript and two copies, with three sets of illustrations, and should retain one complete copy. The Journal is not responsible for losses in the mail.

Requirements of this Journal for Considering Manuscripts, and the Agreement of Author(s) to These Conditions

Decisions concerning editing, revisions, acceptances, and rejections will be made by the editors; editing may include shortening of the article and reducing the number of illustrations and tables, as well as other changes in format. An accepted article may be published with an accompanying discussion if the editors so desire.

Articles are received only for exclusive publication in this Journal, with the understanding that they have not been published elsewhere (in part or in full, in other words, or in the same words) and will not be submitted elsewhere unless rejected by the Journal.

Published manuscripts become the sole property of the Journal and will be copyrighted by the American Society of Plastic and Reconstructive Surgeons.

By submitting an article to the Journal, the author (or authors) agrees to each of the above conditions. In addition, the author (or authors) explicitly assigns any copyrighted ownership he (or they) may have in such article to said Society if the article is published in the Journal.

Preparation of Manuscripts

Copy must be typewritten, double-spaced, on one side only, on 8½ x 11 inch (22 x 28 cm) white bond paper, with 1½ inch (4 cm) margins at the left, top, and bottom and a 1 inch (2.5 cm) margin at the right. All copy must be double-spaced, including text, footnotes, bibliographies, legends, tables, and headings (i.e., all material that is to be set in type, large or small). Text references must be supplied for all tables and figures in order in the text, which will determine placement on the printed page.

The title page carries the full title of the article, followed by the authors' names, degrees,

Fig. 6-5.

and city. Footnotes giving the principal affiliation of each author and where and when the paper was presented must appear at the bottom of the title page. Each page of the manuscript after the title page should carry a running head, which is a shortened form of the title. The first text page is numbered one.

At the conclusion of the text, the name and complete address of the principal author should appear. At the bottom of that page, list three to five nouns that are appropriate key words for indexing.

The references must be typed on separate pages following the text. All references must be cited in the text in numerical order, not alphabetically. References to journal articles should include (1) author(s), (2) title, (3) journal name (as abbreviated in *Index Medicus*), (4) volume number, (5) the first page number, and (6) year, in that order. References to books should include (1) author(s), (2) chapter title (if any), (3) editor (if any), (4) title of book, (5) city of publication, (6) publisher, and (7) year. Volume and edition numbers, specific pages, and name of translator should be included when appropriate. *The author is responsible for the accuracy and completeness of the references.*

Legends

Legends are required for illustrations and should be typed on separate pages following the bibliography. They should be brief and pertinent and need not be full sentences.

Illustrations and Tables

Consider the size and shape of the Journal page when planning your illustrations, and arrange them to conserve vertical space.

Photographs must be selected and prepared with great care. They must be in sharp focus and have good contrast. Glossy prints are preferable, and they should be larger than they will appear in the published article. If the exact arrangements of photographs into groups is important and unusual, the author should so indicate on a separate sheet of paper. Before-and-after photographs of patients must be identical in terms of size, position, and lighting. Backgrounds should be clean and uncluttered (retouching is permitted on backgrounds). Color photographs that significantly enhance the presentation will be considered for publication. If approved by the Editorial Board, a color page containing up to 6 photographs (or occasionally two such pages) may be allowed at a charge to the author of $350.00 per page.

Drawings should be rendered in black india ink on white illustration board. The size of any lettering must be large enough so it wil lbe legible after it has been reduced to the size in which it will be printed. Send originals on pieces of illustration board, along with two photostats, no larger than 9 x 13 inches (23 x 33 cm).

Acknowledgments

Illustrations taken from other publications must be acknowledged. Include the following information in the figure legend when applicable: author(s), title of article, title of journal or book, volume number, page(s), month, and year. The publisher's letter of permission should be submitted to *Plastic and Reconstructive Surgery.*

Correspondence and brief communications will be published as space permits at the discretion of the editors. They should be typewritten, double-spaced (including references, if any), and must not exceed 500 words in length; they will be subject to editing.

Galley Proofs are sent directly to the author from the typesetter. They should be read carefully and returned promptly to the editor with the author's approval indicated by initialing.

Reprints may be ordered when galley proofs are received. A table showing the cost will be enclosed with the proofs. The number of reprints will be limited if it is contrary to the interests of the Journal.

Fig. 6-5, cont'd.

all illustrative material to the editor at the address indicated in the manuscript guidelines. The use of certified mail will ensure immediate confirmation that the package reached its destination. It is most important that you retain a copy of the manuscript and duplicate copies of all illustrative material. Journals rarely take responsibility for losses in the mail.

If the manuscript is rejected by the first journal to which it is submitted, by all means submit it to another. However, incorporate any suggestions the rejecting editor may have and send a clean manuscript to the next publication. Never send a manuscript with editorial comments noted on it to another publication.

DECISION ON PUBLICATION

Once a manuscript is received at a publication office, it will be acknowledged. (If this acknowledgement does not arrive in a reasonable amount of time, contact the publisher; possibly the manuscript never reached its destination.) Normally, this first correspondence is no more than information that the manuscript is being considered for publication. The time lag between receipt of a manuscript and a publication decision varies.

Manuscripts will be judged by one or more individuals. Some publications have a medical editor who alone determines the content of the journal. Others have editorial boards, members of which may read every paper submitted or may be responsible for specific medical fields or areas of expertise within a given field. If a manuscript is judged by two or more individuals, their comments will be compiled when the final determination as to publication is made.

A manuscript may be accepted or rejected; or it may be accepted or rejected with stipulations. In the latter case, the paper may be of interest to the publication but cannot be considered without certain modifications. The author can either comply with these modifications and resubmit the manuscript or remove the manuscript from consideration.

Because of the current copyright law, most publishers require assignment of copyright. This means that the author grants to the publisher the right to determine whether others may reprint all or part of the manuscript. At some journals, copyright is held jointly by the author and the publisher, meaning that any requests to reprint an article must be granted by both. Editors may require completion of the copyright assignment form at the time the manuscript is submitted or at the time of acceptance.

PRODUCTION

Once the manuscript has been accepted for publication by an editor and the author has agreed to any stipulations, it will be placed in the publication's editorial

rotation. This rotation allows time for the staff of the journal to prepare the manuscript for publication; and unless the editor has a specific reason for quickening this rotation (i.e., timely topic, special issue), the staff's average amount of preparation time will lapse before the manuscript is published (see Appendix A-7).

The staff will prepare the manuscript in accordance with the publication's editorial style. Style varies, but an accepted version is that of the American Medical Association. (When an author is in doubt about how to edit the final draft, use this style for any portions of the manuscript not explained in the publisher's guidelines.) Depending upon the publication, significant amounts of editorial assistance may or may not be given during the editing process. In fact, a few editors will turn a badly written manuscript on an interesting topic into a well-written article.

Following editing and prior to publication, the manuscript will be returned to the author for final approval. Depending on the journal, the author will see one or more of the following proofs (see also Appendixes A-7 and A-8).

Edited manuscript: A typewritten copy

Galley proof: A copy of the manuscript that has been typeset for publication

Page proof: The text of the manuscript, typeset and arranged in page format as it will appear in the publication

Whatever the proof, you must read it carefully and make any additions or corrections. Proof copies of any illustrative material will be attached; these also should be checked for accuracy. The staff of the publication will have read the proof before sending it to you and their corrections will be noted.

Publishing is an expensive business. In addition to basic overhead costs of staff, office space, and utilities, printing costs have risen substantially over the past years. Therefore, it is most important that authors not expect to make revisions in a manuscript after submission. Proofs are used to prevent errors, not to provide an opportunity for the author to rewrite a manuscript. In fact, an author may be required to pay for editorial revisions on proofs except for typographic errors. A reminder: often a type change in one line will cause the remainder of the paragraph to be reset.

Note any corrections or additions in the margins of the proof (proofreading symbols are listed in unabridged dictionaries; see Appendix B-8) and sign the proof. This signature indicates that you assume responsibility for the material as written or altered. Do not fault the staff of the journal for an error you did not catch.

Return the signed proof to the publication office as rapidly as possible. Some publications give the author a time limit for response, but no proof should be retained more than two weeks. If the manuscript is held longer, do not be surprised if publication is delayed or the manuscript is printed "as is."

An author may be provided a complimentary copy of the issue in which the manuscript appears or a limited number of reprints of the article. Additional copies of the issue and reprints must be purchased. If a reprint order form is enclosed with the proof, it should be mailed at the time the proof is returned.

After the proof is received at the publication office, the manuscript will proceed through the final production stages. The manuscript will appear as an edited manuscript, galley proof, page proof, and blueline or brownline (final proof in which all illustrations are incorporated) before going to press. With the printing and binding of the issue, the physician becomes a published author.

CONCLUSION

Begin with an idea and compose a manuscript, using various editing styles as aids. Choose carefully the journal to which the paper will be submitted, striving for the possibility of acceptance. Compile the final draft of the paper with that journal's manuscript guidelines at hand, and submit the text and illustrative material exactly as specified.

If the paper is accepted, comply with any requests of the publisher, including reading proofs quickly and accurately. Moreover, do not be discouraged by a rejection notice. Rewrite the manuscript, incorporating any suggestions, and try again elsewhere.

From physician to published author requires many, not-so-easy steps; but the pride of authorship is worth the time and effort. Your paper will remain in the medical literature forever—a not insignificant accomplishment.

CHAPTER 7

Choosing and working with a book publisher

Karen Berger

"Publish or perish" is a familiar saying in scholastic circles; "true professionals" are expected to display their professional acumen through the printed word. Medical Curriculum Vitae are replete with lists of published works, papers in progress, and books that are contemplated. The forces that encourage a professional to engage in professional writing are strong, and physicians are among the most prolific of writers.

The publication of a book begins with an idea and a need. Sometimes the idea is the impelling force; an author has an idea for a book and seeks out the help of a publisher to bring that idea to fruition. At other times it is the need that provides motivation; the publisher, through analysis of the market, perceives that need and finds an author to meet it. Whatever the inception of the book, it is the carefully tuned cooperation of the author and the publisher that brings about the best possible book.*

Writing a medical book requires special dedication and discipline. It is a time-consuming endeavor that entails many late hours and lost weekends. If you choose to edit a book, you must be prepared to cope with errant contributors, personal disappointments, and writing disasters. In either case, you as the editor or author need to realistically assess the amount of time needed for writing and schedule extra time for that purpose. Your motives for writing should also be carefully examined. Scientific writing produces numerous rewards in the form of intellectual challenges, ego gratification, professional prestige, and pride in accomplishment. Few of these rewards are monetary. A writing project motivated purely by financial considerations is likely to be disappointing in

the long run. All the questioning and examination of motives should take place before you approach the practical considerations of writing a proposal and selecting a publisher.

WRITING A PROPOSAL

It is not enough to want to write a good book or to have an excellent reputation. Books are not contracted on whim or admiration. Solid evidence of planning and intent is necessary to write a book and to get a publisher to accept your proposal. Even if a publisher solicits your writing skill on a particular topic, you will be expected to provide a detailed prospectus outlining the scope and sequence of your intended book along with the manuscript specifications, markets, and competition. The publisher may also request sample chapters.

Preliminary decisions

As a prospective author you should have a clear idea of the level of presentation you intend, the markets you are appealing to, and the format (text, atlas, synopsis) that you are planning to use. Other initial considerations include typing, research, and artwork assistance. Do you have the type of support you will need to prepare a manuscript? Will your book be heavily illustrated, and is there an artist available who would be good for the project? Practical considerations such as artist's fees and secretarial charges must also be taken into consideration. If these services are necessary, will you need any assistance with these costs?

It is also advisable to make a preliminary decision about the authorship or editorship of the book. Careful consideration should be given to the advantages and dis-

---

*Mosby Author's Guide, St. Louis, 1981, The C. V. Mosby Co.

SPECIFICATIONS FOR NEW BOOK PROPOSALS

This form provides guidelines for the type of information necessary for a publisher to evaluate a proposed book for possible publication.

1. Names, titles, addresses, and telephone numbers of authors/editors

2. Number of contributors to book

3. Tentative book title

4. Present stage of manuscript: idea ( ) 50% ( ), more than 50% ( )

5. Probable date for manuscript completion

6. Mechanical dimensions of manuscript:

    _______Estimate of printed pages (approximately two, double-spaced typewritten pages to one printed page. Two tables or illustrations to a page.)

    _______Number of tables

    _______Number of line drawings

    _______Number of halftones (photos)

    _______ Number of color illustrations (explain)

7. Description of purpose and scope of the book

8. Listing of primary and secondary professional and/or student markets for which the book is intended with emphasis on the level of readership at which it is aimed

9. Estimate of approximate price range for the book

10. Listing of competing titles: (Include author, title, publisher, date of publication and price.)

11. Comparison of proposed book to competing titles highlighting unique features offered by proposed book

WHEN PROVIDING THIS INFORMATION, THE AUTHOR SHOULD ALSO INCLUDE:

    Curriculum Vitae
    Introductory or Prefatory Statement
    Table of Contents (detailed outline of project)
    Contributor list (if applicable)
    Sample chapter(s)

Fig. 7-1.

advantages of each method of authorship. If the book is going to be an edited work, a contributor list should be decided upon and submitted with the proposal. Contributors should be selected carefully, not on the basis of cronyism, but on the basis of reputation, authority on a particular topic, and geographic distribution. A large, edited contributor work has the advantage of providing information from numerous authorities in the field. Different approaches and perspectives can also be introduced. It has the headaches, however, of many different writing styles, some barely approaching the English language, and the colossal task for the editor or editors of rewriting, checking references, and reminding errant contributors of missed deadlines and forgotten promises. A single-authored text has the advantage of having a coherent, consistent approach but the disadvantage of an arduous writing task without peer support. Other variations on these two alternatives, such as co-edited or co-authored texts, are also possible. Once these preliminary decisions are made, a proposal can be written.

The proposal

The publisher's eventual acceptance of a manuscript for publication is based on a logical evaluation of the author's proposal. Among the factors taken into consideration are the topic (its timeliness and general interest to the markets), the size of the markets, the ability of the company to reach the targeted audiences that have been outlined by the author, expert reviews of the material submitted, the reputation of the contributors and authors, the organization of the proposal, the size and structure of the book, and the cost of producing the book. The more detailed and comprehensive a proposal an author has supplied, the more information the publisher will have to conduct an effective marketing evaluation (Fig. 7-1).

SELECTING A PUBLISHER

After a proposal has been prepared, the next major step is choosing a publisher. There are many publishers to choose from, and frequently it is difficult for a prospective author to differentiate one from the other. In making a preliminary selection of publishers to submit proposal material to, you might find it helpful to check the medical school library and the medical bookstore to see which companies have the most books in your area of expertise. This bookstore browsing will give you an idea about where the different companies' marketing efforts are being directed. It will also provide you with the opportunity to compare the quality and type of books produced by the different publishers. Professional associates are also good sources to check about their experiences with different publishers; satisfied authors often

serve as very positive recommendations. Another source for investigation is your personal medical library; you should reexamine your own books to see which publisher seems to dominate your bookshelf. If you are fortunate enough to conceive your idea at the same time as your medical society's annual meeting, you might also visit the exhibits and see which publishers are represented. You should examine their offerings and meet their editorial representatives.

After all of these factors have been weighed, you will be able to select the names of several different publishers to whom to submit your proposal.

Contacting the publisher

The person to contact about your book proposal is the acquisition editor.*

Acquisition editors are skilled, highly trained persons who have extensive knowledge of the publishing world. They know books and what makes them good or bad, they know the markets, and they know the production procedures and how they can best be utilized for your book. They are usually responsible for a select number of subject areas, a fact that allows them to become specialized. By attending conventions, reading specialty journals, visiting schools, and talking to professional people, sales representatives, and other . . . authors, these editors learn about the subject areas and gain ideas for books and leads to authors.†

Once you have decided which publishers to approach, you should obtain the names of the appropriate acquisition editors from each company and address your proposal to her or him. By personally directing a proposal, you will be sure to receive an answer. Editorial offices of publishing houses are often bastions of old-fashioned courtesy, which requires editors to reply to directed proposals. Unaddressed inquiries do not prompt the same kind of attention that a personal letter does. Letters addressed Dear Sir or Gentlemen are also subject to question, since there are large numbers of women working in publishing houses.

After your proposal has been submitted to several publishers, expect a delay of at least four to six weeks for marketing reviews. If your proposal is submitted in the spring or fall of the year, an extra two weeks should be added, because this is a busy travel time for editorial personnel, who will be attending various professional meetings of the different medical specialties.

The editor reviews your proposal to see how you de-

---

*Acquisition editor is a generic name for the member of the editorial department who works with the author and contracts his or her book. Other titles for this person include: editorial director, senior editor, associate editor, and director of acquisitions.

†Mosby Author's Guide, St. Louis, 1981, The C. V. Mosby Co.

velop the topics in your outline and to evaluate a sample of your writing style.

Your outlines and sample chapters may also be sent to reviewers for their opinions on the subject matter and approach. . . . These reviewers are often your professional colleagues. They are potential adopters (of a textbook) or purchasers of the book. As such, they are representatives of your readership, and the reviews can be very helpful to you*

The acquisition editor's review, professional reviewers' critiques, and marketing input combine to provide the publisher with the information necessary to make a decision about the suitability of your submitted proposal as a company publication.

Some publishers might call and express an immediate interest in your project. This feedback is encouraging but should not lead you to believe that the company has agreed to publish your manuscript.

The response that the prospective author is waiting to hear is a positive one; and when you receive positive responses from several different publishers, you are left with the responsibility of making a final choice. At this time it is good for you to review some of the basic criteria mentioned earlier concerning the initial investigation of publishers. Next, arrangements should be made for a personal meeting with the editorial representative or acquisition editor from each of the companies being considered.

The acquisition editor will be your link with the publishing company, and it is important that you be able to work and communicate with this person. All of your special desires for your book in terms of scope, format, and organization should be discussed with the editorial representative at this time. Any requests for color illustrations and any additional needs for grants, advances, or manuscript deadline delays should be investigated. You should pay attention to see if the person you are meeting with seems to be knowledgeable in publishing matters and in your area of expertise. You should also assess whether the editor's ideas agree with yours. Is your vision of your book the same as the editor's? Are you willing to alter your proposal to meet the demands of the publisher or its reviewers, or are you uncomfortable with their suggested changes? These are all important questions to consider.

A frequent concern of new authors is the quality of editing that takes place in the publishing company. Specific inquiries should be made about company procedures for editing each manuscript. Other areas of concern for you to explore with the acquisition editor include the company's marketing and promotional plans

---

*The Mosby Author's Guide, St. Louis, 1981, The C. V. Mosby Co.

for the book, the company's attendance at medical meetings in your specialty, and the company's access to international markets.

It is usually better for a publisher to have a good line of books in your specialty, but this should not be the sole criterion of judgment for choosing a publisher. A strong company commitment to developing books in your area of expertise might lead to some very promising developments. Future possibilities for growth and development should be considered in this situation.

Making a final choice

After all of this information has been gathered, you should have sufficient data to make a satisfactory decision based on the company's reputation, the quality of its books, its marketing efforts, and its editorial and editing departments. Often, if all points seem equal, a reasonable decision can be reached based on the acquisition editor you will be working with. This method of selection is not necessarily the most scientific, but it does assure that you will have a pleasant working relationship and will be able to communicate on a project that is very dear to your heart.

Contract negotiations

In all contract negotiations with publishers, it is important to have a good idea of your contract requirements (covering such items as royalties, advances, grants, and indexes) before meeting with the publisher. Playing one publisher against another does not necessarily help to secure a better contract and may even serve to discourage the publisher's further interest in your project. The primary consideration in any contract should be that it is fair and equitable and will provide you with the specific considerations that you feel are most important. After the monumental task involved in writing a book has been completed, most authors are primarily concerned that the object of their labor be produced as a quality publication and promoted effectively. In the long run, these considerations should be the major criteria in making your publishing decision.

Signing the contract

The signing of a publishing agreement brings with it mutual obligations and commitments on the part of the author and the publisher. These obligations are detailed not only in your contract but also in your various meetings and correspondence with the acquisition editor. It is difficult to enumerate all the possible obligations of the author and the publisher, but certain basic responsibilities do seem consistent with all publishing agreements and author-publisher working relationships.

Obligations of the author

1. To prepare the manuscript. Usually this means submitting a reasonably clean, typewritten manuscript; this manuscript should be double-spaced with one-inch margins to allow room for editing. Additional expense may be incurred in preparing extra copies of the manuscript (some publishers require several copies) and in preparing charts, illustrations, and tables (some contracts specify the author's responsibility for all or part of the artist's cost). The preparation of the index usually, but not always, is at the author's expense.

2. To deliver the manuscript by a given date. Different publishers allow different periods of time for writing. Usual time spans range anywhere from six months (very short) to two years. This deadline is subject to negotiation, but the date that appears on the contract should be considered a realistic one; a late manuscript can upset the proposed publishing and promotion schedules thus causing unpleasant feelings and much distress on the part of both the publisher and the author.

3. To keep the number of pages and illustrations within the agreed-upon limits. No color illustrations should be included unless originally specified in the contract.

4. To provide outlines with each chapter, which help the editors establish headings and understand the organization of the manuscript.

5. To check and return galley or page proof or both within a reasonable time of receipt; the period allowed for proofreading is short but varies from publisher to publisher.

6. To bear the cost of alterations other than the typesetter's errors above a certain percentage of the cost of typesetting. Variations are found in this percentage, but 10% is a frequent standard.

7. To supply artwork, photographs, and charts in a suitable form for reproduction. This condition is either contained in the contract or agreed upon by the author and publisher before the contract is signed.

8. To obtain at his or her own expense permissions to reproduce previously copyrighted material. It is the author's responsibility to provide complete credit lines for all borrowed information and to provide signed permission forms from both author and publisher for each item that has been borrowed.

Obligations of the publisher*

1. To publish the work at the company's own risk and expense, unless prevented by catastrophe or calamity, such as strikes, floods, fires, or other circumstances beyond control. In many contracts the obligation to publish is further qualified by being subject to approval or acceptance of the finished manuscript. Consequently, the completed manuscript may be subject to final review to ensure that the form and content meet the originally agreed-upon requirements for publication.

2. To agree with the author on an approximate date of publication. Considerable variation exists here. Some contracts include the actual date for publication, and others make no mention of this detail. Many contracts simply include a manuscript deadline date for the author to turn the work over to the publisher.

3. To establish a fair and competitive price for the book. The approximate price is usually agreed upon, but most often the publisher reserves discretion in this matter and does not include the price as part of the contract.

4. To implement the production, advertising, and distribution of the book. Publishers are open to suggestions from authors on these aspects of publishing, but it is unusual for a publisher to accept any specific obligations in these matters.

5. To provide for the payment of royalties. Royalty rates vary greatly according to individual companies. A 10% royalty rate based on the published price of the book is one of the most usual. This royalty is sometimes more advantageous than the rate of 15% of net received, which is occasionally quoted, because the royalty based on published price keeps the author in step with inflation and a higher price means a higher royalty. Other possibilities include escalator clauses, which provide a sliding royalty scale that increases with sales. Grants and advances against royalties are also means of financial assistance included in contracts. Once again, these royalty options vary greatly according to publisher and project.

With these rules in hand you are now prepared to get involved in the actual work of writing your book and the rewarding and challenging experience of working with the publisher.

WORKING WITH THE PUBLISHER
Writing the book

Editorial department. Your first contact and continuing liaison with the publishing company is through the acquisition editor. The acquisition editor is the person who works with you on your proposal, reviews your manuscript, contracts your book, helps answer your questions, and responds to your complaints. Your editor will discuss the book with you frequently, conferring with you about your progress and any problems you may be having. He or she will talk with you about the subject matter and possible approaches you might take in presenting it. If you are serving as the editor of a contributor book, the acquisition editor will also help contact contributors, coordinate schedules, send welcoming letters and manuscript instructions, and provide reminders of manuscript deadlines.

---

*Modified from Lock, S.: SOMA-Society of Medical Authors, Br. Med. J., pp. 312-313, 1979.

The acquisition editor is your advocate in the company. It is his or her job and responsibility not only to contract your book but also to make sure that it arrives according to specifications and on schedule. He or she is your contact with the publisher for all of your problems and interests and is considered the company expert on your book.

Because of the necessity for frequent exchanges of information between the acquisition editor and you, the author, it is important that good communication exists over topics of mutual concern.

Deadlines. Manuscript deadlines provide one of the primary topics of concern and misunderstanding for both author and publisher. Deadlines are extremely important in publishing and determine production schedules, budgeting goals, and marketing plans. Failure to meet a deadline can cause a whole realignment of priorities in many different areas of the publishing operation: typesetting, printing, binding, and advertising and promotion. It can interfere with the release of the book at the most auspicious time of the year—for example, in time to be considered for textbook adoption or to be displayed at the annual meeting of a key national society. Editors understand that deadlines cannot always be met, but realistic planning is essential. Comments like "What's another month!" may be meant to diminish anxiety but in reality reflect an insensitivity to the problems of publishing and a lack of awareness of the importance of meeting commitments.

Promptly met publishing deadlines are also important from the author's point of view. They allow you to see the fruition of your labors more quickly and assure that your book will reflect the current state of the art. Simply sticking to your writing task will also mean that you will complete it sooner and be able to move on to other projects.

Communication. As work on your manuscript progresses, you will be in frequent contact with the editorial department, securing the help you need to put your book together. The publisher's responsiveness to your questions and needs will help to make your writing task a more enjoyable one. It is also important for you to be responsive to the publisher's phone calls, letters, and editorial meetings. For example, reminders of missed deadlines are not meant to inflame errant authors or contributors but to alert them to the fact that the manuscript is behind schedule and that schedules need to be reassessed and redefined.

Realistic expectations about advertising. Even though all authors dream of having a full-page spread advertising their book in the *New York Times* and in all of the major medical journals, this is not economically feasible. Marketing and advertising requests should be tempered by realistic expectations. As an author you need to understand that the publisher is committed to producing and marketing your book as effectively as possible.

Finished manuscript

It is difficult to describe the immense feeling of relief an author feels when the manuscript is complete and has been safely delivered into the hands of the publisher. This relief is sometimes quickly replaced by anxiety over seeming delays in getting the book published. It may have taken two years to write, but many authors seem to feel that the book should be published in a day. The most rational professionals have been known to swear that publishing companies other than their own have published monumental works in a mere six months, while their publisher cannot manage to bring out their book in less than twelve.

It is often felt that a certain mystique surrounds the workings of a publishing house, and most authors are uncertain about what actually happens to their book once it leaves their hands and is delivered to the publisher. Information about the actual workings of the publishing company and what happens to the book once it reaches the publisher may help clear up some of the misunderstandings (Fig 7-2).

Editorial review. The first people to see your manuscript are in the editorial department. After they review the manuscript for content and style, it is passed along for an intensive "processing" to clarify any problems before editing begins. The processors ascertain whether all materials are present, such as illustrations and legends (captions) for illustrations, permission letters, and credit lines for borrowed material. They cross-check numbers of tables and figures (illustrations) with the numbers on legends and in-text mentions. They review the organization and prepare the illustrations for the production process. Although this manuscript check-in varies with each company, it will proceed smoothly if, before submitting the manuscript, you have taken the time to give a final check to see that all information is complete and the manuscript conforms to the guidelines provided by the publisher (Fig. 7-3). Scrutiny of your manuscript before mailing it to the publisher and the publisher's screening procedure after receipt help ensure that all major questions are brought to your attention before the manuscript is edited and sent to the typesetter; they also help the editing process proceed more efficiently. When processing is completed, your manuscript is ready to be copyedited.

Manuscript editing. The arrangements for copyediting your book are handled in different ways by different companies. Some publishers use freelance editors while others maintain an in-house staff of experienced manuscript editors. The role of these highly skilled editors remains basically the same. Manuscript editors subject

1 AUTHOR
Instant book bypass
PUBLISHER
9 FINISHED BOOKS
8A CLOTH MILL
Actual route
1A ILLUSTRATOR (Freelance)
8 BINDERY
Manuscript
Illustrations
Binders board
6 LITHOGRAPHER
Press sheets
2 EDITORIAL
Editorial Director
7 PRINTER
7A PAPER MILL
Printing plates
3 EDITING
Processor
4 PRODUCTION
Production Manager   Designer
5A PHOTOLITHOGRAPHER
Illustration proofs
Reproduction proofs
Illustrations
Editing Manager
Manuscript Editor
5 TYPESETTER
Manuscript
Aspirin
Manuscript
Illustrations
INDEXER (Freelance)
Page proofs
Index
Galley proofs
(To and from author via Production and Editing)
Proofreader
Page proofs
Debbie Fenner

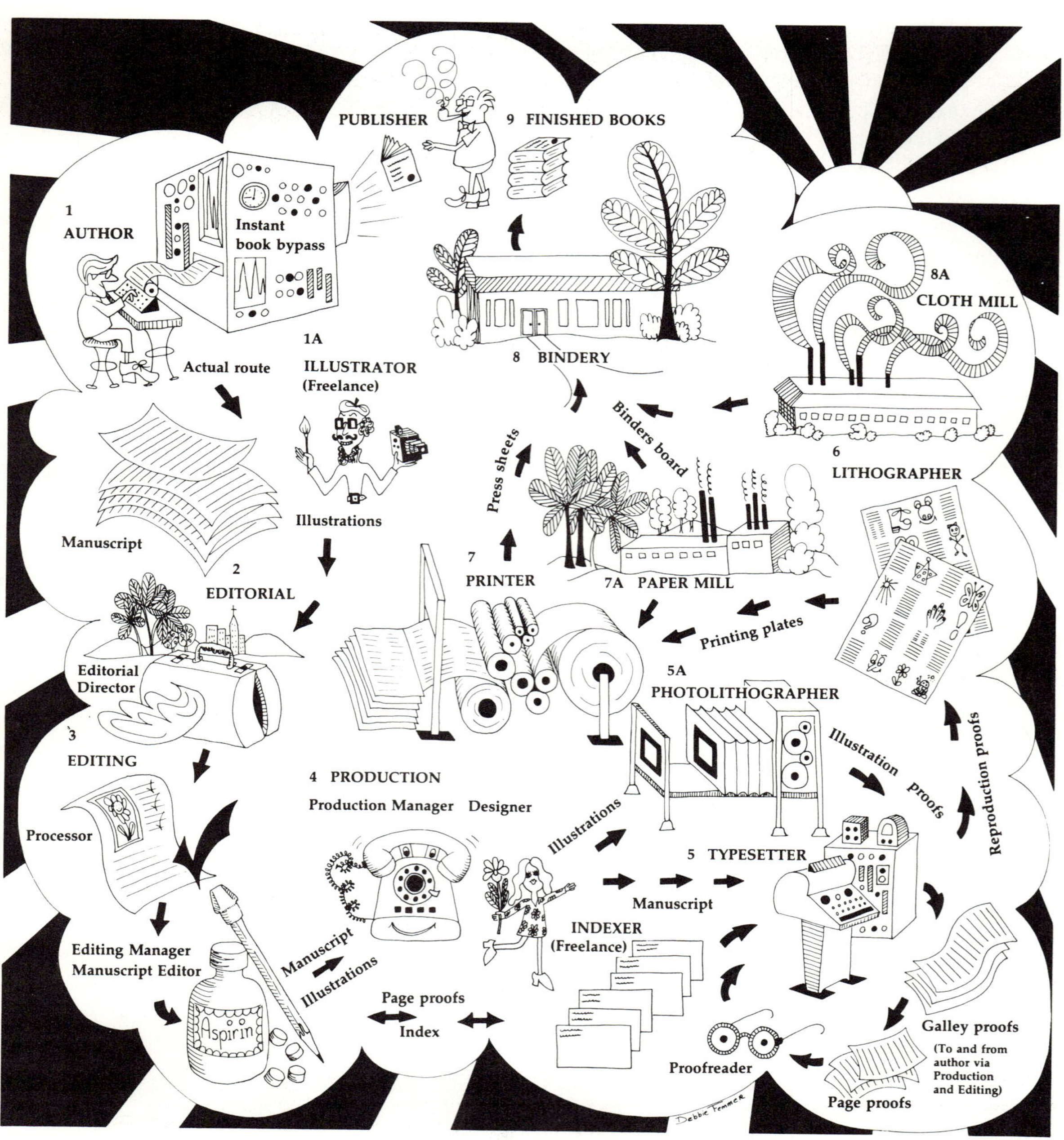

Fig. 7-2.

AUTHOR CHECKLIST

I. The following items should be present before the manuscript is delivered
to the publisher:

Title page	Illustrations
Preface	Legends (to match illustrations)
Table of contents	Credit lines (to indicate when informa-
Contributor list	tion has been borrowed from another source)
Dedication (optional)	Tables
Foreword (optional)	Permissions
Acknowledgments	References
Chapter outlines	Appendices (optional)

Glossary (optional)

II. The following questions should be answered:

Is the manuscript double spaced and typewritten with one inch margins?

Are the pages numbered?

Do the legends match the illustrations?

Are the legends detached from the illustrations?

Are all the illustrations mentioned in the text?

Are all the tables mentioned in the text?

Are all the reference numbers cited in the text?

Are all the illustrations legible?

Are the illustrations numbered to match the legends?

Are cropmarks noted on all illustrations?

Is the top of each illustration marked whenever necessary?

Are all of the tables numbered properly and do they have complete
credit lines where necessary?

Does each borrowed illustration and table have both author and publisher
permission?

Does each illustration which shows a patient who is recognizable have a
patient or parent consent? If the consent is not available, is illustration marked "block eyes"?

Has permission been obtained for and a full credit line given for every
quotation?

Are references in the style agreed upon for the book; e.g., alphabetical/
numerical, author/date?

Are references in the same style in every chapter?

Fig. 7-3.

your manuscript to careful scrutiny; they focus on its organization, logical development, and clarity of expression. They also give attention to more mechanical details, such as spelling, grammar, and reference style. Finally, these editors mark the manuscript for the typesetters so that they can set all elements of the manuscript into the appropriate type.

Manuscript editors frequently confer with you before the manuscript goes to the typesetter. Any major questions that have arisen during editing are checked out with you. Minor questions are usually handled as queries on the proofs of typeset text that are sent to you. After your manuscript has been set in type, the manuscript editor examines the proofs of the type and sends them to you for proofreading.

During the entire editing and proofing process, the acquisition editor or other representative of the publisher is in contact with you periodically regarding the schedule, the progress of your book, and any other questions that may arise.

Production. You seldom have direct contact with people who perform production department functions for your book; yet the work they do is vital to its publication. The editorial and editing staffs are experts in how the book's information is presented, the authors are experts in the book's content, and the people in production are experts in how the book will look and technologically how it gets from manuscript to bound book.

During production, major design decisions are made about your book. The typography for the inside of the book and the cover for the outside are determined. Illustrations are prepared and sent to the photoengravers.

Finally, coordination of the scheduling of your book is done through production; members of the department establish with the typesetter, photoengraver, printer, and binder the times that must be allotted for each stage of production for each book. They are in constant contact with the editing and editorial personnel to make certain that these schedules are met and that all mesh to reach the final publication date for your book.

Finished book

The end result of all this effort is a finished book, a source of justifiable pride for you and your publisher, who have successfully cooperated to contribute another fine piece of scientific writing to the literature. This is the culmination of several years of work and a cause for celebration for every member of the team who made it happen.

SECTION II

Speaking

CHAPTER 8

Putting a speech together

Robert C. Reeder, M.D.

A scientific presentation is, in essence, something worth saying arranged in proper order and said in a suitable way. It must succeed when it is given, since it will be heard but once by the audience. Unlike the author of a printed paper, a speaker does not have the advantages of paragraphing, headings, and footnotes; nor can the audience read and reread the text at leisure until all the material has been comprehended. The speaker must, therefore, prepare material carefully and must develop an orderly approach to its preparation. To a large part, the success of an oral presentation will depend upon the time spent in organization, preparation, and rehearsal.

Before you begin to write the script for a presentation, determine the location, date, and time of your appearance; how much time you have been allotted; the subject about which you are to speak; and the type audience to whom the presentation will be made. Determine, also, what types of visual aid equipment will be provided by the sponsor. After you have this information you can prepare a speech that will be suited to the audience, to the occasion, and to the time limit.

TYPES OF SPEECHES

Having obtained the preliminary information, you can begin to prepare your manuscript. You must first decide which type of speech you will present. Regardless of the type you choose, your speech should have a format similar to a written paper and contain, at a minimum, an introduction, a body, and a conclusion.

There are four basic types of speeches:

1. The *impromptu speech* requires no previous preparation. This is the least effective type, regardless of how accomplished a speaker you are.
2. The *manuscript speech* is written, revised, rehearsed and then read word for word. This type allows you to say exactly what you want, but lacks a lively, direct approach since it is difficult to write a manuscript in the spoken style.
3. The *memorized speech* is similar to the manuscript. It also is written and revised, but is then committed to memory. It, in effect, becomes a public recitation. This type may strain the memory of a speaker and may cause great anguish should he or she lose the train of thought in the middle of the presentation.
4. The *extemporaneous speech* is one in which the material is selected and prepared in advance, but is then expressed in the language of the moment. The preliminary planning includes what to say, but how to say it is left to the discretion of the speaker at the time of the presentation. Notes are used for memory and for quotes, statistics, and accuracy of detail.

You should use the type of speech that is most comfortable for you. If you are inexperienced or if you are presenting a major dissertation to a large group, the manuscript style may be the best. When using this type you are thoroughly familiar with your material because of careful preparation and rehearsal, and you have the manuscript to reinforce your presentation.

Another good method is to write the speech as a manuscript, then prepare an outline for notes during the presentation. The introduction and conclusion may be written completely, and the rest of the speech outlined.

OUTLINE

The outline of a speech is a blueprint or preliminary plan for the manuscript. It places ideas in logical order and systematic arrangement. A good outline should result in a good presentation.

There are two types of outlines: the topical, in which ideas are expressed as simple words or phrases, and the complete sentence, in which ideas are expressed fully. You may prefer to first make a rough outline containing only major topics, then refine this into a final, more complete outline.

MANUSCRIPT

The manuscript for a speech should be prepared in the spoken rather than the written style. The spoken style is direct and personal; it receives and reacts to audience response. On the other hand, the written style tends to be more aloof and impersonal and may sound stilted. Remember, also, that even though you are preparing a manuscript in the spoken style, it must still follow a standard format and have an introduction, a body, and a conclusion. In other words, tell the audience what you are going to say, say it, then tell them what you have said.

If you are going to make your presentation from a manuscript that has been prepared for publication, it will be necessary to rewrite it in the spoken style, not only to make it suitable for verbal presentation, but also to stay within the allotted time on the program. You should prepare a manuscript that follows the general outline of a paper written for publication, but that becomes conversational rather than formal or dogmatic.

NOTES

Regardless of the type notes you prefer, they should be easy to read, easily kept in order, and unobtrusive; they should not detract from your podium appearance. An otherwise perfectly prepared presentation can be destroyed if you must fumble for notes or if you lose your place in the middle of your talk. Avoid, at all times, multiple types of notes such as note cards intermingled with handwritten notes and, perhaps, photocopied pages from a journal.

Note cards. If you choose to use note cards, they should be large, a minimum of 4×6 inch. Use only one side and put only essential information on each. The printing should be large enough to be read easily.

Complete text. If you use the complete text for notes, it should be typed on a standard $8\frac{1}{2} \times 11$ inch sheet in large type, double-spaced with wide margins. Try to make the line width such that it can be scanned with a single glance.

Outline. Outline notes should also be typed on an $8\frac{1}{2} \times 11$ inch page. Like a complete manuscript, these should be double spaced and in large type. You may prefer to use all capitals. You may wish, also, to write the introduction and the conclusion completely.

If notes are typed on standard size paper, they may be paperclipped together, so that one page may be slid unobtrusively aside as you finish with it. Never staple a set of notes together; turning the pages may produce dis-

traction. Another good way to keep notes of this type in order is to punch the pages and to place them in a small three-ring notebook. This assures that the pages will be kept in order, may be followed easily, and will produce a minimum of distraction for the audience.

Regardless of the type notes used, try to give the audience the impression that you are well prepared and well organized.

VISUAL AIDS

We learn 11% of what we know through our ears and 87% through our eyes. We retain 20% of what we hear, 30% of what we see, but 50% to 75% of what we both see and hear. For this reason visual aids can be an important adjunct to a scientific presentation. They attract and hold attention, make the meaning clear, emphasize ideas, prove a point, impress the memory, and make a speech more interesting. In themselves, however, they do not make a good speech. They must be selected, prepared, and used with skill; they must be necessary, should save time, and should amplify the presentation. At the same time, however, they should not be simply a repetition of your text.

Preparation and correlation of visual aids with text

After you have written your speech, you must then correlate the visual aids with the manuscript. The top of your probably already cluttered desk or the bedroom floor at home is not the proper place to do this. You will accomplish the task more efficiently and effectively if you establish a place in which to work. This can be a small room at the office or at home in which you can assemble the materials to prepare your visual aids and to correlate them with your manuscript. Such an area permits you to organize your work and results, ultimately, in a more effective presentation with a minimum of confusion and wasted effort on your part.

Working area. In the working area you can collect all equipment and materials you will need to prepare your visual aids and to correlate them with your text (Fig. 8-1). Even if your visuals are prepared professionally, you still need such a space to preview them and to assure that they are properly integrated your with presentation. You will need, at a minimum, a work table that provides room for planning, sorting, arranging, previewing, and assembling visual aids (Fig. 8-2). If you are going to prepare your own visuals you will also need a drawing table and a taboret for storage of art supplies (Fig. 8-3); also, equipment for photographing the artwork (Fig. 8-4). Other equipment in the working area that is helpful, but not essential, is a storage area for slides and carousel trays and a small file cabinet for pertinent reference material and the scripts of previously prepared or frequent-

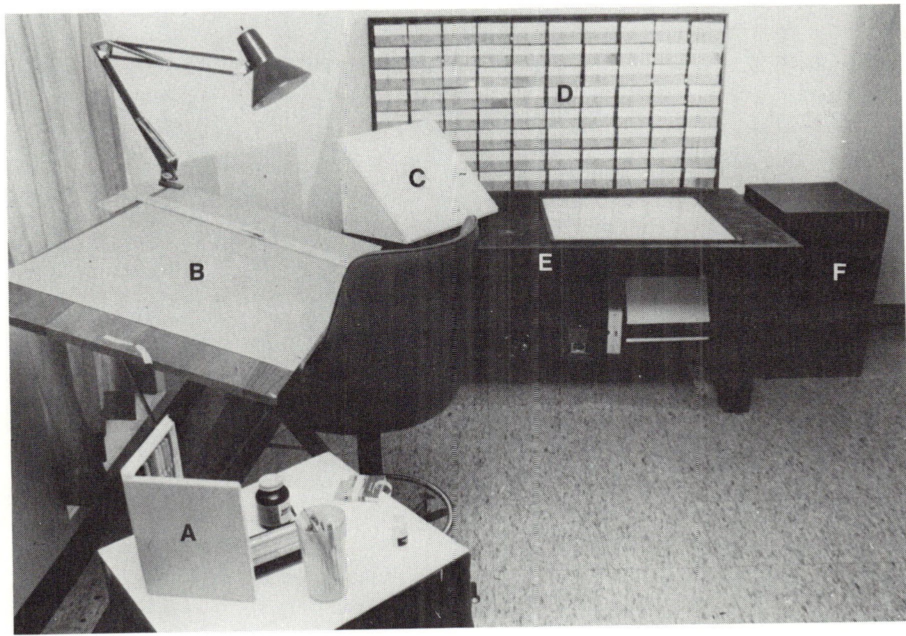

Fig. 8-1. The working area. **A,** Drawing supplies; **B,** drawing board; **C,** slide sorter; **D,** planning board; **E,** work table with illuminated slide sorter inset into top; **F,** file cabinet.

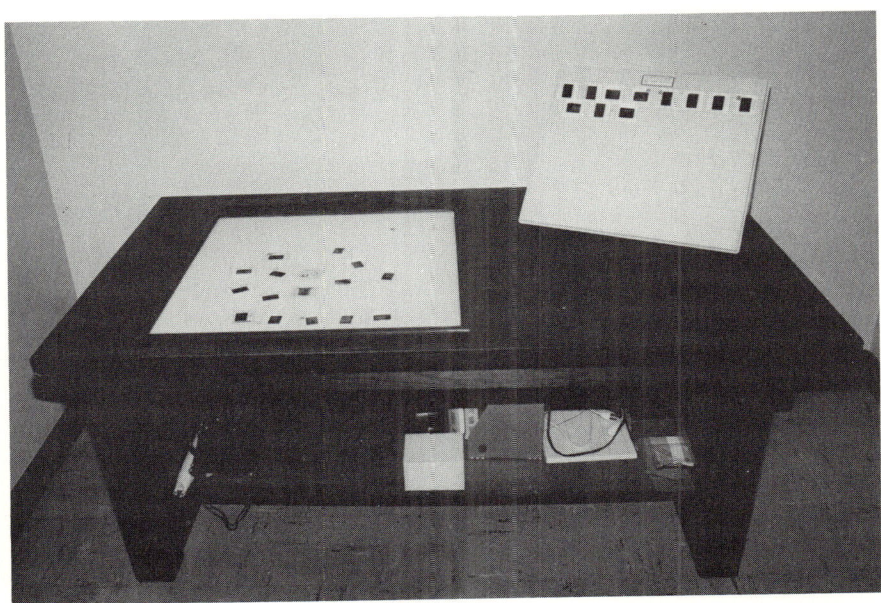

Fig. 8-2. The work table provides a place on which to sort and arrange slides. The lower shelf can be used for storage of supplies and equipment.

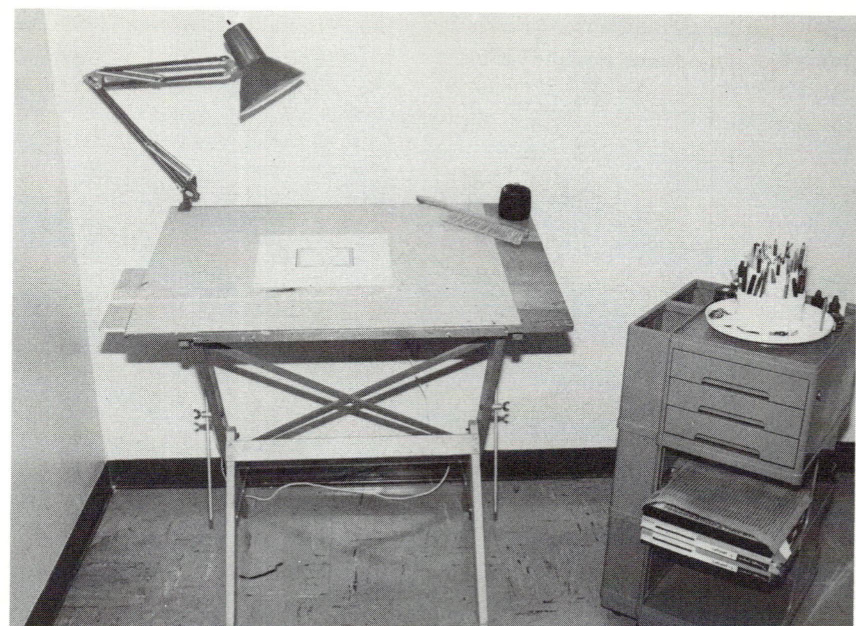

Fig. 8-3. Drawing board and taboret. The type board illustrated here can be folded away for storage, but when set up it gives a sturdy surface upon which to prepare artwork. A clamp-on type light provides good illumination. The taboret is used to store art supplies and equipment.

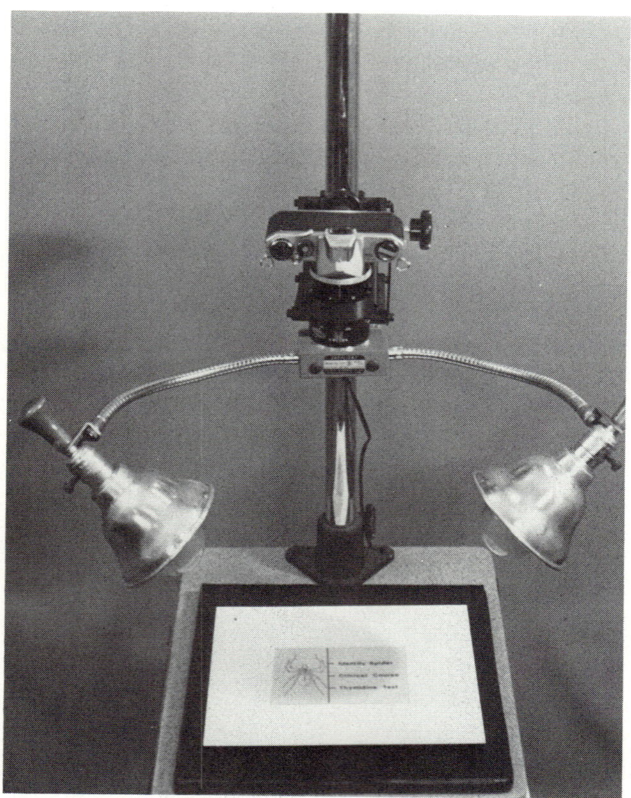

Fig. 8-4. Photographic copy stand. While this equipment is not essential, it makes the task of copying artwork easier. The camera can be adjusted to accurately frame the picture, then fixed securely in place. Also, the lights can be positioned to provide even and reproducible illumination of the original.

ly presented talks. Even if you do not have room for this type arrangement, at least set aside an area in which you can work and in which you can leave your material undisturbed until you have finished putting together your talk.

Planning board. A planning board helps to correlate visual aids with the text of a scientific presentation. These are available commercially or may be constructed very simply from plywood, cleared X-ray film, or clear plastic and suitable molding (Fig. 8-5). Regardless of the type used, there should be eighty pockets into which file cards will fit. This will, then, be compatible with the standard 80-slide carousel tray.

As a decision for each visual aid is made, the instructions are written on a planning card (Fig. 8-6) and this card is inserted into the proper slot on the planning board (Fig. 8-7). These can be rearranged on the board as necessary until the proper sequence is determined. After the final sequence has been decided, the planning cards can be used as a guide to the preparation of the visuals (Fig. 8-8) as well as to assist in the proper arrangement of the completed slides.

Sorting and viewing slides. After all the visual aids have been prepared, they should be previewed on a light box or viewer. This may be as simple as an X-ray view box (Fig. 8-9) or one that is constructed by building a plywood box, painting the inside white, mounting a fluorescent fixture inside and covering the top with translucent plastic. The "homemade" box can be as large as you wish to make it. It may be used either independently or flush mounted in the top of your work table (Fig. 8-10).

After you have previewed your slides on a light box, arrange them in order on a lighted sorter, using the planning cards as a guide. Since the standard carousel tray holds 80 slides, use a sorter of similar capacity (Fig. 8-11). After the proper sequence has been assembled on the sorter, load the slides into a carousel tray in appropriate order.

Occasionally a slide that looks acceptable on the view box will be slightly out of focus or poorly exposed when projected. Therefore, you should project all slides before making the decision to use them.

After you have selected the proper slides, have projected them to ensure that they are acceptable, and have arranged them in proper sequence, each should be oriented, numbered, and labeled. Put your name on them with either a small rubber stamp (Fig. 8-12) or by writing on the mount. Then orient each by placing a mark in the lower left corner when the slide is viewed as it will be seen on the screen. If the slides are then loaded into the tray with this mark in the upper right corner, they will project in proper orientation (Fig. 8-13). Next, mark the slide number on each as dictated by the planning cards.

After the slides are loaded into a carousel tray, project them once again to be sure each is in proper order and is properly oriented. Check again for the quality and sharpness of focus of each. Having done this, project them once again, while following the script. On this, mark the appropriate point at which each is to be shown. This may be done in the left-hand margin or in the space above the text where the slide change is to occur.

Text continued on p. 51.

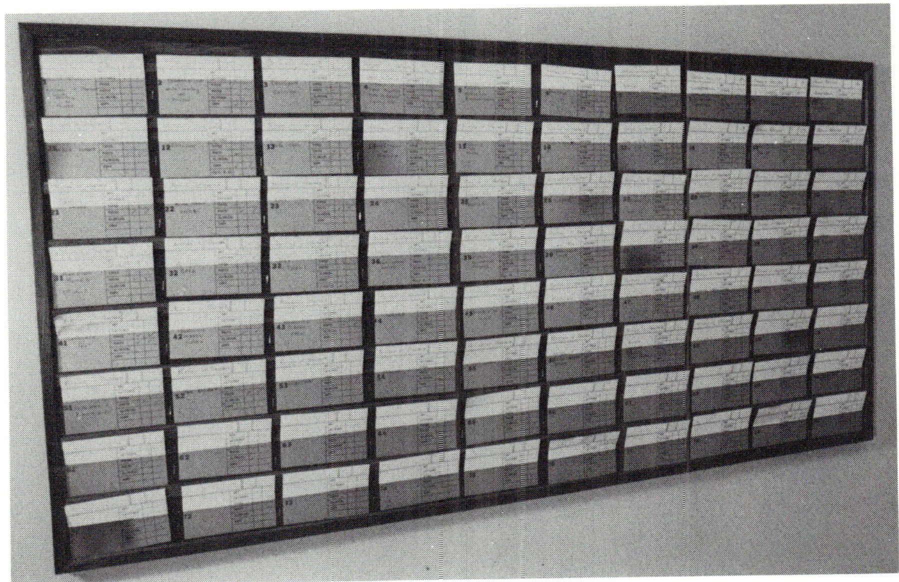

Fig. 8-5. This planning board was made of plywood and cleared X-ray film. Others can be obtained commercially. Regardless of the type used, there should be 80 pockets for planning cards to correspond with the number of slides held by a standard carousel tray.

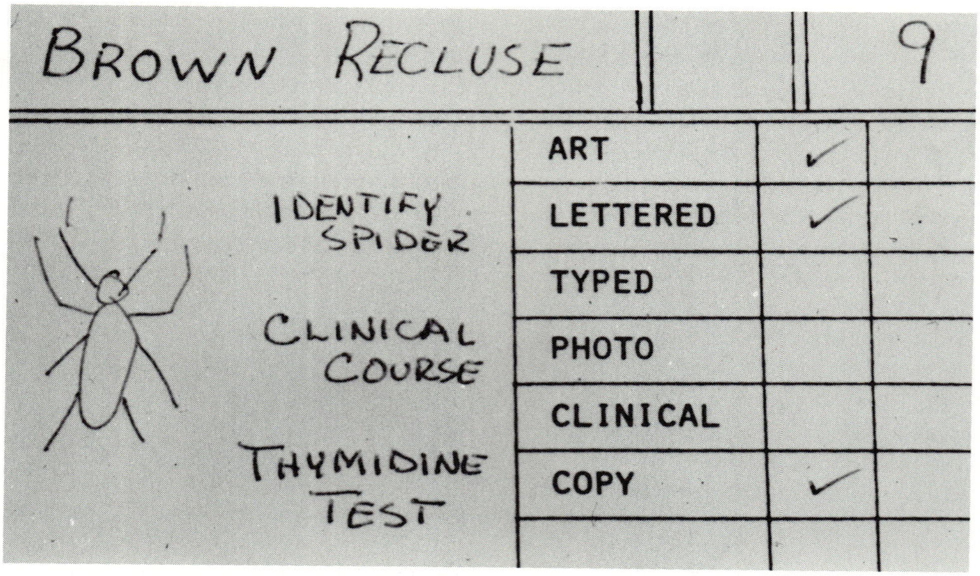

Fig. 8-6. A planning card should be made for each visual to be used. On the card there are spaces to designate the title of the talk, the slide number, a rough sketch or description of the slide, and columns to designate the tasks that must be done and to indicate when these have been completed. A check in the first column designates what must be done and one in the second column indicates that this has been done. Using different colored pens in the two columns makes it easier to determine when all work has been completed.

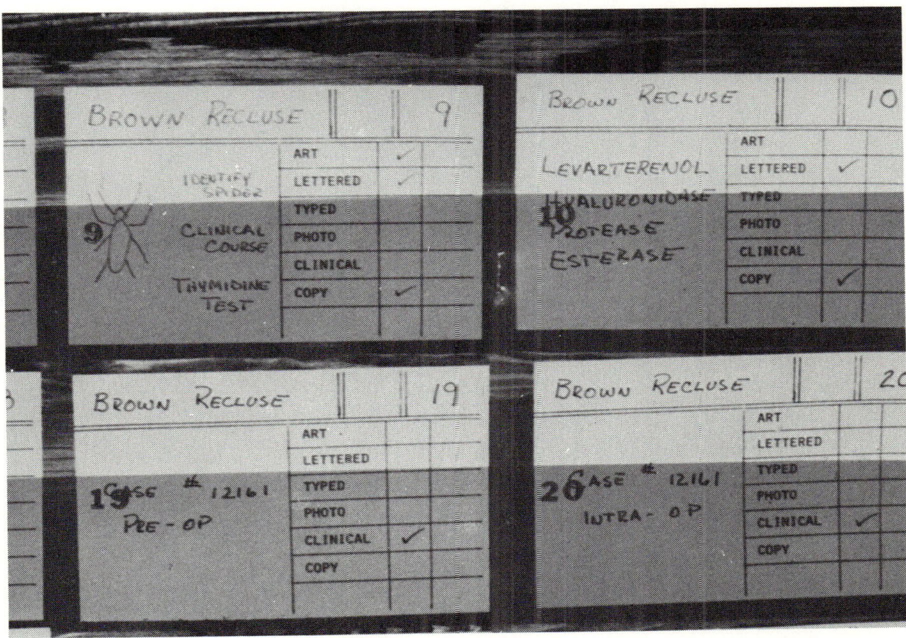

Fig. 8-7. The planning cards are inserted into pockets on the planning board and rearranged until the proper sequence has been determined. When the proper arrangement has been made, the cards may be numbered to correspond with the number on the pocket.

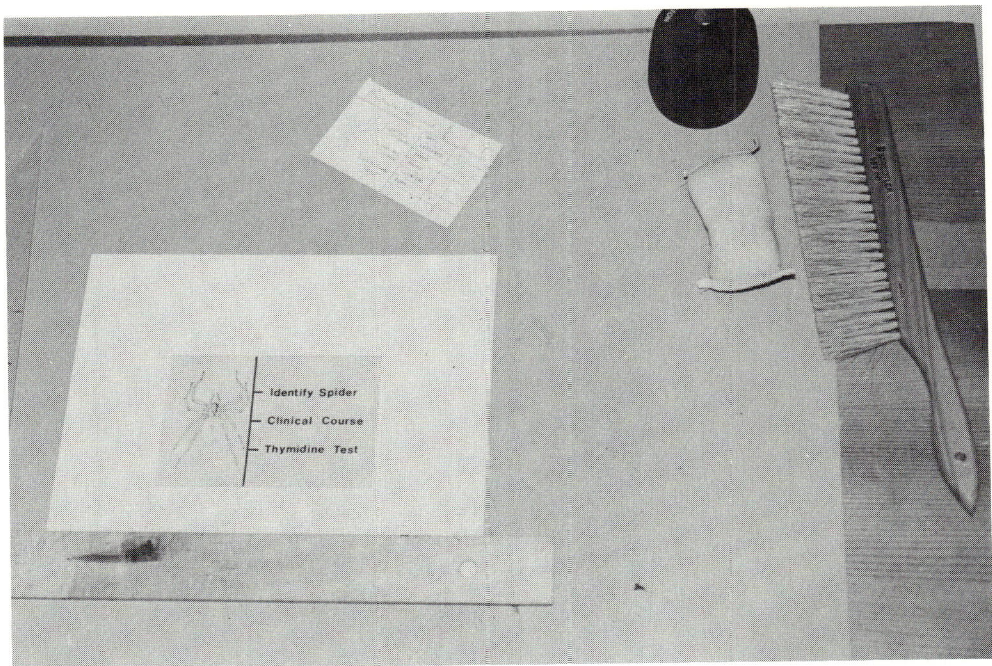

Fig. 8-8. The planning card can be used as a guide to preparation of artwork.

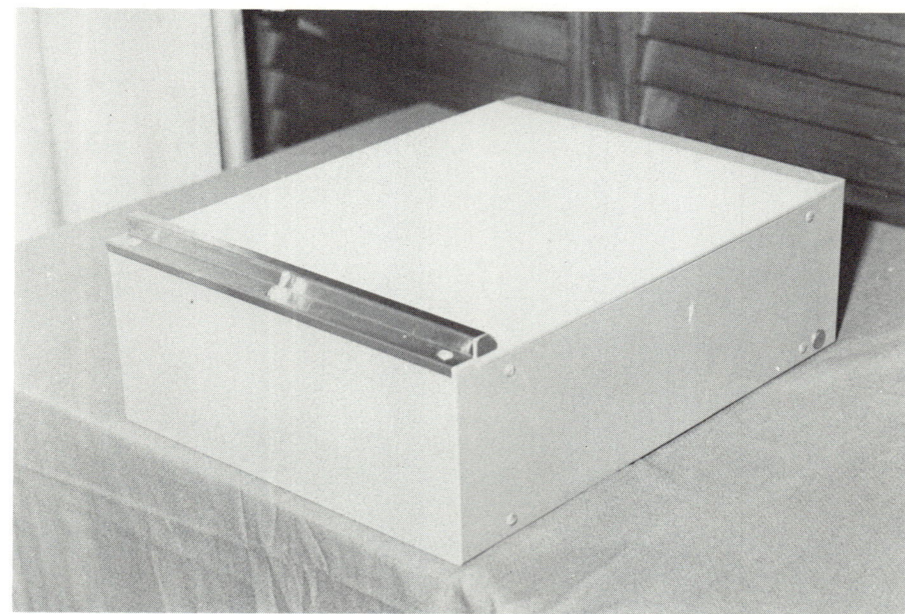

Fig. 8-9. A standard X-ray view box can be used as a tabletop viewer for slides.

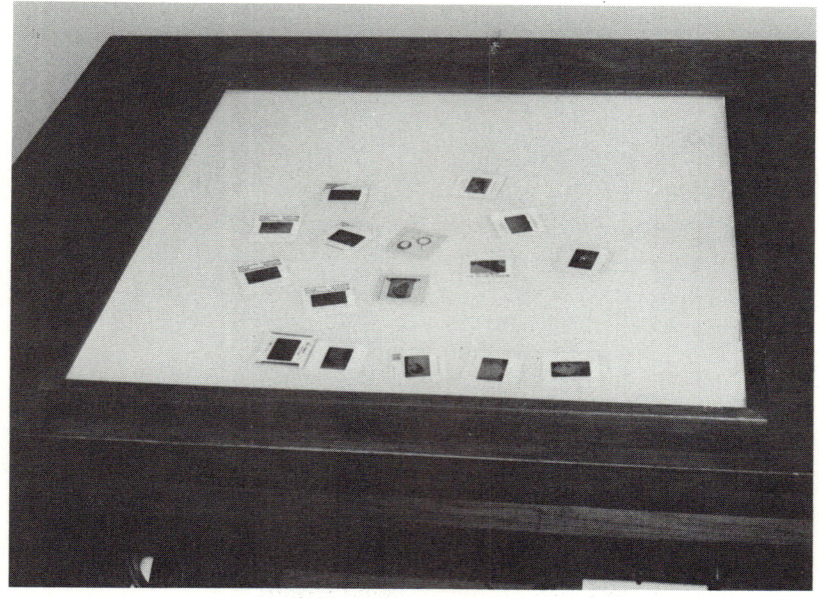

Fig. 8-10. For permanent use an X-ray view box or a specially constructed light box can be flush mounted into the surface of a work table.

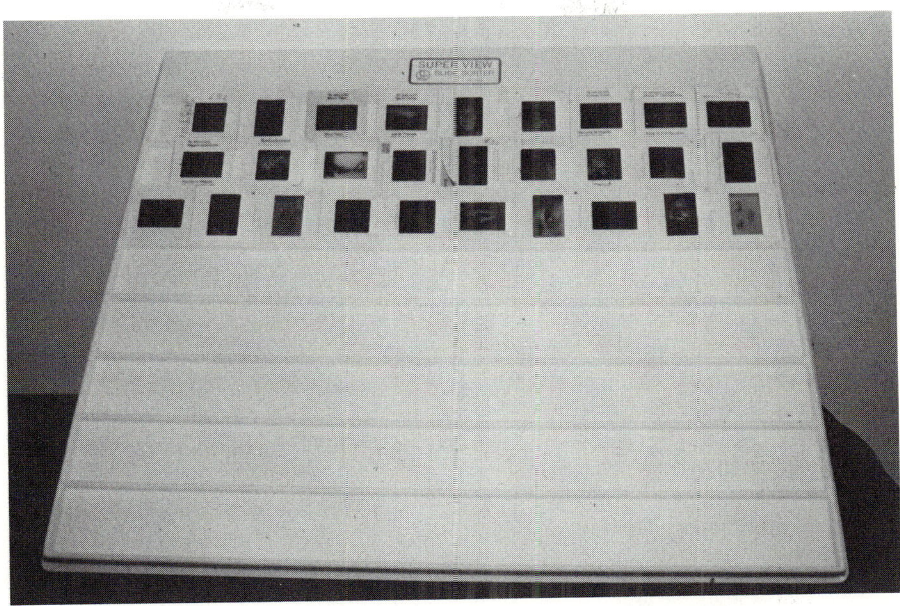

Fig. 8-11. An illuminated slide sorter is helpful to arrange slides in proper sequence after they have been previewed on the light box. Since a carousel tray holds 80 slides, the sorter should have the same capacity.

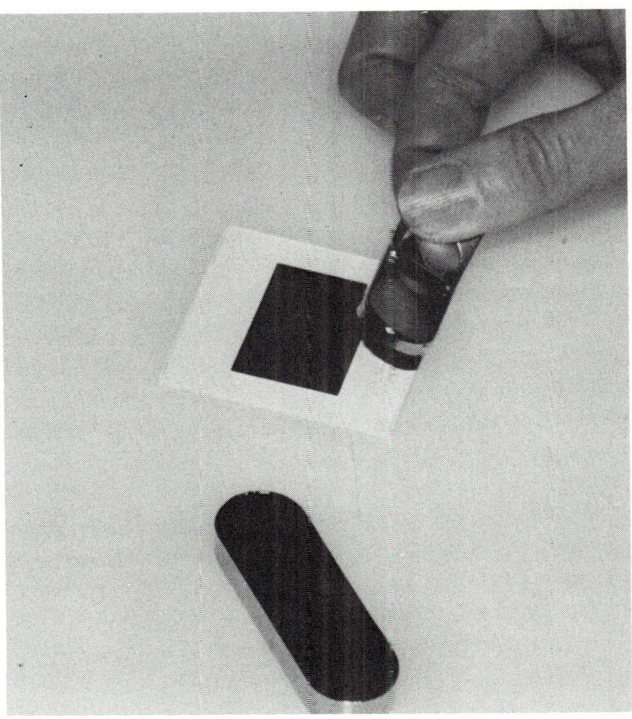

Fig. 8-12. All slides should be identified with the owner's name. This illustrates the use of a small rubber stamp to do this. The owner's name can also be written on the slide mount.

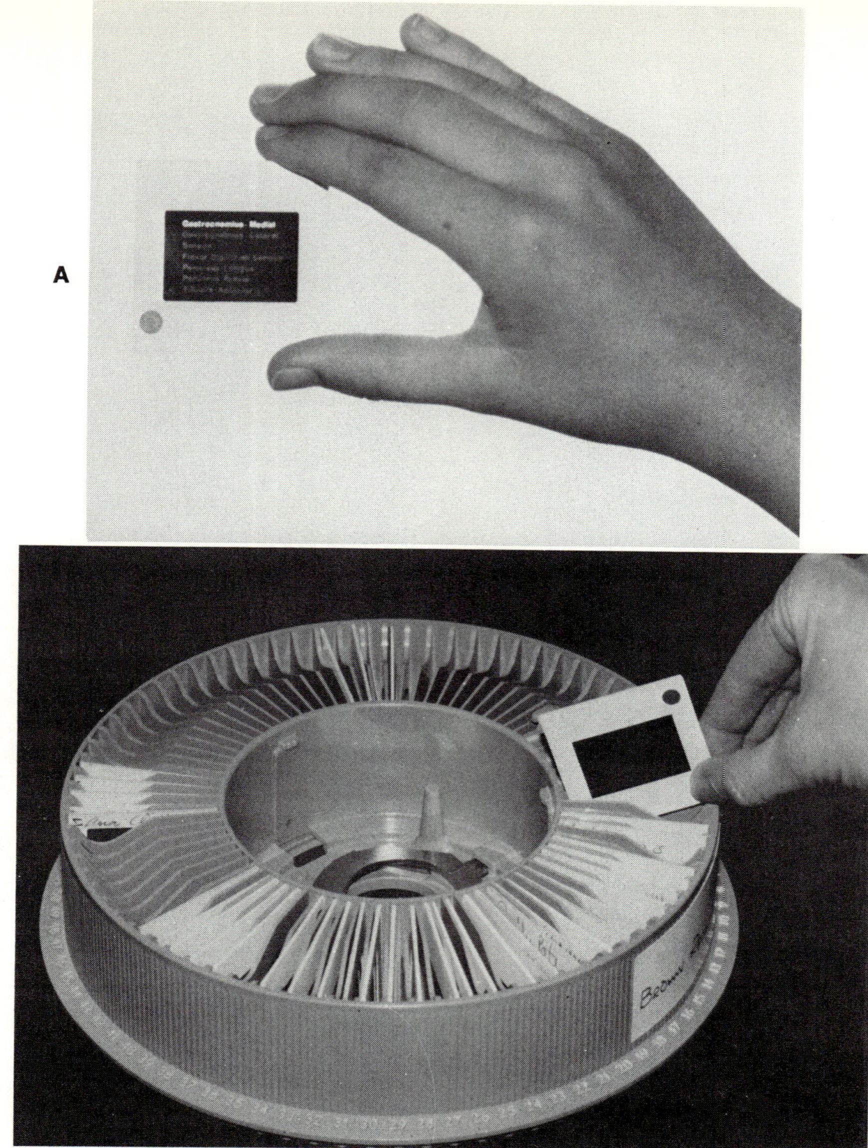

Fig. 8-13. Slide orientation. **A,** When the slide is viewed as it will be projected on the screen, place a dot in the lower left corner. **B,** Place the dot in the upper right corner when loading the slide into the projector tray.

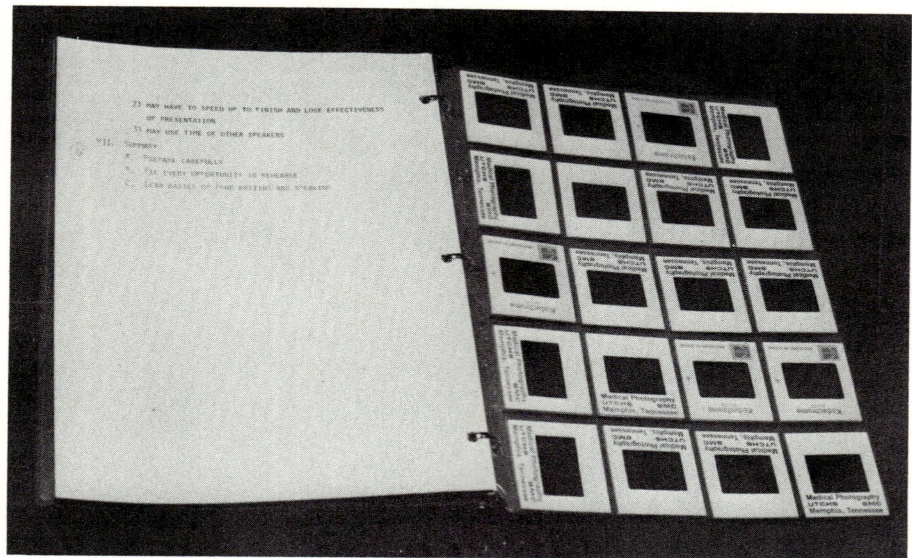

Fig. 8-14. One method of taking slides to a meeting is to place the slides in transparent file sheets and place them in a three-ring binder with the text or notes of the presentation.

Transporting slides

If you are presenting your talk locally or if space is not a problem, load the slides into a carousel tray and transport them this way. This should ensure that all will be in proper order and properly oriented if you have projected and checked them after loading the tray.

If you must travel by air or if you have several trays to take, consider carrying them in a less bulky manner. A small slide file or even the processor's box may be satisfactory. An even better method is to place the slides in order in page-size transparent file sheets and to include them in the notebook with your manuscript (Fig. 8-14). If you use any of these latter methods, it is imperative that each of the slides be identified, oriented, and numbered to prevent confusion when loading them into a tray at the meeting.

Regardless of the method you choose to carry your slides, they should be previewed by projection immediately before you give your presentation. This will avoid the embarrassment of having slides out of sequence, backward, or improperly oriented.

REHEARSAL

The adage that "practice makes perfect" is particularly appropriate when preparing for a scientific presentation. It is during rehearsal that you become thoroughly familiar with your material and bring the speech to perfection. During rehearsal you can improve your speaking technique by relying on self-analysis and on criticism from both yourself and others. You will find it helpful to present your talk not only to a group of your peers but also to lay persons. While the latter may not understand the technical content of your paper, they can, nevertheless, comment on your clarity and method of delivery.

A tape recorder is an invaluable help when rehearsing a scientific presentation. By listening to the recording you can analyze the pace of your presentation, listen to your style and voice inflections, and listen for any distracting habits such as the frequent use of "uh." If you use a portable recorder, you can repeatedly review your material while commuting to your office or the hospital, and you can take it with you to the meeting for a last minute "brush up" in your hotel room.

If you are fortunate enough to have a videotape recorder, you may then see yourself as the audience will. Lacking this, practice in front of a mirror to develop eye contact with the audience and to develop gestures that will help emphasize important points.

FINAL PREPARATION

Take a duplicate set of notes and slides with you to the meeting—one in your briefcase, the other in your luggage. By so doing, even if one of them is lost you will still have a set of notes and slides. If you wear reading glasses, be sure to take an extra pair with you. If you don't, Murphy's law will dictate that your only pair will be lost or broken just before time to go to the podium and there you will be: having written a brilliant manuscript and unable to read a word of it. Be sure to take the proper visual aids for the presentation you are going to make. The slides of your vacation to California add little to a scholarly dissertation about the molecular structure of RNA. Finally, take your tape recorder for a last minute review.

The time is at hand. You are at the podium. If your preparation has been careful, thorough, and accurate, and if you have rehearsed until you are familiar and comfortable with your material, you can make your presentation with the conviction that your message is the result of honest and serious preparation and that it will be of value to those who hear it.

CHAPTER 9

Speaker readiness

Earl Bauer

A speaker should be ready to go when the time for the presentation arrives. The slides should be in order and properly oriented, he or she should know how to advance the slides, where the pointer is and how to operate it, and what type of microphone will be used. How does a program chairman ensure that all of this will be accomplished? Very simply: by providing a speaker ready room.

Every audiovisual coordinator should establish a firm policy of having each speaker report to the speaker ready room to load and preview the slides. I recall an incident when one of the speakers refused to check through the ready room, saying "No, it's not necessary. Everything is fine. I've run through my slides up in my room, they're fine, just take them." He walked up to the lectern to begin his paper. He asked for his first slide and began his presentation. After a few sentences he hesitated and asked for the next slide. Speaking into the microphone to the projectionist he said, "That is the wrong slide. Go back . . . no, go forward. Go forward another one. Wait." There was total silence for several seconds, then, "My gosh . . . that's from my program for tomorrow. I've brought the wrong slides."

In another instance a speaker walked into the ready room, walked over to the table and announced "I am Dr. Good, the first speaker. Here are my slides. They are in the proper sequence, numbered and marked." The technician proceeded to load the speaker's slides. The doctor was right; they were all in proper order with a yellow dot in the corner. The technician then asked the speaker to review the slides with him on the projector. The first slide was projected, sharp as a tack, but rotated 90 degrees to the right. It was rotated in the tray and then projected perfectly. Slide number two: also rotated 90 degrees to the right. With that Dr. Good came to his feet and demanded to see the tray. "No wonder," he

said, "you have them in wrong. The dot should go in the upper left corner." The patient technician pointed out that the thumb mark is normally placed in the upper *right* corner. "But," explained Dr. Good, "I'm left-handed."

The moral to these stories is to always check your slides through a speaker ready room. It is the only way to guarantee that each speaker's slides are exactly as they are to be seen during the presentation. It also gives the speaker a chance to become familiar with the other equipment that will be supplied at the podium in the meeting room.

EQUIPMENT

What goes into a good speaker ready room? To begin with, coffee, juice, and sweet rolls. This is a simple gesture, but it helps relax jittery speakers who may have been up half the night putting the finishing touch on their papers. Equipment includes an X-ray view box on which to check the slides to be certain they are in proper order. Also necessary is a carousel projector or a tabletop audioviewer on which slides can be projected to be sure they are right side up and in the right sequence (Fig. 9-1). Also needed are a table with extra trays, white gloves, tape, marking pens, and gummed labels.

A lectern similar to that being used in the meeting room should be available (Fig. 9-2). The slide change apparatus, a pointer like that to be used, and any other special equipment such as a timer should be on the lectern. The speakers can familiarize themselves with the equipment before going into the meeting room to make their formal presentation. For large meetings a reception desk and typist are also helpful.

The trays should be labeled after they have been loaded—one color label for morning sessions and a different color for the afternoon. The speaker's name, the

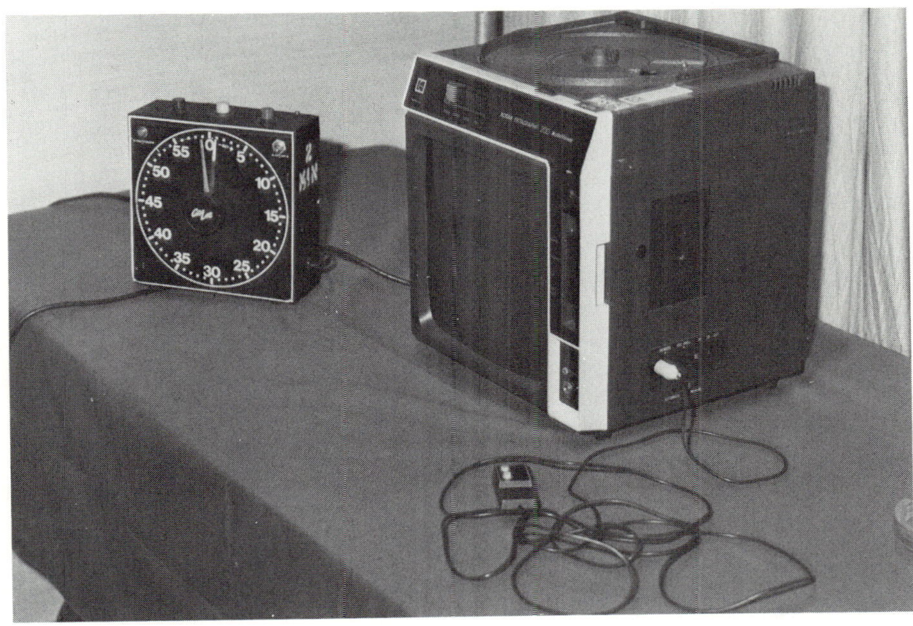

Fig. 9-1. Speaker ready room equipment. A tabletop viewer allows a speaker to preview slides for orientation and proper sequence. The timer can be used to check the length of the presentation.

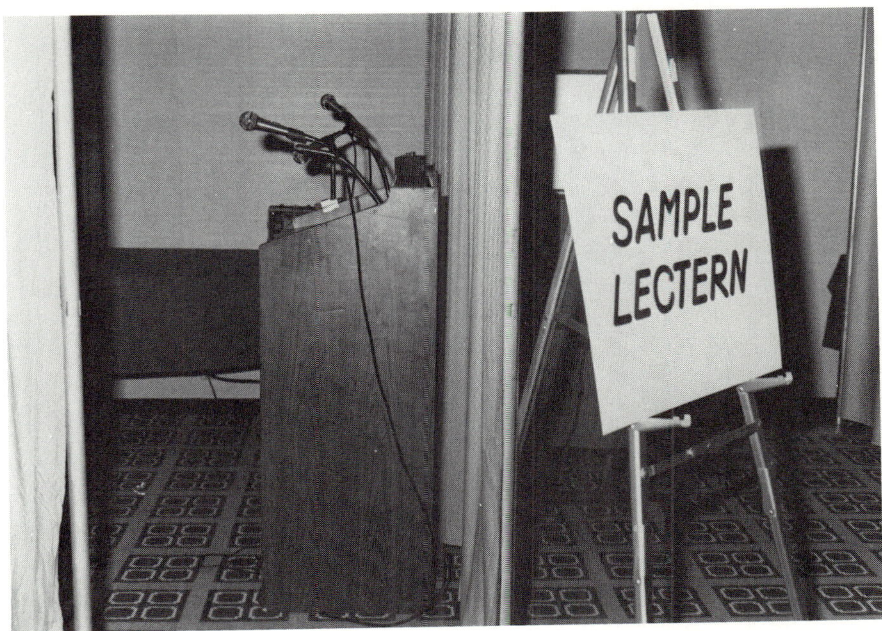

Fig. 9-2. There should be a lectern in the ready room that is identical to that on the podium in the meeting room.

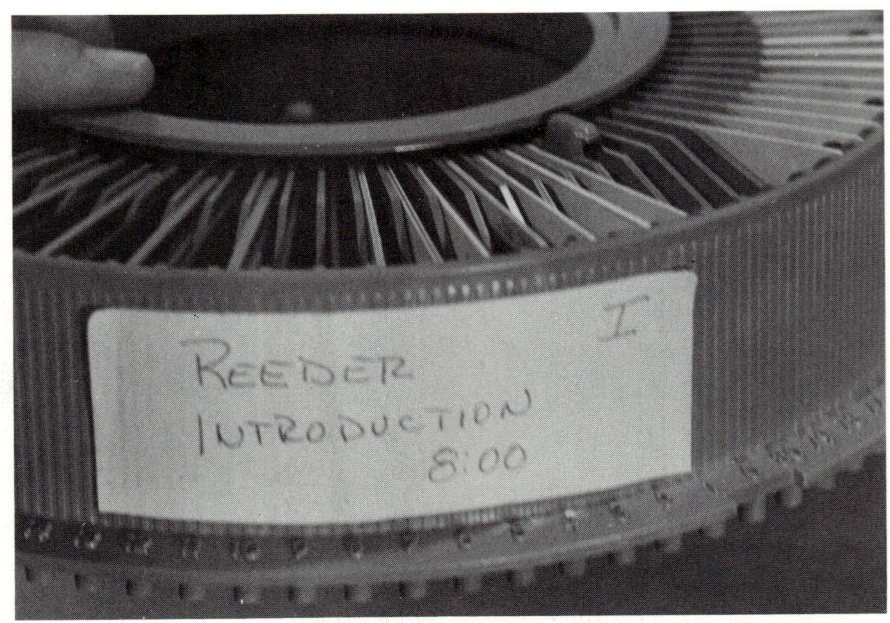

Fig. 9-3. Labeling trays. A label with the speaker's name, time of presentation, and number on the program is placed on the slide tray with the edge of the label on slide 1.

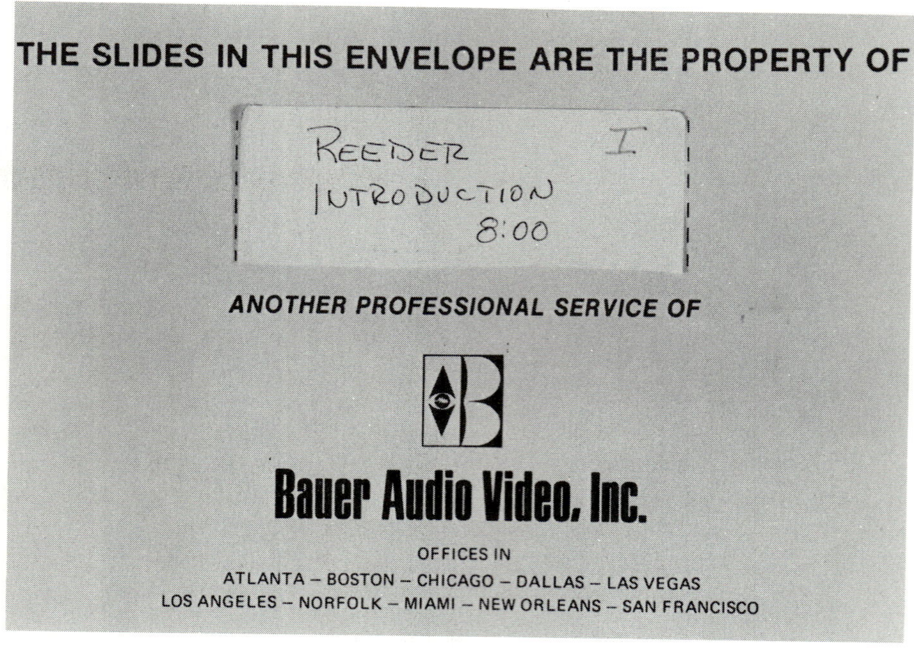

Fig. 9-4. Returning slides to the speaker. After the presentation, the slides are placed in an envelope; the sticker is removed from the tray and affixed to the envelope for identification.

time of the presentation, and his or her number on the program should be written on the label. The label is placed on the tray with the edge of the label on slide 1 (Fig. 9-3). For panel discussions all of the speaker's slides are loaded in the same tray and each identified by placing the label at the location of the first slide. At the end of the presentation, the slides are placed in an envelope, which is sealed. The label is taken off the tray and put on the envelope to identify it (Fig. 9-4).

An opaque slide can be placed as the last in a speaker's sequence. By so doing, the speaker and the projectionist are aware that the last slide has been projected. This can also be a signal to the projectionist to bring up the house lights. It is also a good idea to load a blank slide in slot 80 so that if the speaker is confused and presses the reverse button on the change mechanism, the screen remains dark and is a signal to use the forward button.

POTENTIAL PROBLEMS

Some of the potential problems we look for in the speaker ready room, and ones that you should look for, are the following:

Dog-eared mounts. When a slide in a cardboard mount is projected over and over again, the mount starts to fray and separate. The slide will not drop completely into the projector gate or may jam the projector. The permanent cure for this, of course, is to remount the slide; but a good temporary fix is to simply cut off the bad corner with a pair of scissors.

Metal mounts. We recommend that you stay away completely from metal mounts. They may twist or become distorted and jam a projector gate. They are especially prone to deform in the heat of high intensity projectors and to cause malfunction.

Glass mounts. Never use glass mounts when speaking

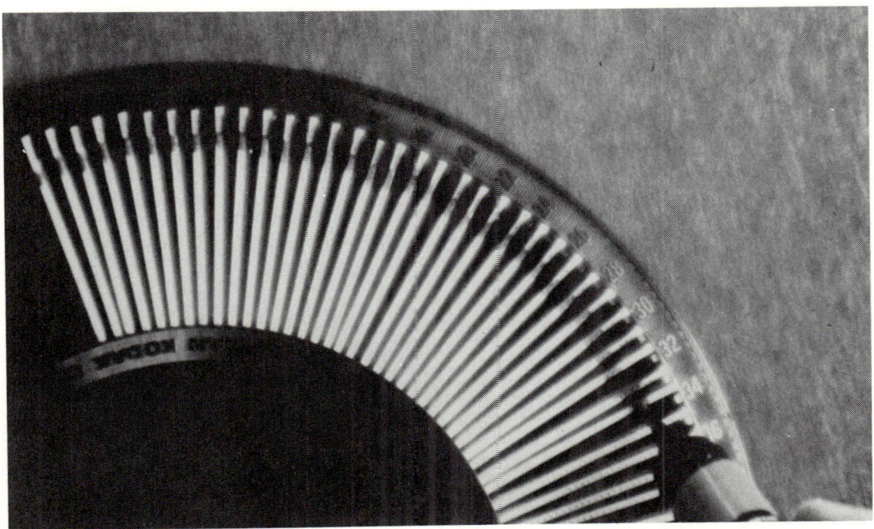

Fig. 9-5. Orienting slides after they have been loaded into a projector tray. After slides have been loaded into a projector tray and have been previewed to ensure that all are in proper orientation, they may be marked in the upper right corner with a felt-tipped pen.

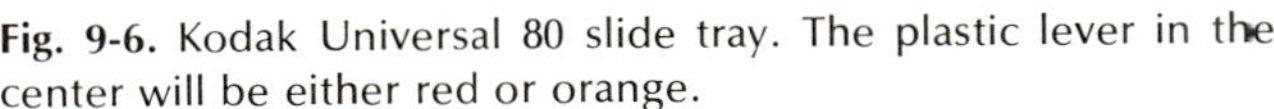

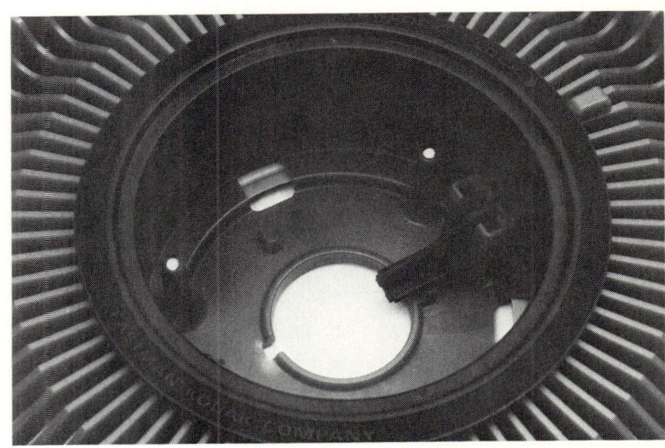

Fig. 9-6. Kodak Universal 80 slide tray. The plastic lever in the center will be either red or orange.

in a large room where xenon projectors will be used. The glass traps the moisture the emulsion has absorbed, the heat of the lamp drives it out of the emulsion, it condenses on the cooler glass facing the lens, and appears as a dark gray or "burned" area. It does not harm the slide but is very distracting to the audience. Glass slides also reduce the image brightness. Also, if there is a fingerprint or any oily substance on the glass, an automatic focusing projector will focus on this rather than the film emulsion, thus causing the projected image to be out of focus.

Original slides. Never project original slides. Every time a slide drops into a projector, the light bleaches away just a little bit more of the color. This is especially true of the high-intensity projectors. Plan ahead for needed duplicates, since they cannot be obtained at the last minute. Try not to mix original and duplicate slides in the same presentation. The emulsion on a duplicate is on the opposite side of the film base from an original. This necessitates constant refocusing.

Marking slides. A slide should be oriented by placing a thumb dot in the lower left corner when the slide is viewed as it will project on the screen. This should be placed in the upper right corner when loading into the tray. Do not use gummed labels or the little colored dots; the glue will soften in the heat of the projector and jam it. A better method is to use a broad felt-tipped pen to mark the corner or use a new pencil eraser and a stamp pad to make a dot. Another good method is to load your slides in the tray in proper orientation, then mark the upper right corner by running a felt-tipped pen along the top edge of the slides after they are locked in place (Fig. 9-5).

Large capacity trays. Do not use 140 capacity slide trays. Because of the limited amount of space allowed for each slide, the slightest imperfection in the mount will cause the slide to jam or fail to drop. The Kodak Universal 80 slide capacity tray is a much more dependable unit. This one has a red or orange lever in the center portion (Fig. 9-6).

Mixing formats. Not all slides mounted in 2 × 2 inch mounts have the same film size (Fig. 9-7). The standard double-frame 35 mm, which is the most commonly used, has an aperture measuring 34.2 × 22.9 mm. The 135 half-frame measures 22.9 × 15.9 mm; the 126 format is 26.5 × 26.5 mm, while the super slide measures 38 × 38 mm. Each of these will project a different size image on the screen. If the projectionist is aware ahead of time that you will be using nonstandard size slides, he or she can select a lens that will fill the screen with the projected image. If, however, you mix the formats, the projected images will be of different sizes, with the half-frame not filling the screen, while the super slide over-

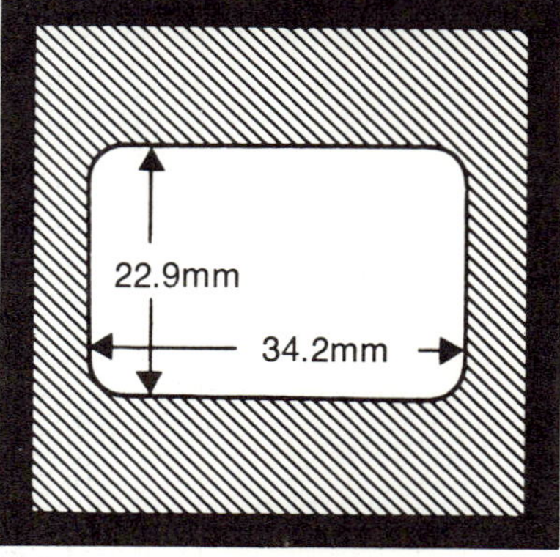

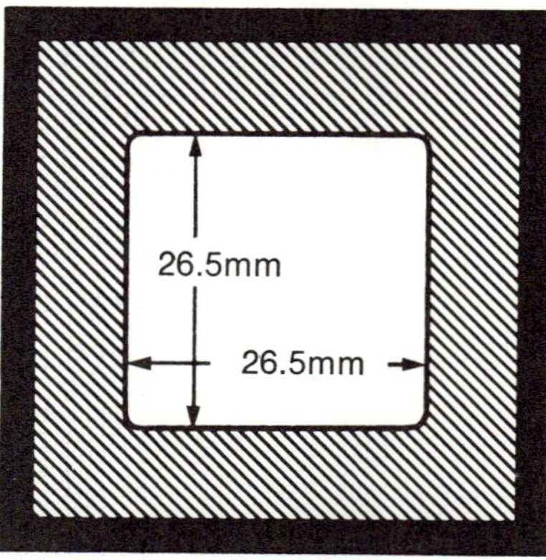

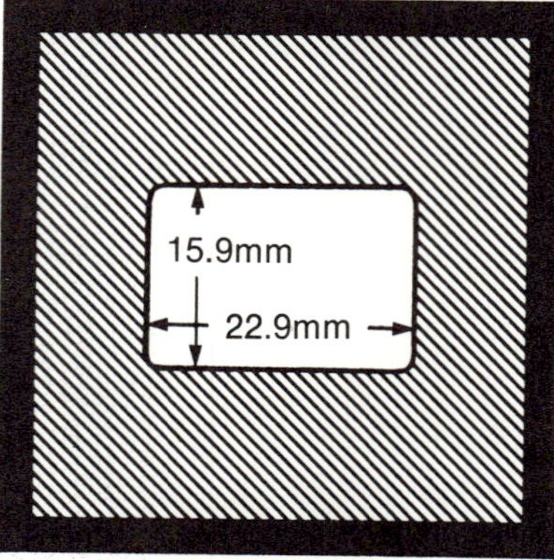

Fig. 9-7. Not all slides in 2 × 2 inch mounts have the same aperture size. (From Kodak Publication No. S30. Copyright 1975 by Eastman Kodak Co. Reproduced with permission.)

flows onto the wall. This can be very distracting and is almost impossible for the projectionist to correct. Therefore, try to have all slides in the same format.

SUMMARY

The speaker ready room is the best way to minimize the risk of a disaster with a slide presentation. Those attending the meeting will soon forget whether they had chicken or roast beef at luncheon. They will forget if the reception lasted an hour, an hour and a half, or two hours. But they will long remember the meeting where the speaker's slides were all upside down or caused the projector to catch fire. Do it the right way. It may cost a few extra dollars, but the ready room can make all the difference in the world to both the speakers and the audience.

CHAPTER 10

The Phoenix Award: a review of the experimental method

Thomas J. Krizek, M.D.*

THE PROBLEM (BACKGROUND)

The explosion of scientific information of the last two decades has been both qualitative and quantitative. The demands of "publish or perish," heretofore the spectre of only those living within the narrow confines of academia, have spread to all spheres of professional life. Contributions to scientific publications, as well as presentations at local, regional, and national meetings, are required for all who would gain access to active membership in our organizations. New organizations proliferate and national meetings now occur with such frequency as to make it possible to completely avoid being at home. The typical plastic surgeon, dutifully attending to his responsibilities for continuing his medical education, might likely belong to some, indeed many, of the organizations in the following list:

Plastic surgery societies
  American Society of Plastic and Reconstructive Surgeons (4½)†
  American Association of Plastic Surgeons (3)
  American Society of Aesthetic Plastic Surgery (3)
  Plastic Surgery Research Council (2)
  American Society of Maxillofacial Surgeons(-)
  Educational Foundation Symposia (6 per year × 2½) days
  Regional society meetings (choose one) (2)
  Military Plastic Surgeons (3)
  Chief Residents' Conference (2)
American Medical Association
  County medical society or state medical society (choose one) (2)
  National meeting (4)

American College of Surgeons
  Clinical Congress (5)
  Spring meeting (4)
  Trauma Symposia (6 per year × 2 days)
  State chapter (choose one) (2)
  Selected special committees
    Committee on Trauma (2)
    Committee on Cancer (2)
    Committee to Study Relationships with Young Surgeons (2)
General societies (including specialties)
  American Surgical Association (3)
  Society of University Surgeons (3)
  American Association of Academic Surgery (3)
  Whipple Society (2)
  Halsted Society (2)
Regional society meetings (choose one)
  New England Surgical Society (2½)
  Southern Surgical Society (2½)
  Central Surgical Society (2½)
Interspecialty societies
  Cleft Palate Society (3)
  Society of Head and Neck Surgeons (3)
  Ewing Society (-)
  American Society for Surgery of the Head and Neck (-)
  American Burn Association (2½)
  American Society for Surgery of the Hand (3)
  American Association for Hand Surgery (3)
  American Association for the Surgery of Trauma (3)
  Association of American Medical Colleges (4)
International organizations
  International College of Surgeons (3)
  Pan American Surgical Association (3)
  British Society of Plastic Surgeons (4)
International congresses
  Burns (every 4 years)
  Plastic surgery (every 4 years)

---

*From Krizek, T. J., and Hoopes, J. E.: Symposium on basic science in plastic surgery, St. Louis, 1976, The C. V. Mosby Co.
†The number in parentheses is the length of each organization's annual meeting in days unless otherwise indicated.

Other activities
- Residency review committee board
- In-service examination committee
- Visiting professorships (3 per year × 2 days)
- Board of directors midyear meetings (4)
- McKorkle Society (½)

It is unfortunate that one cannot attend all of every meeting every year, since, of necessity, some overlap. Active participation could easily result in 90 working days away from home, *not* counting travel. Since at least ½ day of travel each way is likely, another 34 to 36 days may be added, of which at least half are working days. Adding 20 working days vacation a year, the conscientious participant may devote about 127 working days a year to activities away from home. One must assume, of course, that no special extracurricular committee assignments or responsibilities are accepted which would add to this tally. It is clear that at least 50% of the available working day time of the contributing member of organizations is actually spent *at* the meetings, often presenting "work of merit."

If an academician were to devote *all* his remaining time to investigation and not distract his activity with patient care or student or resident teaching and were to assume no administrative tasks within his university, there would still be but 1 work day left to devote to research for each similar day he is away at meetings. However, the facts of life are more complex such that even the most devoted of investigators assumes many other local responsibilities. He operates frequently, takes care of sick patients, and teaches. He probably devotes no more than *10%* of his remaining time to "doing" research, the equivalent of 13 working days per year (even this may be an inflated figure). It is likely that no person is going to present a paper at every meeting, although it seems that some do. We must also recognize that, from a practical point of view, fewer than six presentations (and an equivalent number of publications a year) is unlikely to be impressive to promotions committees. Accepting six therefore as the norm for the academically inclined, the researcher is left with 13 working days available in which to come up with six publications: about 2.16 working days of good solid investigative work per publication. The formula for calculating the time available to the scientific presenter for research and preparation is as follows:

Working days per year	260
Days potentially at meetings	− 127
(plus travel and vacation)	
Subtotal	133
Time spent in clinical care,	− 120
teaching, and administration (90%)	
Time available for research	13

Number of presentations (and publications per year)	6
Time available to devote to each piece of work	13 ÷ 6 = 2.16 days
TOTAL TIME (per presentation)	2 days, 3 hours, 50 minutes

This setting is a difficult one for those who aspire to national recognition. The pressures on all is severe. It is not surprising that with this background and in this setting there has emerged a sort of scientific "phoenix" (Fig. 10-1). Our version of the phoenix appears at each of our scientific meetings with a presentation that is either repetitious, trivial, superficial, irrelevant, or all of the above. Critical discussion from the floor, careful screening of program committees, and, later, incisive editorial review are of no avail. Despite consumption by flames on the scientific pyre, the scientific phoenix reemerges, renewed and undaunted at the next meeting. To the most outstanding of these, the unofficial Phoenix Award is bestowed at each plastic surgical meeting by the Phoenix Award Committee (P.A.C.).* Many of our members are repeat winners of the award. Some have endangered the significance of the award by threatening, by the consistency of their performances, to retire it. However, like the Davis Cup, it cannot be retired; at each meeting, worthy new challengers emerge.

---

*The members of this committee, lest their careers and friendships be threatened, shall be protected by anonymity.

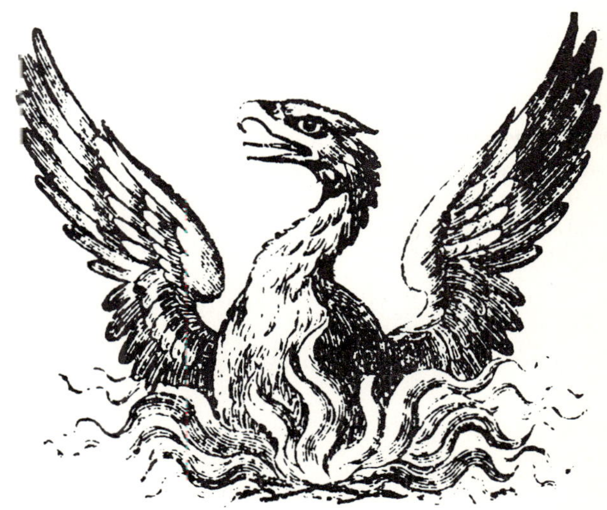

Fig. 10-1. The phoenix, a legendary bird, was sacred to the Egyptian sun-god. When it reached the end of its life span (circa 500 years), it burned itself on a pyre. From the ashes a new phoenix arose, a symbol of death and resurrection. Like the whiffenpoof, it is an imaginary bird, important only as a symbol and significant only to some persons—such as award winners.

Since we have established the scientific climate that has set the stage for the Phoenix Award, we believe that it would be a contribution to our meetings and only fair to the members to outline the criteria whereby the award can be won. The basis for the award is negative adherence to the experimental method. Only negative points may be earned. A perfect score is 100 points. However, this may be exceeded because of the bonus points that may be occasionally earned.

ABSTRACTS

Access to the Phoenix Award requires access to the podium or the pages of a journal. The most direct approach is by way of an abstract submitted to a program committee. As many as 5 bonus points may be earned at this stage. Points are considered "bonus" because they can only be awarded if a member of the P.A.C. is also on the program committee. Points may be earned in the following obvious and not so obvious ways:

1. *Submit only carbons.* This is clear evidence to a program committee that it is only one of a series of committees who are reviewing the same abstract. Recognizing the many organizations involved and the press of time, it is clearly the efficient way for the author. In this day and age, there is really no reason to make the program committee believe that its meeting is a special meeting, deserving of an original abstract typed specially for them.

2. *Submit the wrong number of copies.* A program chairman with a committee of five members will often ask that an original and five copies be submitted. This clearly facilitates ready distribution. Since program chairmen are chosen for their equanimity, they really do not mind having their secretaries make an extra two or four or five copies. It should be noted that this is a tenuous way to earn points, since the program chairman may not be a member of the P.A.C. and is therefore unable to award points, although earned.

3. *Ignore the specified number of words.* The request that abstracts be 200 to 300 words, for example, is probably a frivolous and unnecessary constraint in the first place and may be safely ignored. Understanding committee persons are delighted to interpret the profound and implied significance of meritorious work hinted at in a twenty-word, two-sentence abstract. They are equally grateful for the multipaged, data-laden abstract, which often includes computer printouts. It is a useful challenge for them to interpret and attempt a determination of what the presentation might be about.

4. *Include no data.* "Our series was reviewed; the potential significance will be discussed." There are few phrases more oft repeated, designed to whet the appetite of the committee. These abstracts are occasionally accepted simply to force the author to immediately start counting, in time for the meeting, to see how many subjects there actually were in the series and whether there is really a significance to support the hunch that stimulated the abstract. It is, of course, not appropriate to give too much away in the abstract.

5. *Ignore the deadline.* It is character-building for the inexperienced program chairman to sit with ten abstracts for a national meeting 24 hours before the deadline. He will soon be deluged with telephone calls, telegrams, and special delivery envelopes as 90% of the abstracts arrive *after* the well-announced deadline. We all know that no program chairman worth his salt will deny the stage to the author of a meritorious paper that might add luster to the program, which he shortly before had feared might never occur. Indeed, early submission might well be construed as overenthusiasm on the part of the author.

Following are other minor characteristics of Phoenix Award-worthy abstracts:

a. The abstract is part of a narrative letter to the program chairman.

b. The author failed to include a return address.

c. The proposed presentation is totally irrelevant to the program (e.g., a proposed presentation of finger joint replacement to the Society for Surgery of the Head and Neck).

d. The content of the abstract has been published in a current issue of a major journal (by the same author).

e. The abstract is accompanied by the message, "Please ignore the fact that I am your sponsor for the _______________ Society and consider it like any other abstract."

All abstracts are chosen on the basis of one of the following criteria: (1) it is a super abstract and belongs on any program, (2) it fits well into the overall program, (3) something was needed to fill that slot right before the President's address, or (4) this person just has to be publicly exposed.

Irrespective of how one has made the program, it is the first step to winning the Phoenix Award.

THE PRESENTATION

Since the Phoenix Award is actually earned at the meeting itself, the committee attempts (despite bonus points for the abstract) to give every presenter an equal chance.

The characteristics of a point-earning presentation and the yardsticks employed by the P.A.C. are outlined in the following list. Any good reporter preparing a news article always answers who, what, where, when, and how. The checklist for the scientific reporter is but a slight variation on this basic theme, the order being slightly different as follows:

1. *The question.* What is the problem?
2. *The state of the art.* Why does the literature, the available fund of knowledge, fail to answer this question?
3. *The method.* How did the study intend to solve the problem?
4. *Interpretation of the data.* Where in the data are the answers to the questions?
5. *Significance of the study.* Who is to profit from the results of this study?

Once again, the Phoenix Award is won by earning negative points, received by failing to adhere to these elementary characteristics of the experimental method.

What (the question)

The unsuspecting resident, encountering a case of hemifacial eustomia associated with parahypertrophic syndactylism of the second and third toes in a child with forty-six chromosomes is invited to "look up and report our cases." The situation reflects the common circumstances of (1) the chief doesn't know the answer and (2) the unusual is always good grist for the scientific mill.

This is the germ of the "question," which leads to the eventual scientific presentation. It is the key to all that follows.

Many potential Phoenix points can be won early in the competition related to the question that has been asked. Twenty points can be earned in the *what* phase. Key opportunities for earning points are as follows.

Ask no question at all. It is clear from regular attendance at national meetings that for many presentations, there simply is no question ever asked. It is as though we have been taken on a random walk—like staring at a map.

One of the great pleasures of flying some airlines is that magnificent treasure, the map, to be found in the pocket in front of the passenger. It is filled with extraordinarily fine detail, accurately presented, and usually in nicely shaded colors (Fig. 10-2). It is a delight to the eye and can occupy one's attention for long periods. My gracious, Miami is really closer to being more directly south of Cleveland than of New York; San Diego is really further north than Dallas; Denver is further from Chicago than Chicago is from New York. These are extremely interesting if somewhat trivial and irrelevant

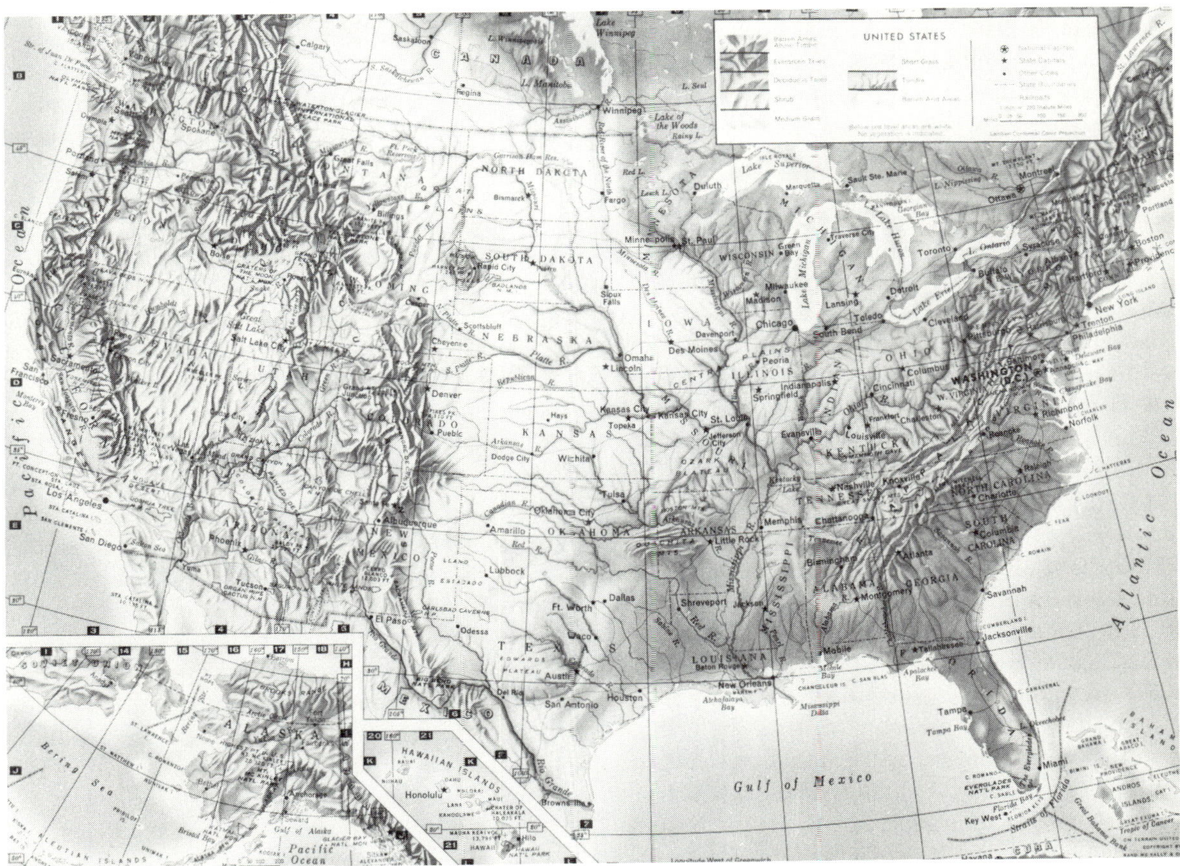

Fig. 10-2. Map of the United States. It is a useless compilation of meaningless, albeit accurate, data reflecting the relative positions of various geographic points. It becomes useful only if one asks, for example, the question of how to get from one place to another.

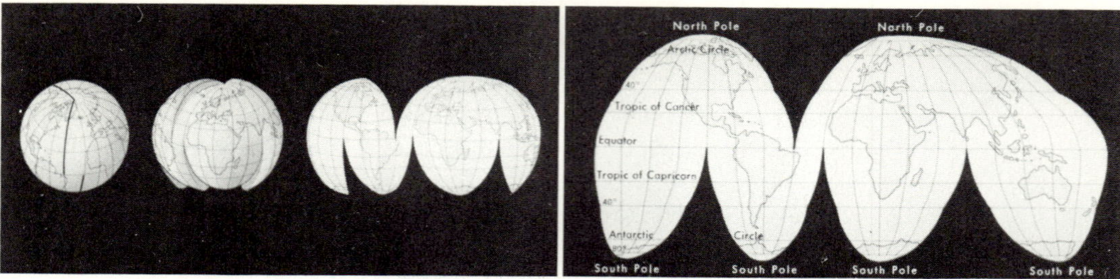

Fig. 10-3. Homolosine equal area projection map—a truly global map. Perhaps this is an unnecessarily broad overview if the problem is how to get from Twentynine Palms, Calif., to Barstow,Calif.

facts. Indeed the map itself is useless except as a diversion, unless one asks a question such as "How do I get to Denver?"

If one is going to take 10 minutes of my life at a scientific meeting merely to show me a map and to tell me a few trivial facts about it, so be it. If, however, he is going to use the map to show me how to get to Miami, then he ought to tell me that this is what is planned so that I will know where to look.

So, too, the tactics may obscure the strategy: "Mr. Chairman, Ladies, and Gentlemen. May I have the first slide please." The lights go out, and we are plunged into darkness. A map appears on the screen (or a flower or the author's name or a picture of the mountains near his home base). So dazzled are we by the colors piercing the darkness and the machinations of the slides appearing that we missed the question. Maybe there wasn't one. He has earned 20 points.

Ask a trivial question. A map of the world appears on the screen, the kind one gets when he unpeels a globe and lays it out flat on a table (Fig. 10-3). The problem is clearly going to be a big one. The oceans and continents are reviewed and orientations made. North America is identified. The close-up is of the United States, east of the Mississippi River. The question is finally asked: "How do we get from Port Allegany, Pennsylvania, to Olean, New York?" The possibilities of air, sea, and land are reviewed in detail. The model is described. The data indicate that the 17-mile distance can be traversed in 1.75 minutes less time by taking the route 446 turnoff instead of continuing along route 305 through Portville. The data are thoroughly analyzed, and the work is nicely documented (p < .001). It is the classic global approach to a trivial question.

The scientific equivalent might be an effort to determine whether the Krebs cycle (Fig. 10-4) really goes clockwise rather than counterclockwise. It is a beautifully orchestrated opportunity to employ obscure biochemical techniques, enzyme chemistry, and many dollars of research money to answer a trivial question.

The global presentation of the trivial question is worth 20 points toward the Phoenix Award.

Ask a global question. This is the converse to the previous example. "How do we manage the patient with cancer?" "Some thoughts on the psychological aspects of aesthetic surgery!" "How do we drive from Hartford, Connecticut to Buenos Aires, Argentina?" These are big questions and they have to be asked. So too, the answers are not simple and, like the trip to Buenos Aires, require a series of detailed maps and travel plans. However, a detailed analysis of the road characteristics, terrain, curves, and undulations of a 1-mile stretch on that road to Buenos Aires is of little value unless we know which of the 5,000 miles it likely represents.

It is clear in scientific inquiry that it is not always possible to know exactly where or even whether the single mile of research related in the presentation fits into the overall picture. This should be made clear to all. It is particularly important when presenting laboratory investigation that the segment represented in the study be clearly related to the big picture and an accurate assessment of its potential significance as part of the big question identified. Failure to try earns 20 points.

Ask a question to which the answer is known. In the press of "publish or perish," it is understandably difficult to always come up with either new questions or new answers. However, points are clearly deserved by a presentation devoted to observations of well-known facts. This is a particularly fine technique if the presenter fails to acknowledge the possibility that others have previously reported identical work. The total unawareness of the literature on the subject is all too often obvious. Guarantee of points can be made if the previous work has been reported by one of the members of the P.A.C.

The major reasons for stepping to the podium should be to present new information or to say something better than it has been said before. The distinction deserves to be made clear.

Ask a question to which there is no answer. There are many problems, in plastic surgery in particular, in which the questions are the scientific equivalent of "how many angels can dance on the head of a pin—a quantitative analysis." Important observations must often be made and accepted on subjective grounds only—it is inappro-

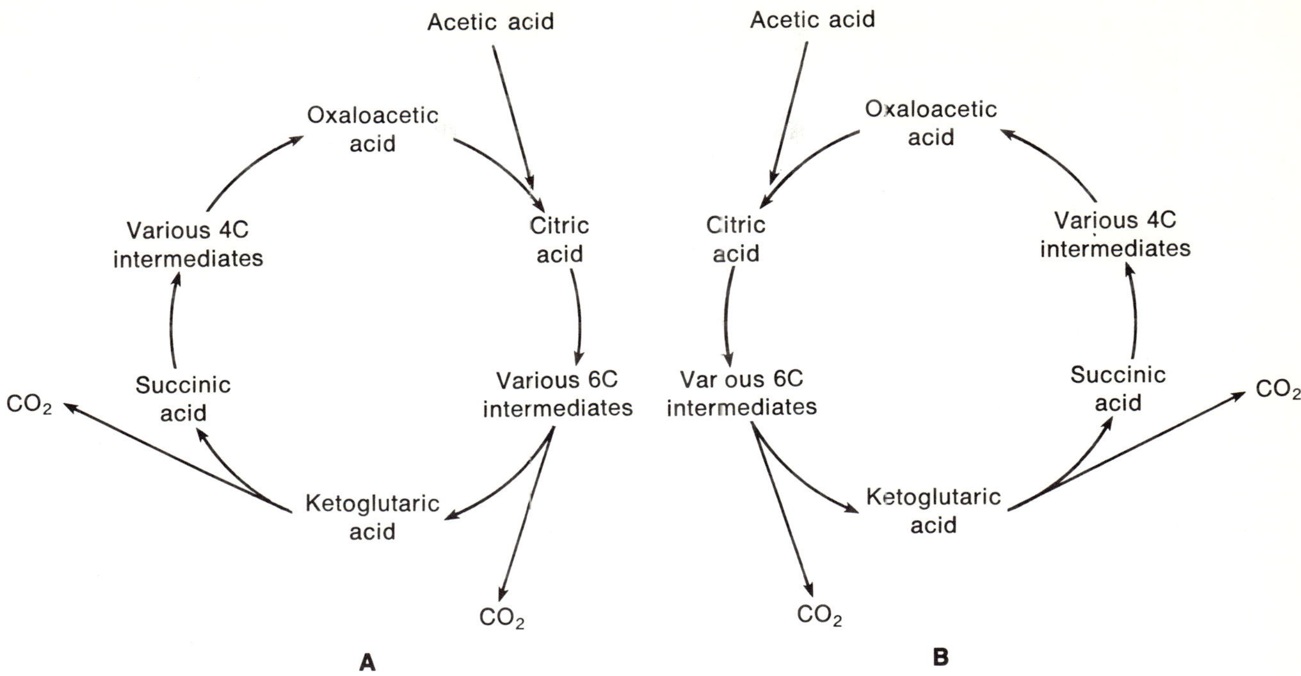

Fig. 10-4. **A,** The Krebs citric acid cycle has been unquestioningly assumed to move in a clockwise rotation. **B,** New data indicate that in actuality the cycle advances in a counterclockwise fashion.

priate to attempt fitting these into a mold which can only be suitably applied to laboratory evaluations. The failure is less in the question itself than in failing to recognize the nature of the question.

Ask a question designed to fit a known answer. Serendipity often provides the investigator an answer to which there may be no specific question. Under these circumstances, there is a temptation to attempt to fit too many questions or perhaps the wrong question to the answer. For example, the observation may be made that penicillin destroys streptococci. This answer is already clear. The appropriate question might be whether penicillin either can prevent or treat streptococcal infection. The mere fact of the answer does not necessarily answer the above questions. If the question were "Does penicillin kill streptococci?" then the answer is "yes." If the question is "Does penicillin prevent or treat streptococci infection? Then the answer is only "maybe" and certainly not proved by the available answer. It has been shown that penicillin prophylaxis may result in the emergence of penicillinase-producing staphylococci. The penicillinase then destroys the penicillin being taken orally, and the incidence of streptococcal infection remains unchanged. It was a good answer, but the question may not be proper.

. . .

The question is really the introduction to a presentation or a scientific paper. It is the attention-getting, stage-setting, first portion of a talk. Although the P.A.C. awards only 20 points for this portion, it sets the tone for winning more points. It should be clear that when one begins with an incisive introduction, clearly outlining the scope of the problem and identifying unequivocally the question that he proposes to answer, the P.A.C. is unable to award points. This early expository portion is best presented in a few clear sentences without the use of slides.

Why (the state of the art)

The introduction of the *why* phase of a presentation was alluded to in the section on asking a question to which the answer is known. It relates to the presenter's failure to share with the audience the current state of knowledge in the area to be discussed. Sad to say, all in an audience may not be equally familiar with the subject and the material as is the speaker. The speaker may indeed hope that this is true and may make every effort to maintain his status by way of secrecy. However, when the question is important enough to be on the program, the audience deserves to have it brought into focus. Twenty points are awarded in this phase by adherence to the following principles.

Failure to relate the question to known information. As just alluded to, the question may have innocently occurred to the investigator as if he were the only one in the world who had ever asked it. If he is truly the first, then a review of pertinent literature is necessarily brief.

Even so, it should be related as follows: "There has been no previous work in this or related areas." However, it is a far more common point-earning maneuver to (1) ignore published material on the same subject or (2) ignore material published by a member of P.A.C. on the same subject.

As in the setting described earlier, it is not surprising that a great many presentations are mere replications of previously published work.

Failure to point to potential significance of work. The question, nicely outlined for the audience, can be rendered meaningless by the author's failure to attempt to put it into context. The audience, tantalized by the interesting nature of the question, is eager to learn how the material to come is likely to be of significance. For example, the audience is told that "the Krebs cycle moves in a counterclockwise fashion, not clockwise as reported in all previous studies" (Fig. 10-4). The question is clear. The answer may turn out to be equally clear. But why on earth did the investigator choose to study it? When one discusses fibrous capsule formation around a breast prosthesis, the significance of the work is so momentous and the problem being challenged is so profound as to require little comment by the speaker. However, the importance of a presentation about an identified defect in the immune response that may dispose the population to cancer may require amplification and clarification of its potential role in clinical practice.

Fragmentation. This particular maneuver is subtle and may go unrecognized. However, when discovered, it is particularly deserving of points—almost a special award. The subtley relates to the fact that the presenter has failed to relate his own previously published work to the question at hand. This may be reflected at any phase of the presentation but is awarded at this point for convenience. It is always interesting to the P.A.C. when a speaker fails to refer to his own work, particularly when the subsequent data are patently at odds with previously published work.

A more common observation, however, is the clearly planned fragmentation of his work. A single nice piece of work has been sliced like a pie into two, three, four, or more individual servings. It is true that each individual piece has all the characteristics of the original pie. Besides, it enables one to make an offering at four meetings instead of wasting it all on one meeting or paper. Each represents a separate line on one's bibliography. The motives and strategy are clear. Finally, when the series is complete, one can put it all together in a monograph, a chapter, or a collective review (of one's own work).

A variation on this theme is multiple authors. By merely altering the order of the authors, one can secure publication of the same data in a variety of scientific journals. It is particularly effective if another slice of the pie is published within a month or so of the date of the meeting.

• • •

It is clear that the P.A.C. considers the first 3 minutes or so of the presentation to be worth 40% of the total value. Failure to ask an appropriate question or to make it perceivably relevant are the most common point earners. It is rarely possible to ask a proper and relevant question and then design a model that is so bad that enough points can be earned to win an award. However, the committee looks for consistency as well. A strong start in the what and why categories puts the investigator in the strongest position for winning points in the *how* phase. It is equally difficult to ask a bad or irrelevant question and not also be in a strong position for gaining additional points during the meaty portion of the presentation—the how.

How (the method)

The experimental method demands a scientific rigor that will provide an answer specific to the question being asked and without alternate explanations. Furthermore, it is relevant, comparable, reproducible, mathematically and statistically valid, and hopefully, biologically significant. Not all data with statistical significance have biologic significance, but all data that are biologically significant can also stand the scrutiny of statistical validation.

This section is devoted only to nonclinical investigative work. It is, however, an inflexible caveat that studies on other than humans are a poor substitute and chosen only when the study cannot be performed and answers satisfactorily obtained clinically. All laboratory studies require final documentation in humans to meet the final test of significance.

The definition of the biochemistry and pharmacologic characteristics of penicillin were almost irrelevant findings that *followed* the only important observation, that penicillin was effective against certain infections in humans. All the laboratory observations, experimental studies, and results of animal studies would have been meaningless if penicillin had not met the test of clinical value.

Much required investigative work cannot appropriately be performed in the clinical sphere. Laboratory studies remain an absolute necessity. Such studies should be designed in such a way as to be most like the clinical circumstances. One should also recognize that the laboratory, as opposed to the clinic, provides the investigator an opportunity to control every conceivable variable other than the single one being studied, an opportunity rarely available clinically. The possible ways of earning Phoenix Award points in this section are legion, and only the highlights will be mentioned. The excitement of being a member of the P.A.C., is the opportunity for observing new and exciting ways of ignoring the experimental method that innovative investigators discover. There are 30 points available.

Choose the wrong model. The key feature of the experimental method is the suitability of the chosen experimental model. Indeed some of the greatest contributions to investigative work have been in the design of an experimental model comparable to the human situation, highly reproducible and available to all. A number of such models have become classic examples: the Wigger's model of irreversible shock, the Brooke model of burn wound sepsis, the McFarlane rat flap design, and Medawar grafts for studying the rejection phenomena. These are only selected examples of excellent models of which there are many others. They have been particularly valuable because they enable many investigators, working in the same area, to accumulate data that are comparable to what others have done. The body of knowledge is increased in an orderly fashion by multiple investigators working in a semiorganized way.

One can promptly earn points by apparently trivial deviations from standard experimental models. For example, when all burn sepsis research is being done on 20% full-thickness burns in rats, a paper that purports to study the same problem but for no apparent reason uses a 30% burn is both preposterous and infuriating.

Such remarks should not be construed as criticism of efforts to develop new models, since new and better models may provide new and better answers. This should be done, however, only when available models do not serve the purpose equally well.

Choose the wrong animal. "Every dog has his day," and the dog has had his. It has been a remarkable transition of the last decade that the "experimental dog labs" of great medical centers have become almost as archaic as tuberculosis hospitals. New technology and microtechniques have made it possible to perform most all experiments in miniature. This represents an economy of space and money. There are few biologically significant facts that are true for humans but not for the rat. All experiments should be done on rats! The rat is cheap in great numbers and readily available.

This statement is made as a challenge, recognizing the exceptions. However, deviation from the rat should be made only because of evidence that a study can be done better or more accurately in another animal. Obviously studies on tendons may be more usefully accomplished in fowl or primates. The perceived comparability of the anatomies and vascular characteristics of porcine skin to human skin requires their usage. These deviations should be thoughtfully planned, since some extraordinary variations among animals may negate the value of

otherwise careful work. For example, the almost unique response immunologically and on a vascular basis of guinea pigs and rabbits to challenges of infection make their value in this area of investigation suspect. Animals with a highly developed panniculous carnosus heal open wounds by an intensity of contraction rarely seen in humans and make comparability of healing phenomena open to question.

The smokescreen of numbers. The clarity and incisive nature of the experimental method is in a way inversely related to the number of animals or experiments necessary to demonstrate the point. There is no critical number of animals that can be sacrificed on the altar of experimentation which can salvage a badly designed experiment.

It is entirely possible to perform a complete experiment on but a single animal if properly designed. Moritz and associates, in an effort to reproduce the phenomenon of the "burned lung," which is the cause of death in patients involved in conflagration, performed the ultimate experiment on but a single animal. An anesthetized animal, laryngoscope in place, received a direct shot of a blow torch down the trachea. Burning could not be accomplished beyond the carina; bronchioles and alveoli were unaffected. The effects of burning on the lung, since heat was so rapidly dissipated by the effective heat-exchange of mucous membrane and evaporation, just had to be due to other factors than heat. An alternate explanation (indeed damage is probably due to incomplete products of combustion) was necessary. This was a remarkable experiment—one animal—not even a control.

More often controls are necessary. They need not necessarily be in great numbers, only appropriate. An equally fine experiment was performed by Moyer. It required 3 animals, 2 of which were controls.* The study was done as follows to evaluate the mechanics of burn wound edema:

Rat 1 (control): The tail was subjected to a scald burn. Later the tail was removed, and the weight gain (edema) measured directly was about 50%.

Rat 2 (control): The tail was simply amputated and buried subcutaneously as a graft. There was no burn. The weight gain from such a maneuver was 7.8%.

Rat 3 (test): The tail was burned, amputated immediately, and buried subcutaneously, and the weight gain was measured showing an increase of 49.6% (p < .01) compared to rat 2).

The conclusion was inescapable that burn wound edema occurs from other than leaking capillaries; indeed an attachment to a blood supply is apparently unnecessary. Injured (burned) tissue must draw fluid into it. This was a most elegant experiment, neatly designed and

---

*He actually reported 9 animals.

demanding of controls. Would the experiment have been any more convincing if there had been 100 animals in each group or 1,000? Numbers may obscure but never totally hide the weakness of a poorly designed experiment.

The magic of technology. Modern technology has outstripped the ability of modern science to respond by finding meaningful uses for some of the advances. The following represent only the most egregious examples; there are many more subtle examples of an experimental method designed totally in response to some technologic advance. The technology is presented as the answer when it is really itself the question. Examples of answers in search of a question include the hyperbaric chamber, the laser, and, to a certain extent, the computer.

The most obvious clue in a presentation that the technology has superseded the question is the showing of pictures of the instrumentation or the technology used in the experiment during the course of a talk. There is no greater giveaway than actually showing the audience a slide with a picture of a computer or the twelve-channel recorder used during the course of the experiment to record only the pulse rate. Of particular excitement to viewers recently has been the variety and complexity of the instrumentation available for and ostensibly necessary to the measurement of neurophysiologic phenomena. Finally, the computer, is a means, not an end.

Controls. A control refers not only to the number of animals but to every variable within the experimental model. Perhaps the single largest point-getter for those aspiring to the Phoenix Award is failure to include proper controls. Methods of ignoring the control in the experimental method include the following:

1. *No controls whatsoever.*

2. *Controls disparate temporally.* Controls that utilize previous experiments and are not performed simultaneously beg the question that all other factors have remained the same. However, it is known from infection studies, for example, that yesterday's virulent *Pseudomonas* may be as harmless as a pussycat today. Yesterday's data are not an adequate control.

3. *Incomplete controls.* This involves the failure to include *all* the experimental steps save the single variable being tested. The influence of anesthesia, for example, on any experimental animal is not clearly understood. Rather than assume that it is a negligible factor, when animals are to be control animals, they should be anesthetized if the test animals were anesthetized. Controls should be completely comparable at each step.

4. *Internal controls.* Although internal controls are seemingly ideal, this may not be true. For example, a wound infection study using paired wounds on the same animal, only one of which is infected, is not a good control. The control wound may influence the reaction of the test wound, by some subtle alteration in body de-

fense mechanisms. An example is the fact that an infection, if present elsewhere in the body, renders a wound, even a perfectly sterile wound, six times more susceptible to infection.

5. *Inappropriate controls.* All that appears to be a control may not be. Subtle variations in the methodology may present the control with a series of unrecognized circumstances that render the conditions different from what they appear. For instance, in operating on a series of 6 animals, that the sixth and last animal in the group always is the control introduces the possibility that the operation may not be done the same as were the previous 5 (it may be better or worse). This can be avoided by randomizing the controls among the 6 animals. A similar subtle and perhaps irrelevant alteration would be drawing cards to see into which of three groups an animal should fit. Unless the card is returned to the pool, the next animal does not really have a one in three chance of falling into each group. This can be avoided by using a series of random numbers.

• • •

The experiment has been completed. The question was appropriate, and the model, the animal, and the controls were all in order. A great deal of data have been accumulated. Despite this extraordinary fine handling of the meat of the presentation, it is still possible to gain Phoenix Award points by data interpretation—the *where* of the experiment.

Where (interpretation)

It is possible at this phase of the presentation to recoup all that has been lost to accuracy and clarity in the beginning. The statistician, the biometrician, and the computer have combined to make it possible to turn even the most insignificant trivia into something of seeming importance. So too, work of scientific merit can be destroyed by poor manipulation and interpretation of the available data. This portion of the presentation is worth 20 points.

All that is significant isn't! There is a profound difference between what is biologically significant and what may happen to be statistically significant. As Gertrude Stein said, "A difference to be a difference, must make a difference." There have been a few major scientific advances whose biologic significance required a t-test, a chi-square, or a p-value to tell us that this was a major event. On the other hand, there have been no major advances that could not stand up to the rigors of such statistical analysis. There is, however, a profound difference between them.

It may be entirely possible to take two groups of surgical patients, each containing 10,000 patients. One group of patients receives prophylactic antibiotics; the other does not. The treated group has an infection rate of

0.3%; the untreated group has an infection rate of 0.8%. Analyzed statistically, chi-square = 22.85 ($p < .00001$). This means there was less than one chance in 100,000 that this difference was due to chance. The antibiotics clearly made a statistical difference. However, whether they made a worthwhile biologic difference is entirely dependent on the circumstances. If the wounds involved were trivial and of no particular danger to the patient, even if infected, and the incidence of side effects from the antibiotics was greater than 0.5%, then the biologic conclusion would have to be reached that their use was not indicated. On the other hand, if the operations involved were life-saving and the difference between the two groups was fifty lives, then the difference is of manifest significance.

Failure to relate statistical significance to potential biologic significance earns 20 points.

Failure to use proper statistical methodology. The more common errors include choosing samples that are not representative of the total population, failure to randomize, and failure to include potential comorbid factors, which might be accounting for perceived differences. The obvious failures are apparent to the P.A.C.; subtle ones require the consultation of the committee's own statistician.

Garbage in—garbage out. The P.A.C. is particularly thrilled at modern investigators who employ computer technology in the design of their experiments and interpretation of their data. We award an automatic 5 points for any who would show us a picture in living color of an IBM 370/158—in action. We particularly enjoy pictures of computer printouts.

We are impressed that one will employ this modern technology for such purposes as randomizing a group of 10 animals, comparing two groups of 6 animals each, or attempting to be objective about what is basically a subjective observation.

There is less here than meets the eye. A profound presentation with visual reference to the animals and instrumentation or the use of a computer to produce a large volume of data may nicely mask an insignificant study. There is a tendency on all our parts to wish to draw a global conclusion from a fairly specific, narrowly focused amount of data. All carefully accumulated data from a well-designed experiment are important but no more than the data allow.

Overinterpretation of correct data leads us to the final portion of the presentation: the author's interpretation of the significance of his work.

Who (significance)

The *who* of the presentation is represented in the audience's behalf by the P.A.C. How is the audience, on the basis of the question asked, the experiment performed, and the data analyzed, to profit from the experi-

ence? It is incumbent on the presenter to summarize the experience for us, to interpret it, to relate it, and finally (and here it is highly appropriate) to be speculative. What is the significance of this work? Granted that the audience can take it or leave it or place its own interpretation on the value, we award 10 points for the wrap-up (or lack of it).

Don't end the presentation—just stop. It is the old military tactic—"this is what I'm going to teach you; this is what I am teaching you; this is what I taught you"—end presentation. Such a format also serves the scientific presenter well. The ending is a grand opportunity to redefine the problem (the question), again to briefly outline the method and the results obtained, and to re-emphasize the points that have been made. Does it have implications for further studies? Does it clarify the work of others? Does it have practical value for the audience at this point in time? Where should we look for further information on the subject. All too often the presentation just stops at the end of the data analysis; it lacks those few important moments of interpretation and reflection. One can receive an additional 5 bonus points by being unaware that he has finished, that he has shown his last slide, particularly if he has to ask the projectionist if there are any more slides.

Don't end the presentation—and don't stop either. Program committees attempt to provide to as many as possible the opportunity of the podium and to leave time for the audience to participate in some critical discussion. A memorable presentation can be even more memorable if it lasts more than the allotted time. There are several causes of running beyond the allotted time; none are excusable.

1. The presentation has never been tried out at home and timed. The audience clearly recognizes that they are the first to hear it (they will also probably be the last).

2. The presenter believes that he is the only one on the program. It is inappropriate that even a single golden word should be dropped. The time constraints were clearly inappropriate for work of this value.

3. He has chosen to make his presentation ad lib. Since he handles this approach so well in an hour lecture for students, he has assumed that it can similarly be done before a large, national audience. Unfortunately the time allotted is 10 minutes, not an hour.

4. The presenter chooses to present a paper twice, repeating the question, the model, and the data, as though searching for a way to say "Amen."

MISCELLANEOUS (BONUS POINTS)

As alluded to earlier, it is entirely possible to earn more than the 100 points represented by a perfect negative presentation. These bonus points are used by the P.A.C. to separate out a winner from among many winners. Five points are earned by each of the following underwhelming maneuvers:

1. *Having slides either out of order or upside down (or backward).* The presenter may earn additional points by putting *all* the data on one slide, making it illegible beyond the second row of the audience. The pressures of a national presentation are great, and since one has only an average of 2.16 days to devote to the research and preparation of each paper, this aspect may be easily explained—but 5 points anyway.

2. *Reading a paper instead of giving a talk.* We write in compound, complex sentences that flow and become beautifully balanced. What is missed while reading can be reread. However, the same sentence presented orally, if missed, is lost forever. We simply do not talk (and should not present) the way we write.

3. *Attempting to be humorous and failing.* Humor is a delight in any presentation, if deft and timely. However, here it is not better to have tried and failed than to have never tried at all. The presenter should make sure that others besides his wife and residents think it funny.

4. *Failing to speak about either the subject agreed on with the program committee or failure to cover the subject.* Nothing teases an audience more than to find out at the end of 10 minutes that "the data and the discussion will be thoroughly treated in the final manuscript."

5. *Intangibles: the unknown.* Plastic surgeons remain the most innovative and imaginative of surgeons. New and previously unrecorded ways of earning points are discovered at each meeting. It is difficult to predict.

SUMMARY

The surgical phoenix will probably be with us as long as scientific meetings are held. The proliferation of meetings, organizations, and special interest groups make it unlikely that he who strives for recognition can withstand the temptations and opportunities offered by frequent public exposure. Until such time that there is but *one* plastic surgery meeting a year, representing the broadest interests and only the best work of all, this fragmentation of information transmission will continue.

The Phoenix Award is never bestowed unless earned. If one adheres to the following simple steps, he will not be a contender:

1. Submit an abstract that incisively relates the material in the format requested
2. Begin the presentation with a clear definition of the question being asked
3. Expand the question, explaining how experience and the pertinent literature have failed to answer it
4. Describe a well-thought-out, appropriate, experimental model
5. Present data that are tight and accurately interpreted
6. Draw conclusions and make recommendations that are an honest reflection of the material presented
7. Sit down on and in time

At such point in time *the phoenix will permanently self-destruct.*

AMEN

CHAPTER 11

The podium presentation

Ross Musgrave, M.D.

"Doctor, your time is up!" A rather bone-jarring phrase if coming from your oncologist, but also a somewhat nasty psychic trauma if you hear this phrase from the moderator (accompanied by a blinking red podium light) and you still have two or three more pages of your prepared paper to read before a national meeting!

We have all been subjected, in our scientific lifetime, to a great many presentations from this or that podium. Certain of these we recall vividly because of the smooth delivery and the nice, delicate, deft touch of the presenter. We were sometimes further impressed by how he or she made the presentation seem almost casual and unrehearsed.

While it would be ideal for all speeches and presentations to be given "off the cuff," this is not feasible for a tightly scheduled and structured scientific program where there is usually a severe time limitation. Therefore, for most of us, the script should be written and edited in such a way that the material is presented in a straightforward manner, with illustrations (*only* when indicated) properly scattered throughout. The illustrations should not only be pertinent and meaningful but also readable.

THE MANUSCRIPT

While there are many techniques to make a podium presentation more palatable for the audience, there is no substitute for having a well-thought-out and well-developed paper. The paper that will appear in print is *not* the same as the paper you give from the podium. You must write two papers. One you submit to the journal editor. This contains bibliography, footnotes, graphs, and charts conforming to the editorial guidelines of the journal in which the work will be published. The other is the paper you are going to give from the podium. Both papers contain much the same material but are structured differently. The one you deliver is annotated with signals and, incidentally, is typed differently. It is frequently condensed to stay within the allotted time on the program.

When writing a paper you start with a general outline or blueprint of what you wish to convey. After you have such an outline you must work hard to obtain some sort of catchy phrase, punch line, or description of the specific point you are trying to make and build from there. Your paper must have a goal, other than enhancing your diet-slim curriculum vitae. You must know reasonably well to whom you are aiming. In other words, whom are you addressing? What is your target? Dr. William White always gets a laugh from his aphorism, "If you aim at nothing, you'll hit it every time."

Once you have the paper written and you think you have made all the points, you are only about one fourth of the way home. After you have it written and you think it is in absolutely final, polished form, you sit down with the best friend any speaker ever had—a tape recorder. You talk into the recorder just as though you were giving your presentation at the lectern before a national meeting. Then you rewind the tape and you listen to yourself, watching the typed script carefully as you listen to the recording of your voice. Even though you thought you had a finished paper, you will be astounded at the number of flaws present—not only in language but also in vague reference, duplication of words, and confusing terminology. As you listen to yourself, you change a word here, substitute a synonym there, and eliminate any sing-song, choppy cadence of consecutive sentences. More often than not, you will be surprised to find that a point you wanted to make early in the paper has, for some unknown reason, been buried deep in the latter paragraphs. In your next draft you may wish to transpose an entire paragraph or an entire page, inserting these in the proper positions. Having done that and having had your script retyped, you go back to the tape recorder and tape the new version. This process may have to be repeated several times.

When you have illustrations, you must decide where in your presentation these will be used. Set up the projector and run through the slides while listening to your recorded voice on the tape. As you come closer and closer to the final version, decide exactly where your visuals are to be located and place the word "slide" above the typed line of script. Some people use asterisks for this purpose, but you may not have control of the slide projection and you may have to ask for each slide. It is therefore a good idea to know exactly where you want each one projected. (It is preferable for slides to be changed between sentences.) It is also wise to have your slides numbered and the number noted in the script, in case the carousel gets upset.

Summation

You should have a summary near the end of the paper into which you lead by saying "in conclusion" or "finally" or "in summation." It is usually at this point you may wish to have the house lights come up, preferably by a manual, automatic, or prearranged signal (not by a voice signal). Do not cry wolf with your audience by lulling them with several "Concluding" phrases. If you say "finally" mean finally; if you say "in conclusion," mean you are concluding. The audience, who may be wearing thin in patience, attention, and gluteal comfort, distrusts an untruthful speaker as a con artist and may lose its confidence in what he or she is presenting.

In your summation you should reiterate the main points you have made and want to leave the audience thinking about. It may be only a single thought or it may be three or four special points. Do not restate the paper in abbreviated form.

If you are a football fan you will know what a two-minute drill is. Somewhere on the next to the last page of your printed or typed script, you should have such a two-minute drill built into your paper. Hopefully you will not need to use it. But if the chairman signals you with an amber warning light before you are ready—which can happen easily if your slides jam in the projector or there is a disturbance in the audience or your microphone does not work—go immediately to the two-minute drill and finish your presentation with the same ending and proper conclusion. By so doing you will appear more professional than if you simply ended when the time ran out.

Rehearsal

There is no substitute for rehearsal, more rehearsal, and then more rehearsal.

To reiterate, your absolutely best friend is the tape recorder. Most of them run on batteries and you can take one, complete with your taped speech, in the car with you as you drive to the hospital or the office in the morning, or as you drive home in the evening. You listen to the tape over and over until you have familiarized yourself with which phrase follows which phrase. Do not attempt to memorize your entire presentation. You may wish to memorize the opening sentence or paragraph and the conclusion, but that should be the limit.

After you have rehearsed until you have practically worn out your tape recorder, you sit down with your script and listen to your taped voice again, this time with a timer. Always plan for one minute less than you are allocated, for something is bound to go wrong. For instance, if you are allotted a ten-minute time slot, be sure that you can deliver your paper in nine minutes from your opening sentence to your final "thank you."

Typed script

A speech should be triple spaced. Although some people like to have their scripts typed in all capital letters, many find this annoying because very little that we read, other than telegrams, is in all capital letters. Maintain a very wide left-hand margin on each page. Most manuscript pages are 8½ inches wide. Your typed script should never be more than 5½ or 6 inches in width, which is the amount your eye can comfortably scan at a quick glance. Two or more scans of a single line of typing can be confusing. Be sure that the pages are in order and be certain that they are numbered so that if you unconsciously slip or lose your place you do not meander from page 3 to page 6 and back to page 5. Incidentally, it is a good idea to number pages at both the top and bottom right-hand corners.

In addition to indications for changing slides, the script should be marked with "roadmarkers." You can have markers throughout your script to indicate where to speed up, where to slow down, where to pause, when to raise your inflection, where to lower your pitch, what words to emphasize, where to repeat, and above all, where to swallow (Figs. 11-1 and 11-2).

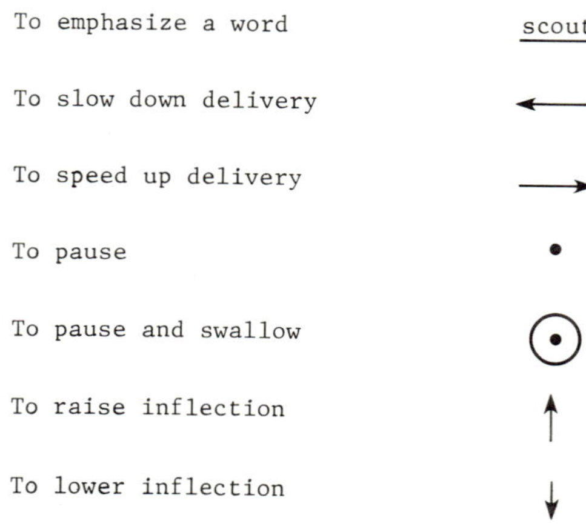

Fig. 11-1. "Roadmarkers."

Again, let me reiterate, your absolute best

friend is that tape recorder! Most of them

run on batteries and you can take it,

complete with your taped speech, in the car

with you as you drive to the hospital or

office in the morning, or as you drive home

in the evening. SLIDE 16 You listen to the tape over

and over again until you have almost

mesmerized yourself about which phrase

follows which phrase. Do NOT attempt to

MEMORIZE your entire presentation. You may

wish to memorize the opening sentence or

paragraph and the summary, but that's the

limit, in my opinion.

Now, on the day of your presentation

and before the meeting starts (or at the

coffee break), scout the turf. Let me

explain. Go up to the podium, check out the

Fig. 11-2. Script annotated with "roadmarkers" and notations for slide change.

THE PRESENTATION
"Scouting the turf"

On the day of your presentation and before the meeting starts or at the coffee break, scout the turf. Go up to the podium, check out the lectern, check the microphone, determine whether or not there is a glass of water in case you get a dry throat. Ascertain where and who the projectionist is. Find out in advance where the slide control button is located and whether or not you have control of forward and reverse. Also determine who is going to focus the projector if slides are not in focus. Also find out where the pointer is and make certain that it works. In the midst of a speech it is unforgivable to search forlornly under the lectern mumbling something like: "There should be a pointer here someplace."

As part of your preparation, always count the steps up to the platform. Carry a small flashlight in your pocket because, as you come up or go down from the podium, the lighting may not be adequate and you may ruin the entire effect if you stumble either approaching or leaving the lectern. Also, should the lectern light suddenly fail, you can use your pocket flashlight and hardly miss a beat.

Personal preparation

When giving a paper, always down-dress. The podium is no place for a peacock. Never wear a shirt with a tight collar or a tie that is too tight. It has been said clothes have a silent language all their own. Unless the meeting is very casual, the scientific podium is no place for the open neck shirt and the protruding macho-type chest hair with golden spangled chain. If it is a black-tie affair be sure that your tux collar is not too starched or too binding. Women lecturers should avoid sequined or frothy bodices.

If you smoke, be very careful not to oversmoke just before you go to the podium. The temptation will be great, but that is a quick way to get hoarse. Instead, use a Lifesaver or a lozenge and have a sip of water just before you start toward the podium. (If you are really hoarse, there is a fine old actors' cure that works: hot tea laced with honey. Of course, you can not take this concoction up to the lectern with you. Another recommendation, besides voice rest, is to take a steaming bath or shower.)

Nervousness will probably make you want to go to the bathroom, so be sure to attend to that chore at the same time you recheck your tie and collar and comb your remaining locks. You have a lot of things to attend to at the coffee break, the least important of which is coffee.

As you approach the podium, get your throat scraping done before you are in range of the microphone. Above all, as you begin your "thank you" to the moderator, be sure that you begin with the lowest pitch you can regis-

ter. Since you will be somewhat nervous, your voice will unfortunately rise to the next higher pitch, and if you start high, you are going to end even higher.

Presenting your paper

Once you are at the lectern and you have the typed paper or notes in front of you and you have addressed the moderator and are ready to give the paper, be sure to thank the person who introduced you. Failure to do so is unseemly and makes you look either pompous, nervous, or rude. You can write a reminder across the top of your script ("Thank you, Dr. Johnson"). At the same time surreptitiously remove the paperclip from the upper left corner. Do not staple manuscript pages together because when you turn them it produces microphone rustling. Unstapled pages slide, hopefully gracefully and unnoticeably, from right to left.

Look around the room and try to establish eye contact with at least some of your audience. Then try to build some sort of rapport with as many people as possible. One columnist recently wrote that no longer should people hide behind the lectern; yet that is where you and the script and the light and the microphone all happen to be. So you must project—or leap across the gap—not only with your voice, but also with your eyes. There is an old theatrical term about listening with your eyes. Watch your audience. The audience can talk back to you in nonverbal ways. They can concentrate on what you are saying; they can smile or frown; they can squirm or look bored; or, heaven help you, they can even fall asleep. You may have to alter your cadence or change your volume to recapture their attention, so work on eye contact if you are to win over the audience.

Do not be afraid of a pause. A pause is the most important form of emphasis we have in the English language, but you have to know how to use it. The well-trained British actors are pastmasters at this sort of thing. It is called timing. Try it on your tape recorder first and observe how different it makes your presentation. Another effective trick is to repeat a word for emphasis. In normal conversation we frequently, yes frequently, repeat a word for emphasis. You can write this repetition into your text.

Be careful about a squealing mike, which is particularly prone to happen if there are two microphones, such as a gooseneck and a lavalier. Be cautious about turning away from the microphone, thus losing your volume, if you turn to peer at the screen. Do not muffle your voice by putting your hand over your mouth.

A disturbing habit of many speakers is to show a few slides, then request the house lights to come back up, then one paragraph later to ask for the lights to be dimmed and go on to the next slide. This is not only amateurish but also disruptive and breaks rapport with the audience. Almost as amateurish is the essayist who gives an entire paper and then shows slides, almost as an afterthought. Slides should be clustered in such a way that the lights are dimmed only once and brought back only once, preferably when you are giving the conclusion or summary. This may mean that you have to put in some filler slides in order to keep the visuals moving along in some sort of orderly progression.

Never leave a single slide on too long; the audience gets fidgety and starts watching to see if your slide will "broil" in the heat, and they stop listening to your message. With a little practice you can work out just how your slides are to be inserted to illustrate, to plump out, to complement your address.

THE "-ATION" SYSTEM

How are you going to remember all this advice? Below is a scheme, which for lack of a better term, is called the "-ation" system:

1. *Inspiration:* If you do not have a good point to make, or your results are incomplete or inconclusive, then defer giving a paper. If the idea for the paper is good this fall, it should be even better next fall after you have an extra twelve months to rethink and reevaluate not only your material, but also your method of presentation.

2. *Preparation:* Preparation includes—aside from writing the paper—rehearsing, listening to your delivery on the tape recorder, scouting the turf, and proper preparation of visuals.

3. *Organization:* The organization of your paper should be logical so that the audience can easily comprehend your message. It should include a short introduction, a methods and materials section, report of the re-sults, discussion, and a conclusion or summary. Although this arrangement is hardly original, its use will help the audience follow what you are saying.

4. *Separation:* This can be spotty on the first or second or even fifth draft, but you had best do some energetic pruning as you approach the final draft. Go over the script as you listen to yourself on the tape recorder. Analyze each phrase. Is this word or this term or this paragraph really necessary? Most neophytes find this pruning to be the most difficult phase of all. It is so much easier to add than subtract.

5. *Declaration:* In broadcasting parlance this is what is known as the "grabber." You have to get the audience on your side in the first three paragraphs, but beware of using humor or the unexpected funny story unless you are experienced. It can ruin you. Try, instead, to make you and your audience be on the same side. In other words, try to convince them of some mutuality of purpose. Otherwise, they will resent your talking down to them.

6. *Oration vs narration:* The difference between the two is a very fine line. If possible, stay on the side of narration. You will find a much more receptive audience. Speak directly to someone you pick out in the third or fourth row. If there is a balcony do not forget to sweep it periodically with your eyes.

7. *Summation:* Spend a lot of time polishing and repolishing this segment of your paper and then be able to give the summary practically with your eyes closed. Remember to be able to go into a "two-minute drill" if necessary.

8. Now, if all goes well, you get the final "-ation"—an *ovation!* Remember, however, you can not possibly earn this "-ation" without much attention to the first seven.

CHAPTER 12

Media and press encounters

Mary Mendelowitz

Nothing in human relations is as important as communication: communication between friends, between colleagues, between physician and patient, and increasingly, between physician and the media. In the past there was a mystique about medicine which the press rarely sought to invade. Recently, however, the public has become interested in medicine, prompting the demand for press, radio, and television coverage not only of new developments, but also of health care in general.

Although most of us consider ourselves articulate and are at ease speaking to a group of colleagues or at other public gatherings, an appearance on television or an interview with a writer may be an uncomfortable experience. By developing a few skills and learning a bit about the news media, we may enter this type situation with confidence.

TELEVISION

Television is the principal source of news for most Americans. Although television was once described by John Mason Brown as "chewing gum for the eyes," it is, nevertheless, an important medium and we should take advantage of its potential for public education.

The product of television is frequently illusion rather than reality. Image, not substance, is often the goal of the television producer. While Johnny Carson may appear to be the epitome of spontaneous wit, the suave, clever image he projects is the product of writers and ingenious direction.

An individual reading a newspaper or magazine can vary the reading time depending on his or her ability to comprehend. An article can be read once or reread as often as the person wishes. The viewer of television does not have this luxury. If the information is not absorbed when it is presented, it is lost. With the exception of sports, there is no instant replay. Therefore, since television is more image than substance, more illusion than reality, the audience's perception of the communicator is the key to success or failure.

First impressions

What factors create a favorable perception? Facial expressions, voice, body language, and clothing style may be more important to the viewer than the substance of what is being said. Therefore, before appearing on a television program you should decide how you want to be perceived by your audience.

Dress. Dress is one of the most important means by which your image is projected. If you want to appear responsible and professional, then dress in a responsible, professional manner. The woman who wants to appear the complete professional should avoid false eyelashes, dangling earrings, and low-cut dresses. The man who wishes to appear dignified and professional does not wear socks that fall down or a casual, open-necked shirt and gaudy medallion.

In general, avoid light clothing or jackets, shirts, or dresses that are checked, patterned or "busy." If you can do without your glasses and can be comfortable without them, do not wear them; but if you need them, wear them. It is very distracting to the viewer to see someone squint and strain, knowing that he or she is not wearing glasses because of vanity.

Makeup. In most major television studios, someone will help you with makeup. The professionals wear makeup whenever possible. If makeup is not provided by a professional, men should apply tan aftershave powder before going on the air. This makes them look healthier and more robust. Women, of course, usually have the advantage of already being made up. Carry a tissue into the studio with you to blot perspiration from your face during breaks in the program.

Behavior on camera

Do not worry about your appearance once you are on camera. Your zipper should have been checked, your socks pulled up, your tie straightened, the spray net used, the makeup applied before you entered the studio. The monitor is no place to check all this after you are on the air. Once you are on camera, forget it and relax.

Although it is easier said than done, try to ignore the camera. Your answers should be directed to the interviewer, not to the camera. Think of yourself as being in your living room talking to a friend. The studio director, by selection of camera angles, will make sure that the home audience is getting a good look at you. If, however, you have a very important point you wish to emphasize, answer directly into the camera—but be sure you know which of the studio cameras is on.

Swivel chairs are often used on television sets and can be your downfall. Nothing is more distracting to an audience than watching someone swivel back and forth. Sit still and upright; try to relax, but not to the point that you appear casual and disinterested.

You may have a short and usually friendly conversation with the host before the program. At that time he or she may discuss much of the subject matter that will be covered during your interview. When the program begins the interviewer may ask the same questions you previously discussed. Avoid the tendency to preface your answers with such phrases as, "As we discussed earlier" or "Well, as I told you before . . ." An interview should give the impression it is happening for the first time. If you do have a preinterview discussion, once you are on the air, act as if it had never taken place.

Personality

All of us have different personalities and personality traits, some of which must be compensated for if we are to project well on television. Consider the quiet introspective person. Since the television camera is instantly on, there is no chance for this type of person to warm up or to get into the mood after the red light has come on. This person must acknowledge his or her shyness and must make an all-out effort before the show begins to raise the level of energy and "get up" for the appearance. Accomplishing this is not unlike preparing oneself for an important meeting or for a final examination. The introvert should try to ignore the television audience and approach the interview as if it were a one-on-one situation involving only himself and the interviewer engaged in a friendly conversation.

The extrovert has a different problem. He or she is usually well received by the audience, but may tend to overreact to the interview situation. Television is not a stage in the theater where one must project to reach the person in the last row of the balcony. It is, rather, a close

medium in which motion or loudness can become magnified and thus distracting. A loud or overwhelming voice, a hearty laugh, or a giggle can be irritating to the audience. The extrovert may also have a tendency to interrupt, to correct others, or to elaborate unnecessarily, all habits that should be tempered during a television interview.

What we are talking about is making subtle, but conscious adjustments to your personality when you appear on television. Keep answers simple, keep statistics to a minimum, eliminate as much technical terminology as possible, and avoid long qualification of every statement. Do not try to dot every *i* and cross every *t*.

Beware also of the "I disease." The viewing audience knows that the statements or opinions are yours; it is not necessary to preface each answer with "I believe" or "in my opinion" or "I think." Avoid self-aggrandizement; do not elaborate on your achievements. The moderator will have covered this in the introduction.

Preparation

Preparation for a television appearance will, of course, depend upon the type of show on which you are to appear. If you are to just make a statement before a camera, no preparation is needed. If, however, you are going to be a participant on a panel show or if you are to give an hour interview on a talk show, your preparation must be more extensive.

Although you should not give an interviewer a list of questions in advance unless requested to do so, it is permissible to ask if some background material would be helpful in preparation for the show. Most interviewers will accept this offer. By the type of material you provide, you may be able to direct the emphasis of the interview.

The first rule of preparing for any type of television appearance is to know your material. Naturally, you will know the technical material, but you may not be prepared for some of the questions that may be asked of you. Remember that a television host wants to attract and keep the attention of the audience, which he or she may do by asking controversial questions, using sensationalism, or gossipy tidbits. It is not unusual, for instance, for a plastic surgeon to be asked about some of the famous people he has operated on.

Do your homework. If possible, watch the show you are to appear on and try to determine the interview techniques of the host. Also, watch the politicians and other public figures on such programs as "Meet the Press" to see how they handle themselves in difficult or embarrassing situations. It may even be a good idea to have some of your colleagues simulate an interview situation. Let them drill you on the questions that may be asked and on issues that may be raised.

In your advance preparation do not lock yourself into a rigidly memorized scenario. Be flexible; be able to "roll with the punches." Answer only the question that is asked unless you feel obligated to expand upon it in order to present the full picture. Be as factual as possible. Do not make exaggerated claims about yourself or your profession. Do not try to impress your audience by using a complex or technical word when a simple one will suffice. Do not ever be afraid to say "I don't know." Remember that the impression you leave behind is more important than any particular detail that surfaces in your interview.

There may be unexpected and distressing surprises in an interview. Before going on the air you met your hostess and she is charming and sweet. You have the feeling that she respects you and that your appearance is going to be a breeze. You feel relaxed and comfortable with her. Then comes the opening camera shot and she says with a tinge of biting sarcasm in her voice, "Isn't it true, Doctor, that all of you make just lots and lots of money?" Panic!!! How do you respond to a question such as that?

There is the *counter attack* response in which you say, "I am certainly not here to discuss the financial situation of my colleagues." This is not the best response in this situation.

There is the "happy, Hubert Humphrey" stance, where you say, with a big grin on your face, "I am delighted that you asked me that question." You then relate a folksy tale about your life on the farm when you were a little boy walking barefoot in the snow. This is a poor response because it is evasive.

Then there is the "not me" approach in which you get an extremely painful look on your face and say to your hostess, "Money! That is complete exaggeration and government distortion." A response such as this, which is a flat denial without evidence, wins no points.

The way to handle a hostile or embarrassing question is to keep cool. Do not allow yourself to be drawn into a hostile exchange with an interviewer. This may well be his or her technique to achieve a goal. Television is like a headline in a paper: the headline may not reflect what is in the story, but is a "grabber." One way to win sympathy and respect from the audience is to remain calm, friendly, and poised in the face of hostility. Try to avoid controversy and stay on safe ground on which you have the facts and on which you have done your homework. Remember you are a spokesperson not only for yourself, but also for your profession.

Bridging is an excellent technique to use in the face of hostility or embarrassment. By careful and skillful use of this technique the person being interviewed can assume a role of leadership and direction of the interview, rather than simply being led along by the interviewer. You first answer the question, then move on to the point you wish to make or in the direction you wish the interview to take. For example, in response to the question, "Isn't plastic surgery all about making people pretty?" you may bridge by saying, "Yes, one part of plastic surgery is to make people look younger or better, but a great deal of plastic surgery is devoted to reconstruction in which the plastic surgeon is involved with burn patients, those with injuries of the face and hands, the repair of birth defects, and reconstruction of patients deformed by surgical operations for the removal of cancer of the head, neck, and breast." Answering the question and then expanding on it, as illustrated above, is an excellent technique that should be mastered.

Another technique is known as "no comment." This should be used rarely. If you do not want to answer a particular question, give the reason why rather than simply saying "no comment." For example, if asked the question, "What did you think of the Playboy interview given by your colleague Dr. Tom Smith?" you can answer, "I haven't seen the article so I don't have adequate information to comment." Then, very subtly, you can make an important point by saying, "Playboy, of course, is not a scientific journal." With this type of reply you have avoided directly answering the question, have appeared professional, and did not denigrate your friend nor did you allow yourself to be drawn into a discussion about which you may not have adequate information.

To summarize:
1. Learn the basic techniques of television.
2. Know your subject.
3. Prepare yourself before the interview.
4. Know your interviewer.
5. Be candid and brief.
6. Be adept at handling tough questions.

RADIO

Many of the suggestions regarding the television interview also apply to radio. Radio is usually more casual and relaxed than television and, of course, you do not have to worry about your personal appearance. The discomfort many people feel when before a television camera causes them to lose much of the warmth, spontaneity, and uniqueness of their personality. Because radio is not as frightening, the warmth and sincerity of the person being interviewed usually projects better.

The technical side of radio is not as hectic as that of television. Since you are not being seen by the audience, you can use notes or even a prepared script. Again, as in televised interviews, do not try to impress the audience with technical or multisyllabic words, but at the same time do not talk down to either the interviewer or the audience.

As in a television inteview, be wary of being led astray into subjects you do not want to cover but which the interviewer may think exciting and controversial. If your interview is taped, you may have an opportunity to listen to the tape and, perhaps, rerecord any material that is less than satisfactory. Even if you cannot change any portion of the interview, listening to the tape may help you to prepare for subsequent interviews.

WRITTEN MEDIA

The journalist traditionally uses the "five Ws": who, what, when, where, and why. When you are to be interviewed for a newspaper or magazine article ask yourself these same questions. *Who* is doing the interview? *What* is that person after? *Where* will the interview appear in print? *When* will it be published? And, most important to you, *why* do they want this story and *why* do they want to interview you?

Before the interview ask the writer if you can review what he or she has written before it is published. Most will say that this is not allowed, but do your best to review the material if you can. Even if it is only read to you over the phone, you may get a chance to correct any misquotes or misleading material.

The journalist who interviews you considers himself a professional. He has a way with words and questions. His job is to interview you and to write a story that will attract readers. Since it is easy in any medium for the reporter to place you in a position of self-aggrandizement, try to use the "royal we"; share the credit with your colleagues. A newspaper interview is usually a casual one-on-one situation in which you may be relaxed and less attentive to keeping your guard up. The same rules for a good interview apply in the written press as in the spoken; be honest, avoid controversial subjects, keep it simple, and remain composed. Above all, do not discuss your private life style; this can be embarrassing not only to you, but also to your colleagues.

If there are any drawings, diagrams, or photographs to be reproduced in the story, have signed releases for them. It is too late to do this after the story is published, and you may face litigation if proper releases have not been obtained.

The writer of the story does not write the headline. This is done by an imaginative person whose job is to write a headline that will attract the attention of the reader. The headline may have little to do with the total content of the story, but unfortunately you have no control over this aspect of your interview.

SUMMARY

In summary, do not be afraid to accept an invitation for an interview. It is your opportunity to get the message of your profession to the public. If you do your homework, spend some time thinking about the image you wish to project, and master the techniques of the media, you can approach an interview with assurance and will appear the distinguished professional that you are.

Artwork, photography, and audiovisual aids

CHAPTER 13

Legibility

Earl Bauer

Legibility of visual aids is a function of four factors:
1. Image size projected on the screen
2. Size of detail in the original artwork
3. Image contrast
4. Image brightness

IMAGE SIZE

The size of the projected image is a function of the focal length of the projector lens and the distance from the projector to the screen. Varying either of these will alter the size of the image. For maximal legibility we obviously want to use as large a screen as possible and to fill the screen with the projected image (see also Appendix C-8).

A good rule to use when determining the size of screen needed for maximal legibility is that no one should be seated further from the screen than eight times its narrowest dimension (Fig. 13-1). For large meetings or for maximal legibility, a figure of six times is better. The important factor is not the total height of the image, but the height of significant image detail. Projected letter height should be no less than 1/50 the vertical dimension of the screen; a height of 1/25 is even better (Fig. 13-2).

To choose the maximal size screen that can be used in a given meeting room, a simple formula can be used. Divide the room length by 6 and subtract 4 feet, which is the distance from the floor to the bottom of the screen, which would be obstructed by the audience. For example, in a room 60 feet long:

$$60 \div 6 = 10 \text{ feet (suggested screen height)}$$
$$- \ 4 \text{ feet (unusable)}$$
$$= 14 \text{ feet (minimal ceiling height)}$$

When setting up a room for projection the most effective place for the screen is in the corner of the room to the audience's right. The lectern should be located in the center and the projection platform in the rear corner to the audience's left.

The selection of the appropriate lens to fill the screen can be determined by referring to the published tables (Fig. 13-3) or by using the formula below:

$$\text{Lens focal length} = \frac{\text{Aperture width} \times \text{Projection throw}}{\text{Screen width}}$$

The aperture width of a standard 35 mm slide is 1.35 inches and the height 0.902 inch. For example: If the screen is 120 inches wide and the projector is 60 feet (720 inches) from the screen: $1.35 \times 720 \div 120 = 8.1$. Therefore, an 8 inch projection lens would be needed to fill the screen from that distance. Remember, the critical dimension in most screens is not width, but height, since this is often limited by ceiling height. Always use a

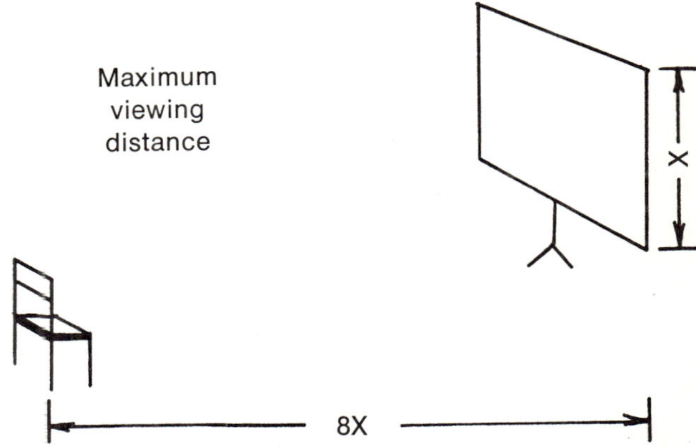

Fig. 13-1. For maximal legibility, no one should be seated more than eight times farther from the screen than its narrowest dimension. A figure of six times the narrowest dimension is better.

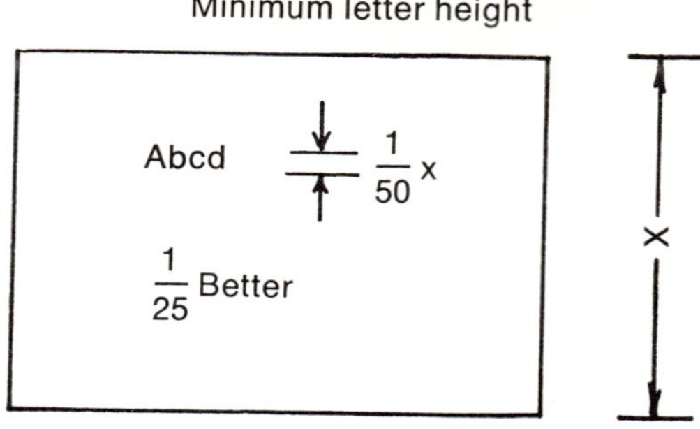

Fig. 13-2. The height of significant image detail should be no less than 1/50 the height of the screen. If lower case letters are used, the ascenders and descenders of such letters should be not be included when making this measurement.

2″ x 2″ Double frame — 35mm slides —APERTURE WIDTH—1.35″

Lens focal length		40″	50″	60″	70″	84″	96″	9′	10′	12′	14′	16′	18′	20′
								Screen width						
3″		7.9	9.8	11.6	13.5	16.1	18.3	20.5	22.7	27.2	31.6	36.1	40.5	44.9
4″		10.6	13.0	15.5	18.0	21.4	24.4	27.3	30.3	36.2	42.2	48.1	54.0	59.9
5″		13.2	16.3	19.4	22.4	26.8	30.5	34.2	37.9	45.3	52.7	60.1	67.5	74.9
5.5″		14.5	17.9	21.3	24.7	29.4	33.5	37.6	41.7	49.8	58.0	66.1	74.3	82.4
6″		15.8	19.5	23.2	26.9	32.1	36.6	41.0	45.5	54.3	·63.2	72.1	81.0	89.9
6.5″		17.1	21.2	25.2	29.2	34.8	39.6	44.4	49.2	58.9	68.5	78.1	87.8	97.4
7″		18.5	22.8	27.1	31.4	37.5	42.7	47.8	53.0	63.4	73.8	84.1	94.5	104.9
7.5″		19.8	24.4	29.0	33.7	40.2	45.7	51.3	56.8	67.9	79.0	90.1	101.3	112.4
8″		21.1	26.0	31.0	35.9	42.8	48.7	54.7	60.6	72.5	84.3	96.2	108.0	120.0
8.5″		22.4	27.7	32.9	38.2	45.5	51.8	58.1	64.4	77.0	89.6	102.2	114.8	127.4
9″		23.7	29.3	34.8	40.4	48.2	54.8	61.5	68.2	81.5	94.8	108.2	121.5	134.8
9.5″		25.1	30.9	36.8	42.6	50.9	57.9	64.9	72.0	86.0	100.1	114.2	128.3	142.3
10″	Projection distance in feet	26.4	32.6	38.7	44.9	53.5	60.9	68.3	75.8	90.6	105.4	120.2	135.0	149.8
12.5″		33.0	40.7	48.4	56.1	66.9	76.2	85.4	94.7	113.2	131.7	150.2	168.8	187.3
15.5″		40.9	50.5	60.0	69.6	83.0	94.4	105.9	117.4	140.4	163.3	186.3	209.3	232.2
20″		52.8	65.1	77.4	89.8	107.1	121.9	136.7	151.5	181.1	210.8	240.4	270.0	299.7

16mm Motion pictures —APERTURE WIDTH—.380″

Lens focal length		40″	50″	60″	70″	84″	96″	9′	10′	12′	14′	16′	18′	20′
								Screen width						
1″		8.9	11.1	13.3	15.5	18.6	21.2	23.9	26.5	31.7	37.0	42.3	47.5	52.8
1½″		13.4	16.7	20.0	23.3	27.9	31.8	35.8	39.7	47.6	55.5	63.4	71.3	79.2
2″		17.9	22.3	26.7	31.0	37.2	42.4	47.7	53.0	63.5	74.0	84.5	95.1	105.6
2½″	Projection distance in feet	22.3	27.8	33.3	38.8	46.5	53.0	59.6	66.2	79.4	92.5	105.7	118.8	132.0
2¾″		24.6	30.6	36.6	42.7	51.1	58.4	65.6	72.8	87.3	101.8	116.2	130.7	145.2
3″		26.8	33.4	40.0	46.6	55.8	63.7	71.6	79.4	95.2	111.0	126.8	142.6	158.4
3½″		31.3	39.0	46.6	54.3	65.1	74.3	83.5	92.7	111.1	129.5	148.0	166.4	184.8
4″		35.8	44.5	53.3	62.1	74.4	84.9	95.4	105.9	127.0	148.0	169.1	190.1	211.2

Fig. 13-3. An example of a table showing the focal length of a projection lens needed to fill different size screens at various projection distances. (Copyright DaLite Screen Co. Reproduced with permission.)

square screen if slides are to be used, otherwise you will be limited to an image size equal to the smallest screen dimension.

ORIGINAL ARTWORK

No amount of superior projection equipment can compensate for poorly planned and executed original artwork. The projected image can be only as good as the original copy. When preparing your artwork, do so with the people in the last row in mind. If they can read the projected image, so can all others in the room.

The dimensions of the artwork should be consistent with the format in which it is to be copied. Since the most common format is the 35 mm slide, which has a height-to-width ratio of 2:3, original artwork should be prepared in the same ratio. As much as possible, all artwork should be done on the same size stock. By so doing, selection of letter sizes is simplified, as is copying and filing. We prefer to use 10 × 12 inches as the standard for artwork. This allows an information area of 6 × 9 inches and margins large enough for notations, guidelines, registration marks, and attachment of overlays. The usable area of the artwork should fill a space slightly larger than the information area so that background edges, registration marks, and guidelines will not show when photographed. This part of the artwork should ex-

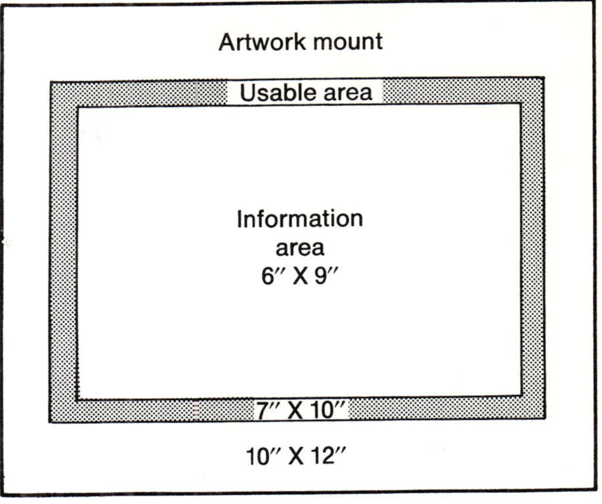

Fig. 13-4. 10 × 12 inch artwork stock showing the usable (7 × 10 inch) area and the information (6 × 9 inch) areas. The usable area should be at least ½ inch larger than the information area. One inch is better.

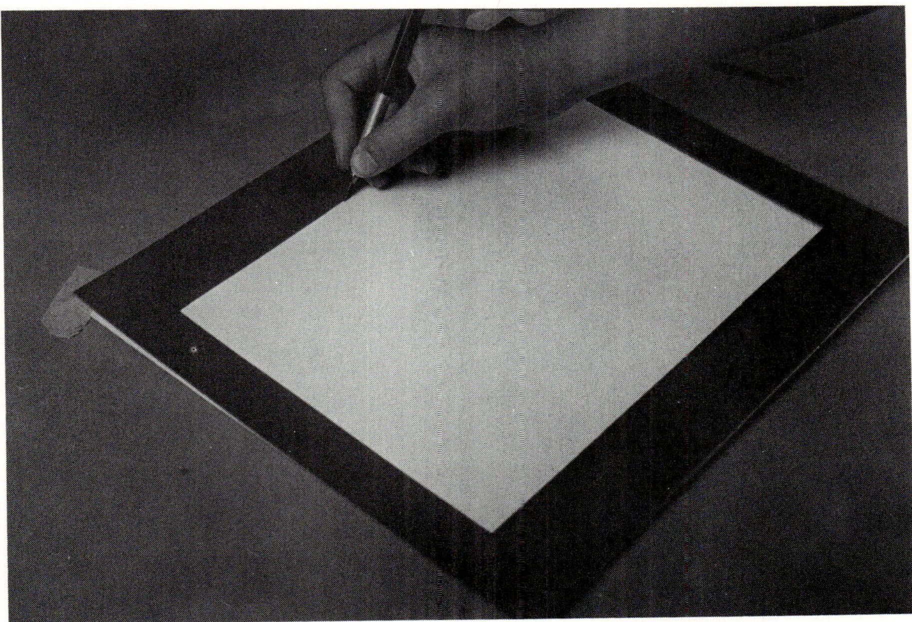

Fig. 13-5. A template is helpful to outline the information area when preparing artwork. This is constructed by cutting a 6 × 9 inch section from the center of a 10 × 12 inch piece of card stock.

tend at least ½ inch (preferably 1 inch) beyond the information area on all sides (Fig. 13-4). A template outlining the information area is useful in planning and layout (Fig. 13-5). This can be constructed by cutting a 6 × 9 inch section from the center of a 10 × 12 inch piece of heavy paper or lightweight card stock.

The minimal letter height should be 1/50 the vertical dimension of the artwork. Larger size letters increase legibility and should be used whenever possible. If lowercase letters are used, the body of these should be 1/50 the height of the vertical dimension. For average viewing, when a 6 inch vertical height of the original artwork is used, minimal letter height should be ⅛ inch.

Lettering should be bold, clean, and without ornamentation or small openings, which tend to fill in when copied and projected. Printer's type and dry transfer letters come in a variety of styles and sizes. Size alone does not determine legibility. Some typefaces are significantly more legible than others, even though the size is the same (Fig. 13-6). Printer's type and dry transfer letters are measured in points (Fig. 13-7). A point is roughly 1/72 inch, since there are 12 points per pica and 6 picas per inch (Fig. 13-8). When judging which size type to use this can be a helpful guide, but the style of the type must still be considered for greatest legibility.

Line weight on graphs and charts should be as care-

24 Point

24 Point

24 Point

24 Point

Fig. 13-6. All of these lettering styles are the same size, but note how much more legible some are than others.

12 Point

18 Point

24 Point

30 Point

Fig. 13-7. Examples of the sizes of printer's type or dry transfer letters, measured in points.

1 Point = $\frac{1}{72}$ Inch

12 Points = 1 Pica

6 Pica = 1 Inch

Fig. 13-8. Printer's measures showing that a point is roughly 1/72 inch. This should be used only as a guide when selecting type, since the style will also determine the size to be used to give maximal legibility.

fully planned as lettering styles for maximal legibility. The information lines should be the most prominent and the axis or grid lines clearly visible, but not distracting. The minimal line width for axis lines on 6×9 inch artwork is 0.9 mm. Graph lines should be at least 1.9 mm.

Try to limit each slide to one significant point. Several simple slides are more effective than a single complicated one. Use no more than fifteen to twenty words or twenty-five to thirty elements on each slide. Leave a space at least the height of a capital letter between lines and use no more than nine lines of copy per slide.

A typewriter can be used to produce copy for slides, but you must use a smaller information area for preparing the original artwork. For a 2:3 ratio the information area should be $3 \times 4\frac{1}{2}$ inches. As with other types of artwork, there should be a minimal usable area of at least an additional ¼ inch on all sides. You may find it helpful

to construct a template of onionskin or clear plastic as a guide to the copy area (Fig. 13-9). When preparing typewritten copy, use a carbon ribbon and clean the type before beginning. Typing should be double spaced with a maximum of nine lines per slide (six is better). Use pica type or larger and limit information to forty-five characters per line.

Regardless of the type of original artwork you have prepared, "come in tight" when copying, so that the information fills the slide. Try, also, to balance the artwork on the slide so that it is centered or has a pleasing appearance when projected.

There are several ways to test the legibility of artwork before it is copied. One way is to view the material from a distance equal to eight times its smallest dimension. For example, if you have a table 6×9 inches, view it from 48 inches. If you can read it easily, the type size and graphics are suitable for copying and projection. Eastman Kodak has developed a legibility calculator that can help you determine the minimal artwork letter size for viewing at various distances. This is reproduced in two Kodak publications, "Planning and Producing Slide Programs" (S-30) and "Legibility—Artwork to Screen" (S-24). Here is an example of the information it will give you: Assuming you are using artwork of 10×12 inches and the screen size will be 10×10 feet, then:

Distance of farthest viewer (feet)	Minimal letter height (inches)
32	3/32
64	3/16
96	1/4
128	5/16
160	7/16
192	1/2

From this you can see that a slide that can be easily viewed on a 4-foot screen in a classroom may be totally illegible when projected in a large meeting hall.

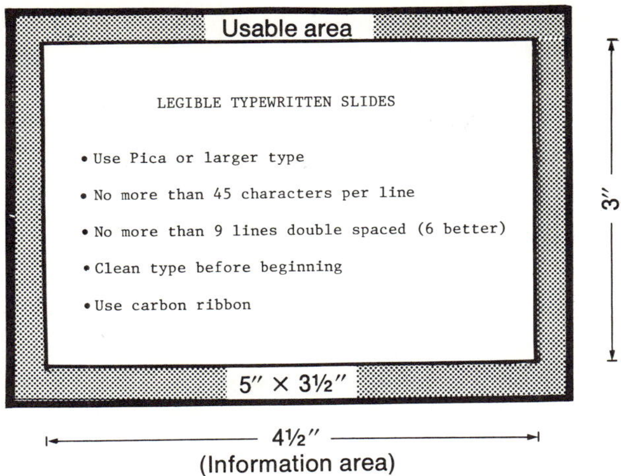

Fig. 13-9. Information area for typed slides. Note that there should be a minimum usable area at least ¼ inch larger on all sides. Use pica or larger type for maximal legibility.

A good method of determining whether or not a slide will be legible is to hold it against a well-lighted wall or view box. If you can read it at arm's length, the chances are that the people in the last row of the audience will be able to read it when it is projected on a screen of sufficient size.

IMAGE CONTRAST

Just as you must pay attention to the size of type and graphics when preparing your original artwork, so too must you consider the contrast of the artwork and background. An improper choice of contrast can ruin an otherwise well-prepared piece of artwork. To be legible, lines, symbols, or letters must have distinct contrast with the background.

You should choose colors that harmonize and work well together. The darker, richer colors show up best, although all of the cool colors, most reds, and some shades of brown are effective. If there is a question about how certain colors will photograph and project, shoot some test exposures. Generally accepted good color combinations for illustrations are:

White on blue	Red on white
Black on yellow	Black on white
Black on orange	Blue on white
Orange on blue	Orange on black
Green on white	White on black

For slides containing copy or lines only, such as graphs and charts, the diazo process is by far the most effective. Never use black letters on dark blue, green, or red. However, if you have no alternative, the letters should be large and bold and the slides must be correctly exposed.

IMAGE LUMINESCENCE

Just as a duplicate slide can be only as good as the original, a projected image can be no better than the projection techniques being used. Those factors affecting image brightness are the projector lens, the type lamp used and its color temperature, the line voltage, the type of screen, and the amount of ambient light falling on the screen.

Most photographers know that changing the focal length of a lens changes the amount of light that reaches the film, thus exposure must be changed to compensate for this. This is also true with lenses on projectors; a shorter focal length lens transmits more light from the lamp than does one of longer focal length. Since long focal length lenses are necessary in large meeting rooms and since these also give better resolution and image sharpness, a lens with a larger aperture must be selected to assure adequate image brightness. For example, changing from a 5 inch f3.5 lens to a 5 inch f2.8 lens will project 27% more light on the screen.

The color temperature of the projector lamp will determine how accurately the colors of the original artwork are projected. Color temperature is recorded in degrees Kelvin (K) and is a measure of the color quality of a light source. Sunlight at noon has a color temperature of 5400 K. This temperature gives pure whites, clean blues, vivid reds, and reproduces realistic color. The ideal projection lamp should, therefore, have a color temperature close to this. In general, the longer-life incandescent bulbs have a color temperature in the range of 3000 to 3300 K and in average use tend to produce colors that are dull, with poor color saturation and poor delineation of tones. These are usually in the D series (DEK, DAH, etc.). The newer quartz bulbs in the E series (ELH, ENG) have a somewhat higher color temperature, ranging from 3250 to 3500 K. Even an increase of 150 to 200 degrees K will improve image brightness and color saturation. Even so, the higher temperature quartz lamps lose their effectiveness when projection distances are long. When a room setup requires long projection throws, the xenon lamp should be used. This type lamp has a color temperature of 5400 K, the same as sunlight, and gives the best color saturation and image brightness of all types of lamps.

The line voltage supplied to a projector lamp will significantly affect both the life of the lamp and its light output. For efficient use of a selected lamp, the line voltage should match that specified by the manufacturer. When setting up projection equipment for a meeting, specify that a separate circuit be made available, so that as near the recommended voltage as possible is supplied. Be sure, also, to use an extension cord of sufficient size to prevent a drop in voltage between the receptacle and the projector.

The matte white and the glass beaded are the two

screen surfaces that are commonly used. Of these the matte white is far superior. It maintains acceptable image brightness over a 100 degree viewing angle, while there is a sharp drop off in brightness with the glass beaded screen as one moves away from the axis of projection. For example, image brightness on a glass beaded screen is reduced 550% when viewed 45 degrees from the projection axis, while there is only a 25% loss from this angle with a matte white screen.

Ambient light coming from open doors, inadequate room darkening, or task lighting, which is necessary for note taking, reduces screen effectiveness. As much stray light as possible should be eliminated. Overhead lights should be extinguished near the screen and dimmed in the rest of the room. Windows should be draped or covered with blackout shades. If there is still too much light falling on the screen, it will then be necessary to increase the lumen output of the projector to compensate for this.

SUMMARY

To ensure maximal legibility of slides, prepare the original artwork properly, select colors wisely, and use projection equipment that provides sufficient light of proper color temperature and a lens that will give maximal projected image size.

CHAPTER 14

Graphics

Hale Tolleth, M.D.

The ancient designs on rock walls scattered over the world suggest that graphics were early recognized as a useful communication tool. It is easy to imagine how a simple pictograph, a stick drawing of a figure, could become the Chinese character for woman (Fig. 14-1). Our own written language had its beginnings in the needs of the Phoenician trader, at least 3500 years ago, to represent ideas and sounds by symbols (Fig. 14-2). And now we are constantly exposed, even inundated, with signs, symbols, drawings, diagrams, and pictures that attempt to influence or express a concept. Nevertheless, effectiveness of this communication will vary, depending on presentation and audience.

The lifeblood of medicine is communication: professor to student, physician to physician, physician to patient. Graphics have an almost unlimited capability to explain, clarify, illustrate, or emphasize, but badly done they can confuse, obfuscate, or distract. In medical communication the need is most often to inform and, on occasion, to convince.

The method and need for graphic illustration will be determined by subject, audience, time, medium, space, and budget available. The strategy chosen will be determined by available resources. Of the many ways to present information—article, essay, book, movie, multimedia, lecture, slide show, or video cassette—graphics can make some contribution in most of them. Surprisingly, the basic processes in graphic production are similar in the various media, although special considerations may be present.

In material to be published, for example, there may be space limitations, style requirements, or special rules by the publisher. The number of illustrations, photographs, or graphs may be limited, but they may be more detailed and complex since they can be studied at length by the reader. Carefully reading the publisher's directions or advice to authors before beginning will save expense and time.

A graphic to be projected, however, has few limitations relative to its color or design, but there are stringent limitations as to type of material, length, and complexity. The slide shown at a lecture will usually be displayed for a very short time; lengthening the time does not allow the addition of excessive material since legibility and boredom both must be considered (Fig. 14-3).

The purpose of a graphic must be carefully thought out and the smallest possible number of graphics chosen, if only because of expense. There is no need to put an entire talk onto slides, nor should every thought in an article be illustrated. Boredom is an enemy of communication. Repetition and trivialization can be major sources. Requirements of a graphic that performs well include irreducible simplicity, attractive design, and readability. The sins of unnecessary information, distracting color, poor layouts, and illegibility must be avoided. A plea could be added to avoid questionable taste or attempts at humor. It is a rare audience in a cold, dark auditorium that is amused by cartoons or pictures of nude ladies. (One might add that the entertainment value of slides of your grandchildren or your most recent overseas sunset photograph is uncertain.)

Budget will be a major concern, especially if many illustrations or slides are to be made. If artwork is to be done by you it will cost at least ten times the price of making a photographic slide. A slide made professionally from copy supplied to an artist may run two or three times that amount, depending on how complicated the design is. Obviously, limiting the number, increasing effectiveness, and producing some of the work yourself are mandatory. Your time, however, should be considered as part of the cost. In the long run it may be

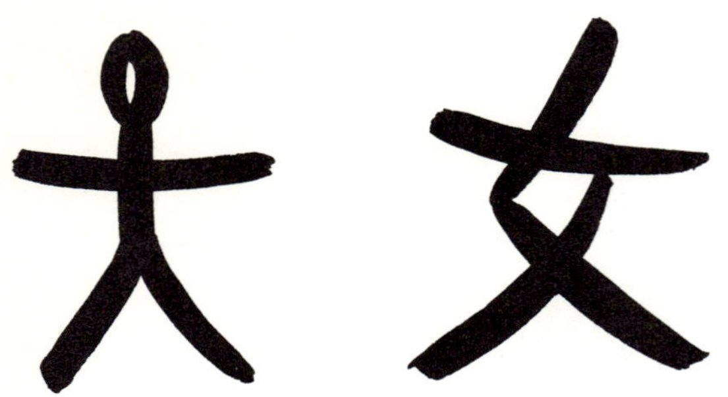

Fig. 14-1. Stick drawing of a woman and the modern Chinese character for "woman."

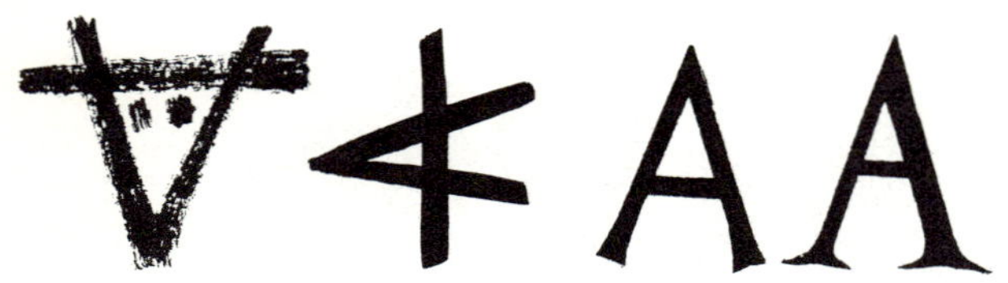

Fig. 14-2. A drawing of an ox or "aleph" became the Phoenician letter "aleph"; aleph became the Greek "alpha" and finally the Roman "A."

This material is set up to be absolutely illegible to the majority of the audience unless they are sitting immediately in front of the screen. There is too much on this slide and in the back of the audience it will be only a blur. Aside from that the time it takes to read will be too long. And more important it is dull and uninteresting to look at even if it were printed in the boldest type with the brightest possible colors. We have all been victimized by this thoughtless kind of poorly designed presentation.

Fig. 14-3. An example of unsatisfactory material set up for a slide.

cheaper to hire an artist or printer than to do it yourself.

A word of caution; sometimes a talented amateur can produce an illustration of sufficient quality. However, the embarrassment of badly done artwork that is published will last much longer than concern for the cost. Anything that diminishes your presentation should be avoided. If there is any question, get professional help.

LETTERING AND TYPE

There is no magic in producing letters on a piece of artwork, but there are many choices to be made, depending on where the material is to be used (see also Appendix C-1). For example, uniformity throughout a

HAND LETTERED WITH A PEN
LETTERED WITH A TECHNICAL PEN
THIS WAS SET-UP BY THE PRINTER.
THIS WAS TYPED ON AN IBM
SET-UP WITH TRANSFER TYPE

Fig. 14-4. Various methods to produce lettering.

book may require that labels on diagrams be set up by the publisher. In this instance your responsibility is to present typewritten copy, carefully indicating special needs. In other cases, you may be able to place the labeling on the artwork to suit yourself prior to submission of the manuscript.

If the artwork is to be projected, all choices are yours, and various methods can be used, depending on your skills, experience, time, and budget. Simply stated, lettering can be done by hand, drawn with a pen or brush; done with a mechanical aid such as a stencil and technical pen; or set up using transfer letters (Fig. 14-4). Solid block letters can be set up on a suitable background and photographed. Mechanical methods include using the typewriter or having a printer do the work.

Handlettering by any method is somewhat slow and requires skill and practice. Mistakes are easy to make and it is difficult to make the work look professional. A technical pen or Rapidograph (a fountain pen that comes with a variety of tip widths) can be used, either with a stencil or lettering device called a Leroy, to make lettering, which if well-spaced, looks neat; it resembles that on a blueprint. The alphabets are limited in style but come in various sizes with both uppercase and lowercase.

Solid block letters are available in photography shops. They come in only a few sizes, colors, and styles and most often are used for setting up titles. They are not very useful if any amount of material is to be shown, and they have a tendency to look somewhat amateurish.

A great boon for those who wish to produce very professional, even handsome, layouts is transfer or pressure lettering. Essentially, these are alphabets silk-screened onto a thin sheet of plastic and then backed with a wax pressure adhesive. Register marks are printed below each letter, allowing even registration, spacing, and lining up of the letters, which are then burnished onto the artwork with a small tool. The choices of alphabets and size are almost unlimited, and there is an extraordinary number of symbols, devices, borders, decorations, texture, and shading sheets available (Fig. 14-5). A few alphabets come in red, blue, yellow, green, and gold, and with special techniques any letter can be made al-

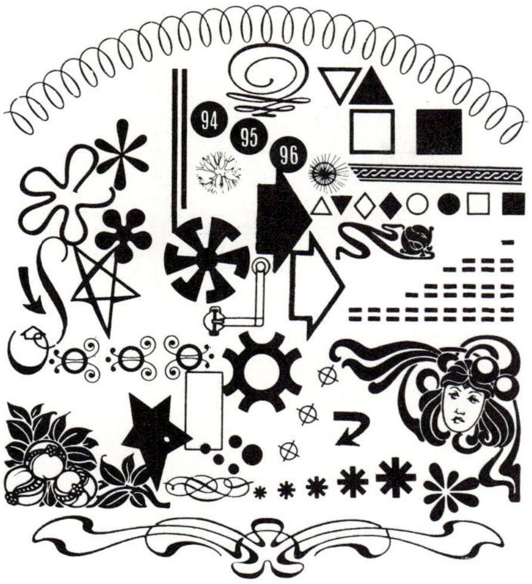

Fig. 14-5. Many devices and designs are available for use in graphs and illustrations.

TYPEWRITER.

Fig. 14-6. Typewritten work when enlarged by projection may appear ragged, irregular, or askew.

ROMAN roman

SANS–SERIF sans-serif

ITALIC italic

SCRIPT script

DECORATIVE

Fig. 14-7. The five basic alphabet families. Note the illegibility of the uppercase script.

most any color. With practice and a little care, the absolute novice can produce very professional work. However, the job becomes somewhat burdensome if there is a large amount of copy to be set up.

By far the easiest and least time-consuming method is to have the work done mechanically by a typist or printer. Typewritten work will be suitable for slides if the typewriter is a good one, with the ribbon carbon and the typeface sufficiently bold. For jobs needed quickly, this method works well, but there are disadvantages, including an almost irresistible tendency to put too much on the slide. Word, letter, and line spacing may be faulty and, when projected, the enlargement of the letters often reveals them to be somewhat ragged, irregular, slightly askew, or out of alignment (Fig. 14-6). Artwork using type from the typewriter normally is not sufficiently tasteful or professional to be published.

A printer can be your best friend for making type look good, especially when there is a lot of it. He or she may set type for letterpress printing, in which each letter is hand set, but more likely a sophisticated phototypesetting machine will be used, much like a typewriter. A printer will have many (but not unlimited) numbers of typefaces available in almost any size. Even better, the problems of letter, word, and line spacing can be solved. You will often be provided multiple copies, which you can cut and paste up yourself to solve special problems. You will be charged by the hour; generally this is a bargain since your own time is likely to be limited. However, be sure to get a cost estimate.

Even with the aid a typist or printer can give you, there are choices to make, including arrangement, typeface, and type size. Native taste and judgment will be

helpful but there are guidelines—not absolute to be sure—that will assist you in creating work that communicates well because typeface, message length, legibility, and attractiveness have been considered.

There are essentially five families of alphabets: roman, sans serif, italic, script, and decorative (or display) (Fig. 14-7). The novice will often opt for an exotic or interesting typeface, not realizing that unusual faces are often hard to read, particularly if the words are long or unfamiliar (Fig. 14-8). The most easily read is the roman face, chiefly because of familiarity but also because the letters are rather easily recognized and a flow of line is created by the serifs. Similarly, lowercase is the most legible because of the strong differences created by the varied letter sizes and shapes (Fig. 14-9). Sans serif, letters without serifs, are very common, but note that, although sans serif headlines are bold and easily read, the body face of a newspaper is usually in roman. Italics are used to indicate special emphasis. Scripts are basically decorative or used for special situations as varied as a wedding announcement or a product label. Do not use uppercase scripts (see Fig. 14-7). Decorative types have obvious wide use but only rarely should be chosen when legibility is a concern, and then chosen with great care. However, decorative faces can create mood, often without any other artwork.

Type, aside from the family it comes from and the name assigned to it, is described in other terms. "Boldness" is self-explanatory and is created by the thickness of the strokes (Fig. 14-10). A very light face or a too bold one creates a legibility problem in body text and should be reserved for headings and other special uses. The "medium" or "standard" face should usually be used. A

Ecumenical

Fig. 14-8. Decorative types are sometimes hard to read if the words are long or unfamiliar.

design using only lower case
DESIGN USING UPPER CASE ONLY
Design using upper and lower case
Design Using Upper Case for most Important Words

Fig. 14-9. Short phrases may be set up in uppercase but for a longer text, lowercase may be advantageous.

ABC	Helvetica extra light
ABC	Helvetica light
ABC	Helvetica medium
ABC	Helvetica bold

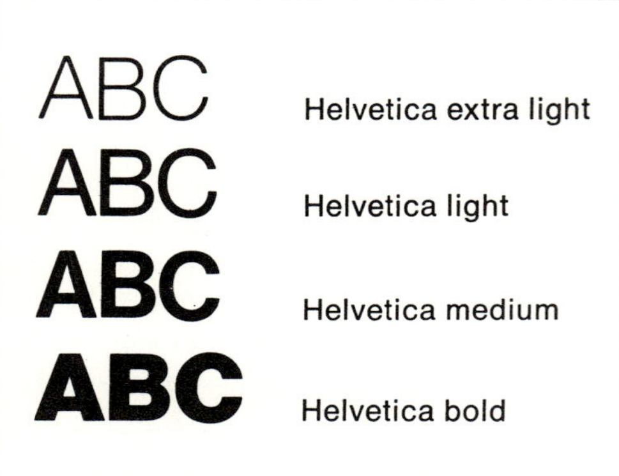

Fig. 14-10. Same style, same size—only the boldness varies.

letter face that is condensed or extended is often used because of space requirements or for special design purposes (Fig. 14-11).

Type size is measured vertically in points, 72 to the inch. One cannot measure a given letter and determine point size since the point measure refers to a letterpress type slug, which includes the top margin, the highest point of the highest letter (such as an *h*), the lowest point of the lowest letter (such as a *y*), and the bottom margin (Fig. 14-12, *A*). In addition, some alphabets have only uppercase and some only lowercase, in which case measurements will be applied differently. The typefaces illustrated in Fig. 14-12, *B*, are all the same size according to their point measurement. Therefore, if you wish to match typefaces by size, comparison is best made by looking in a catalog at the art store or printer's shop.

STANDARD
CONDENSED
EXTENDED

Fig. 14-11. Condensing or extending a typeface is useful in space or design problems.

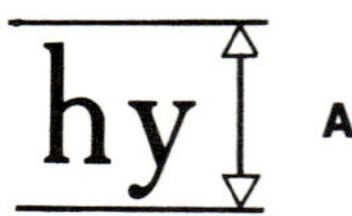

A

AAAAAAA B

Fig. 14-12. A, The method by which point size is determined. **B,** These decorative faces all have the same point size but not only look different in size, they measure that way also.

Spacing letters mathematically leads to a choppy, unattractive appearance (Fig. 14-13, *A*). Letters should be spaced visually, taking into account letter shape and open spaces surrounding them. Letters such as *C*, *A*, *L*, and *T* require less space between letters than closed letters such as *H*, *M*, *N*, etc. The general rule is to match the open space between letters as illustrated in Fig. 14-13, *B*.

To center a line exactly, count the letters and spaces, and divide by 2 to find the center of the line. Start from the center point and letter from the middle of the line, proceeding right toward the end. The line is now half set up; proceed to letter from the middle of the line in reverse toward the left. (Be very careful not to misspell if you use this method) (Fig. 14-14).

Usually space between words should be about 1½ capital letter spaces. Punctuation marks such as periods and commas should not be given a full letter space. If words are too close, they run together and irritate the reader; when too far apart, especially with multiple lines, rivers of white space will dissect the paragraph (Fig. 14-15).

Distance between lines is called "leading" (pronounced ledding), and is critical when there are more than several lines of type. The amount of space between lines is related to point size, boldness, and whether up-

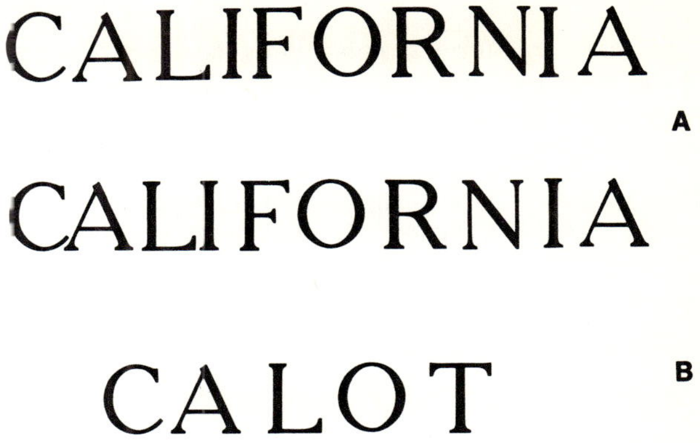

CALIFORNIA

A

CALIFORNIA

CALOT

B

Fig. 14-13. A, Spaced mathematically, the word "California" is much less attractive than when spaced visually. **B,** The letters C, A, L, O, and T all have space around them that must be taken into account.

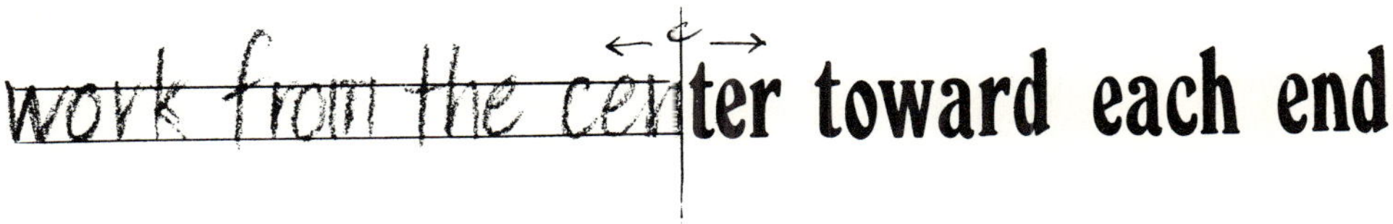

work from the center toward each end

Fig. 14-14. To center a line, count the number of letters, divide by 2, begin at the middle, complete the line, then letter from the center toward the left.

The space between words is critical for readability

The space between words is critical for readability

The space between words is critical for readability

Fig. 14-15. The space between words is important.

the space between lines (leading)
is critical for readability

the space between lines of type (leading)
is critical for readability

the space between lines
of type (leading) is
critical for readability

the space between lines
of type (leading) is
critical for readability

Fig. 14-16.

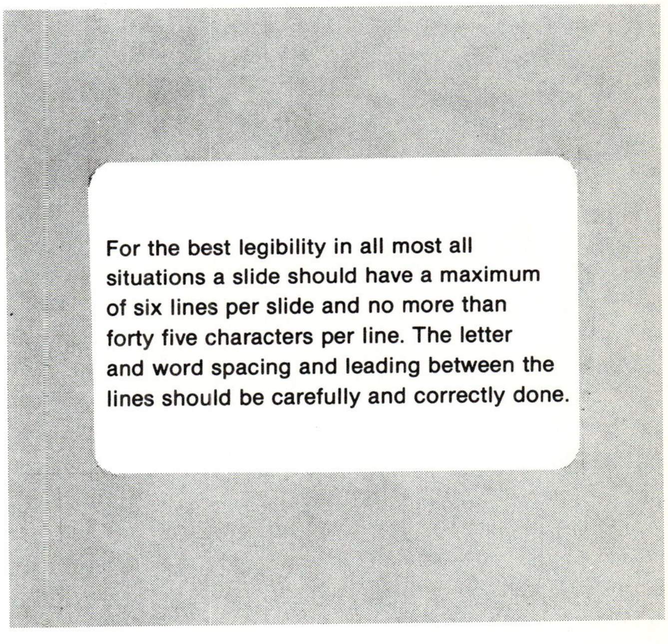

For the best legibility in all most all
situations a slide should have a maximum
of six lines per slide and no more than
forty five characters per line. The letter
and word spacing and leading between the
lines should be carefully and correctly done.

Fig. 14-17.

percase or lowercase letters are used (Fig. 14-16). An easy rule is to leave the distance of the height of the tallest letter, plus the depth of the lowest letter, plus a little bit. If you spread the lines too far apart, the white spaces overwhelm the lines of type.

Line length is very important in readability. Lines that are too short do not allow proper flow; lines that are

Surprisingly there are only a few ways that type can be arranged. This layout is one in which both sides are justified. It is very easily read.

This type is arranged symmetrically but neither margin is justified. It is difficult to read because the eye has to find where the line starts.

These lines are set up to be justified on the left, ragged on the right.

These lines are set up and justified on the right. It is often satisfactory for certain design purposes.

The least legible is type which is both unjustified and asymmetrical since it is very difficult and even irritating to read.

Fig. 14-18.

too long require too many eye movements as the eye travels across the line. The printer and designer have formulas for this but for the amateur there is a good rule to follow: Never use more than six lines on a slide, and never use more than forty-five characters per line (Fig. 14-17). Type for publication is not constrained by this since the material can be studied at length.

It would seem that there would be almost unlimited ways to arrange a line of type on a page. Surprisingly, there are but a few and the choices that you have are limited if you covet maximal legibility (Fig. 14-18). The margins, right and left, can be straight (justified) or ragged. Arrangements of the lines can be symmetrical or asymmetrical. Combining these possibilities provides only a few choices. Of these, margins that are ragged on the left are the hardest to read because the eye has to search for the beginning of the line. Readability is not affected by having the margins ragged or straight on the right side of the column. Asymmetry is used as a design feature and when readability either is less important, as in a title, or can be sacrificed for a special effect, as in some poetry.

DESIGNING WITH TYPE

There are some basic clues that may be of assistance. Stick with only a few styles or typefaces for a given series of slides or illustrations. Clarity and flow of thought are maintained by consistency of style in presentation. Create emphasis or importance by altering the point size or the use of italics (many typefaces have a parallel italic alphabet). Use the "drop-out" subtraction or addition techniques when a line is added or deleted in a series of slides. A similar technique, coloring the line of the slide that you wish to emphasize, may be used. Unity is created by using symmetry or justified margins. An asymmetrical arrangement ought to be balanced; boldness or size is not necessarily equivalent to legibility.

COLOR

Most graphic artwork can be produced in black and white with relatively inexpensive materials. In fact, most professional graphic work, during its preparation, is in black-and-white form and does not gain color until the presses are inked. Illustrations, diagrams, and tables published in professional journals are almost always black and white since color printing is expensive.

Gray as color. The addition of "color" to a black and white illustration is done by creating gray tones obtained either by mixing black and white pigment or otherwise combining black and white. The visual process allows a combination of black and white spaces to look like gray, such as cross-hatching or the use of small dots; the degree of grayness is a function of how much of the white paper is left (Fig. 14-19).

The engraving method determines how the grays are made. If it is an expensive halftone process or the offset printing method, any gray in the artwork or photograph will be reproduced as intended. If the less expensive line engraving method is used, the photoplate will register only black or white and the grays will be dropped out. Grays will have to be made with cross-hatching or dots. Fortunately, there are sheets of dots, lines, and other textures available commercially that can be applied to artwork to create almost any gray tone (Fig. 14-20).

Professional artists give the engraver or printer artwork with a separate overlay sheet, indicating the gray areas by solid black, with a notation that this is to be printed as a certain gray, expressed as a percentage or a screen line value. The screen, which is engraved with a varying number of lines or dots, is used in the photographic portion of the engraving process.

Fortunately, many publications are now printed by the offset process in which an entire page is photographed and made into a "plate." Halftones made by any method will be reproduced satisfactorily.

If a photograph has been previously printed, the grays have been broken down into microscopic dots; rephoto-

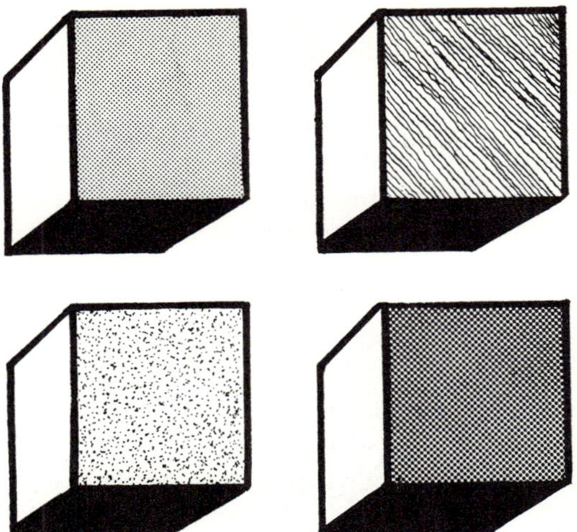

Fig. 14-19. Grays "created" using black-and-white pigment, cross-hatching, dots, and commercially available shading sheets.

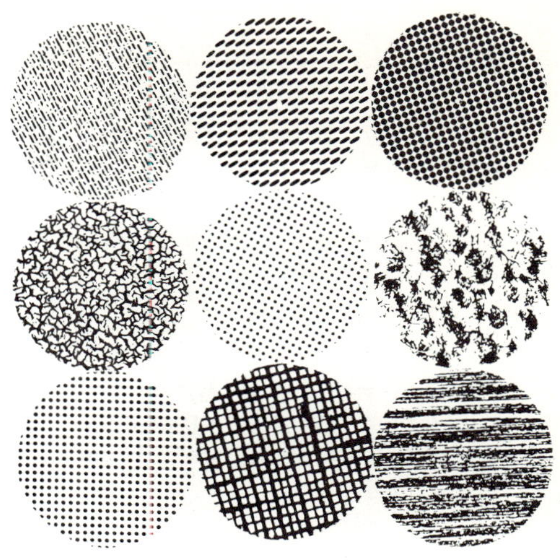

Fig. 14-20. A small sample of the many shading or texture sheets available.

graphing with a screen will result in another pattern of dots. This results in a pattern in large areas of gray called moíre, which looks like watered silk fabric.

Color. Color is a major way to create interest and emphasise, especially on material to be projected. Unfortunately, it may be chosen haphazardly or because a certain process is available. Even worse, colors are chosen as though the slide were a road sign indicating great hazard. A common misconception is that a slide should "show up" like a commercial neon sign. Certain color combinations may give rise to negative feelings, vague irritation, or even outright discomfort. For example, white slides with black letters in a dark auditorium may have a dazzling, overbright appearance; consider using pale gray or blue. Black slides with white letters may tend to sparkle; consider coloring the letters.

Almost any black-and-white artwork can be converted to a color slide photographically. There are at least eight processes available (see Kodak reprints on this) but since not every photographer or processor can do them, a consultation before the photography is done will save time and money. Special film, filters, and processing are required.

A simple and inexpensive way to give color to a slide is to color the negative of the artwork with felt-tip pens after it has been mounted. However, excessively strong color and a certain garishness can be a problem here. A neat trick is to make multiple copies of the same slide, then color the lines of type on each slide in a progressive fashion.

The list of currently accepted satisfactory color combinations is based on "effectiveness"; from the most to the least legible, they are as follows: black on yellow, black on orange, orange on blue, green on white, red on white, black on white, blue on white, white on blue, orange on black, and white on black.

Again, tastefulness and flashiness may be a problem (imagine death statistics presented in orange and blue).

White on muted strong colors such as green, red, blue or brown is a good compromise. White on pastels does not work well but black on pastels may be very attractive.

Adding color before the artwork is photographed is not done as often as the simplicity of the method would suggest. The possibilities are endless; you can use watercolors, colored pencils, felt-tip pens, acrylics, pastels, or color overlay sheets. Photographic reproduction is a simple matter of shooting the artwork with standard color film and flash, although improved quality can be obtained with tungsten light, special film, and a copy stand.

EQUIPMENT AND MATERIALS

How much equipment you need to acquire depends on how much you will do. The better the working conditions, including working area, equipment, and material, the easier it is to do the work. A simple inked circle is hard to draw without the proper compass.

The expensive ideal is a well-lit working area furnished with a drafting table, proper stool, and materials cabinet called a taboret. Most of us compromise with less, settling for the kitchen table, a drawing board (there are many sizes), flexible light (preferably fluorescent), tackle box for tools, and an adjustable stool. A light box or X-ray viewing box is available to many physicians and is a great help.

T squares are made of wood, plastic, or metal. Plastic or metal-bound are best. Triangles are usually plastic and come with angles of 30, 60, and 90 degrees or 45, 45, and 90 degrees. The 12 inch is a good size. Colored plastic triangles are easier to find in the confusion of a project.

A French curve is made from a sheet of plastic punched out with a die and shaped with various guides used to draw nonstandard curves. They come in many sizes and shapes. You will likely acquire them one by one according to the problem to be solved. A similar tool is a plastic template, which also comes in a great variety of sizes and shapes for drawing special forms including letters.

Inking a drawing or lettering requires the use of a pen; the usual fountain pen or ballpoint is not a satisfactory substitute (the ink is not black enough). Many pens are available to solve special problems, such as ruling pens to draw clean lines, technical pens for lettering, and simple nibs for lettering or drawing (Fig. 14-21). The minimum needed is an assortment of simple nibs, which are inexpensive and require little practice to use. The other pens mentioned are used by architects, draftsmen, and commercial artists and are considerably more expensive but often do the job with great ease, saving time and effort.

The compass, which we all had in our pencil boxes at school, is a tool to make circles. To make circles with a pencil is not much of a trick; however, to make them with watercolor, ink, or even to cut an accurate circle requires a more expensive instrument, which is well worth it when the need arises.

A metal rule to cut against and a simple ruler will be needed. (Do not cut against a plastic T square or triangles.) Cutting tools to acquire include a matte knife, scissors, X-Acto knife, and single-edged razor blades. If you use transfer letters, a burnishing tool and small forceps will be useful. Small camelhair brushes will be used for inking, touch-up, and even some drawing. Buy the best available since cheap brushes will not last; they will make easy work hard and your artistic career miserable.

Materials to obtain will vary with the work you must do. However, you will always need layout paper, tracing paper, and drawing tablets. Matte finish acetate sheet comes in either tablets or rolls and can be very useful.

Learning about the wide variety of art papers and illustration boards available is not necessary for our purposes. Simply stated, illustration board is good quality paper backed up with varying thicknesses of cardboard. The surface of the paper varies with whether it is cold-pressed (a matte surface), or hot-pressed (smoother, shinier surface). Illustration board may also be coated with ink, paint, clay, or color for special purposes. You need only to get a good quality board faced on one side,

which will take ink well and can be erased without becoming frayed and fuzzy. These boards usually come in sheets 40 × 60 inches, or 20 × 30 inches. The store will often use their paper cutter to cut them down to a 10 × 10 or 10 × 15 inch size, making them much easier to handle and store. Buy more than you need.

Papers and boards with texture will be used only for certain effects and are usually inappropriate for reproduction.

Pencils you need include simple graphite pencils varying from very hard (9H) to very soft (6B): the larger the lead, the softer the pencil. Very hard pencils make very light lines but if pressed too hard they will scratch or mar the paper. Too soft pencils used for preliminary lines are difficult to erase and may make the work messy. Colored pencils are very handy, especially light blue. A blue pencil line, if not too heavy, will not be picked up in the photo process so need not be erased from artwork.

Erasers, too, come in a great variety for special uses. Get soft rubber, kneaded rubber, ink, and art gum erasers as a minimum. Be very careful using the eraser on the ordinary lead pencil because they vary greatly in abrasiveness and will sometimes even leave a pink stain. Other methods of erasing include scraping with a blade, erasing fluids (made with acid or hypochlorite), cotton swab with rubber cement thinner, special abrasive powders, and an electric eraser.

If you plan on using color, simple watercolors, artists' acrylic colors, poster paint, colored inks, colored pencils, sheets of color, or marking pens can be obtained. Pastels and oil pastels will occasionally be useful. There is an indispensable white paint that comes in small jars

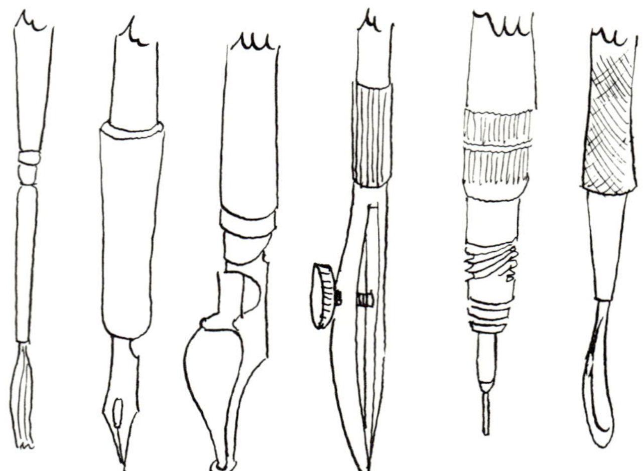

Fig. 14-21. Necessary tools include small sable brush, crow quill pen, drawing nib, ruling pen, technical pen, and burnishing tool.

and is used for touching up, blocking out, or covering small errors.

Finally, remember to buy fixative, which you will spray on completed work. It comes in several types for specific uses. You need adhesives including cellophane tape, drafting tape (used instead of tacks), and rubber cement. Rubber cement thinner is very handy since the glue always seems to be older or thicker than you remembered.

DESIGN AND PREPARATION

The design and completion of your graphic is a matter of progressively refining a rough idea into a finished piece.

1. Read your presentation through and jot down ideas or rough sketches for graphics on 3×5 inch cards (see Fig. 14-22).

2. Lay the cards on the table, arrange them in a reasonable order, and eliminate those that are too trivial, simple, or unnecessary. Pare the number as much as possible.

3. Consider each idea card carefully to determine whether it would best be a table, graph, illustration, diagram, or photograph.

4. Collect the written material for each card. As much as possible simplify by shortening sentences and words. Sometimes a complex idea can be broken down into two or more illustrations.

5. With the decisions made, determine the material that must be produced as lettering or type and make up the copy on $8\frac{1}{2} \times 11$ inch sheets in the arrangement you desire. The amount to be done, difficulty, and time available will suggest whether you can set it up yourself or have it done by the printer. For the latter, write any directions or specifications in blue pencil on the margins, otherwise a very literal typesetter may also set up your directions.

6. Photographs to be published should have good contrast and be printed on glossy paper. Wide margins can be ordered and are very useful. Consider cropping unnecessary portions. In some cases retouching is very desirable to improve quality (as in an equipment photo); in other cases is absolutely forbidden (as in showing the results of surgery). Adequate retouching requires a very skilled person.

7. Tables may be converted to graphs and vice versa. A drawing may be easier to understand than a photograph (as in some anatomy illustrations). Avoid complexity or a plethora of information on a graph or diagram unless it can be studied at length (Fig. 14-23).

8. With the idea card at your side, the light over your left shoulder, and the T square on the drawing board with the T on your left, tape layout paper to the board (Fig. 14-24). Carefully draw the diagram you wish, con-

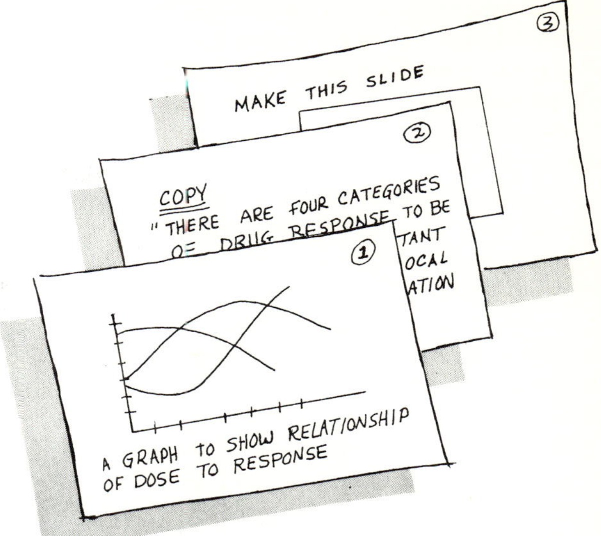

Fig. 14-22. The handy 3×5 inch card planning system.

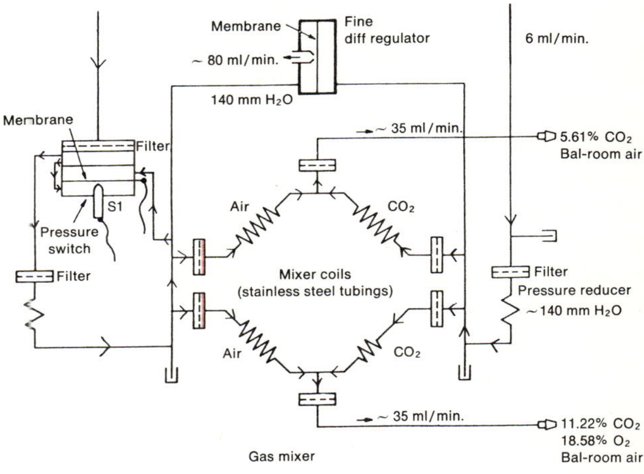

F g. 14-23. A diagram of this complexity makes a poor slide.

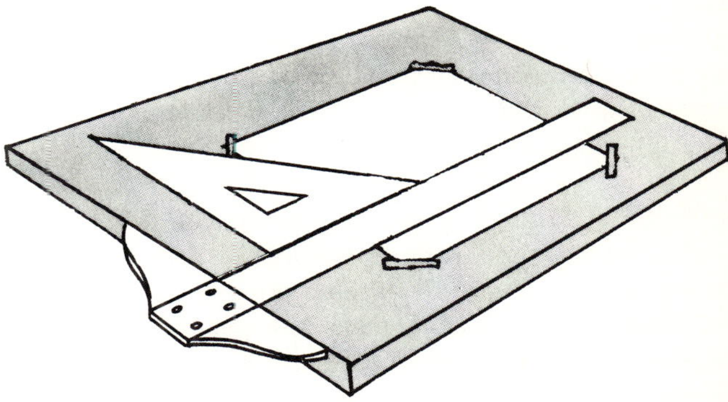

Fig. 14-24. Minimal equipment includes a drawing board, T square, and triangle.

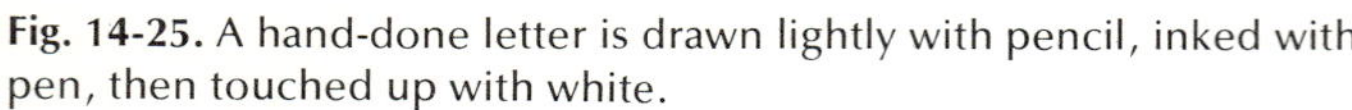

Fig. 14-25. A hand-done letter is drawn lightly with pencil, inked with pen, then touched up with white.

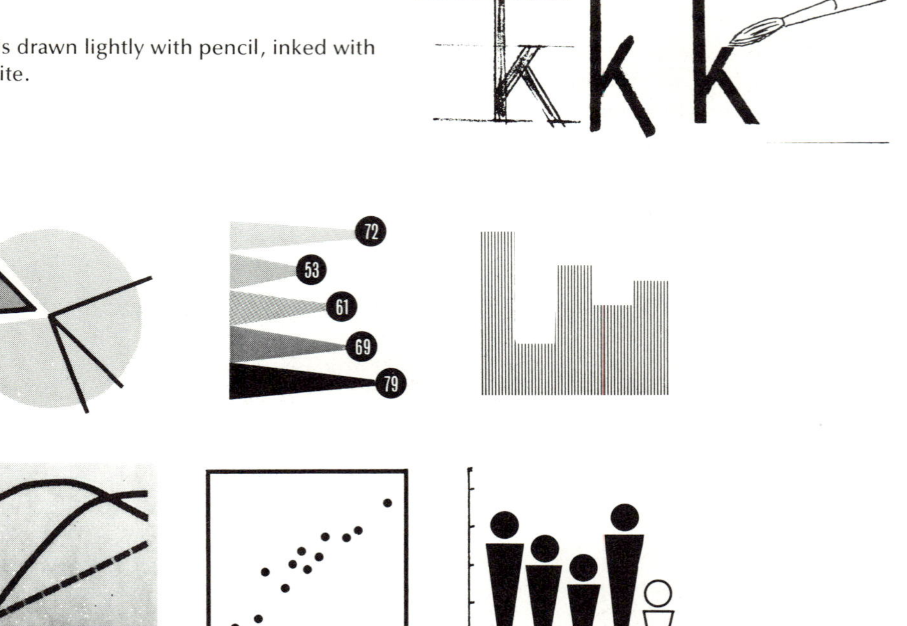

Fig. 14-26. The simpler the graph the better; simplicity does not preclude attractiveness.

fining it within 6 × 9 inch rectangle. When it is complete, trace it onto tracing paper. On the reverse of the tracing paper rub either graphite pencil or blue pencil. This will function like carbon paper. Do not use ordinary carbon paper because it will be difficult to erase and creates smudged, dirty artwork.

9. Remove the rough diagram and place a piece of illustration board approximately 10 × 10 or 10 × 12 inches squarely on the board and tape it in place. If all illustrations are of this size they are more easily photographed and later can be stored in an ordinary file. Using the T square again, carefully position the tracing over the illustration board and tape it down. When you have completed the tracing, ink in the drawing and apply shading film, color, or transfer letters and labels. Clean up and cover up any unwanted marks by erasing or covering with white paint (Fig. 14-25). After removing the illustration from the board, spray it with fixative.

GRAPHS

If there is an endeavor where your best artistic creativity can shine, it will be in the making of a graph. Your imagination is the limiting factor since varying materials are available, including ruling pens for clean lines, French curves for bent ones, and special adhesive tapes of various widths and colors, some of which are flexible and can be formed into curved lines.

Collect the information you wish to illustrate, recalling that the graph's purpose is to clarify (eliminate the nonessential). Graphs can be made as line graphs, cluster graphs, bar graphs (either vertically or horizontally oriented), or the dissected pie shape favored by financial types (Fig. 14-26). They can be fancied up, with color and special devices, or presented in perspective or three-dimensional forms. Dull ink graphs with a dash of imagination can become an interesting illustration— witness the graphs drawn for *Time* magazine by Nigel Holmes.

Transfer the rough to the illustration board with tracing paper. Ink in the straight lines, complete with graph tapes, shading sheets or color overlays.

LABELING AND PROTECTION

As you work on the "final," protect it as you letter or touch up by using a piece of paper under the heel of your hand to protect it from the moisture and oil in your skin. Avert disaster by keeping coffee cups, ink bottles, glue bottle, and pens wet with ink away from the immediate work area. Never lay anything on artwork. Handle all work by the edges; your thumbprint is an unsatisfactory addition. After cleaning up smudges, extra pencil marks, and ink spots, gently and carefully spray a fixative, especially if pencil shading, pastel, or charcoal has been used. Check with an art supply store as to the type of fixative you need since the wrong one could cause running or slow destruction. Read the directions. A heavy spray may cause a problem, remedied only by redoing the artwork.

Artwork that is piled or stacked will be damaged by pieces abrading each other. Lettering will get scratched, glued material will come apart, and colors will smear. In short, the work may be ruined. Apply an overlay sheet of tissue paper, acetate, or tracing paper cut to the size of the work and attach to the top with rubber cement or cellophane tape.

Photographs for reproduction should be labeled on the margins using a stabilo pencil. If you have ordered wide margins this is very easy. Alternatively, instructions can be written on the board on which the photo is mounted, or on the overlay sheet. Some publishers require unmounted pictures with information written on the back. *Never* write on the back of a photo with a ballpoint, marking pen, or heavy-handed pencil since you may emboss the photo or the colors may bleed through photo paper.

Prepare artwork for mailing by cutting corrugated cardboard larger than the artwork and placing the corrugations at right angles on the top and bottom to minimize bending. Write your name, address, and the name of the article or paper on the back of each piece before packing or sending it to the printer or mailing to the publisher.

SUMMARY

Producing a graphic may seem to be an esoteric art but in fact can be successfully accomplished by the inexperienced amateur who is willing to use some judgment in the kind and amount of material he or she wishes to present. By carefully sifting and paring information, then proceeding in an orderly manner and utilizing professional help appropriately, informative and interesting graphics can be economically produced.

CHAPTER 15

Choosing and working with a medical illustrator

Peggy Williamson

MEDICAL ILLUSTRATION

In his biography of Max Brodel, who is considered the father of medical illustrating, Cullen wrote: "Good illustrations are to a fine medical article what windows are to an outstanding department store. People walking along the street stop and look at the window display and enter the store. So medical readers are attracted to an article by the fine pictures and they linger to scan the medical treatise."* Frank Netter considered medical illustration "the accurate transmission of one man's thoughts to another man not only in a different part of the world but also at a different time."† Medical illustration should both attract the reader's eye and communicate information through pictures that can be understood in any language and at any time.

A few years ago, Dr. James Lieberman, in his opening remarks to a meeting of medical illustrators used this story, which is appropriate:

I am reminded once again of the first grader who was sitting in a corner drawing a picture. His teacher came over and asked: "Peter, what are you drawing?" Peter replied: "A picture of God." "Well, you really can't do that," the teacher remarked, "because nobody knows what God looks like." Whereupon Peter said: "Well, they do now."‡

This is the assurance you are looking for in illustrating scientific writing. You know what something looks like, but how can you best communicate it? "A poetic ex-

planation of a surgical procedure in vague, obscure but beautiful words"* would no more accomplish a factual description than would a fuzzy, wide-brush attempt at painting an intricately detailed picture. The final judgment of the proficiency of a medical author or artist is in his or her ability to present factual information in a meaningful manner.

According to Robert Dermarest, "Scientific journals have been pictorial wastelands for too long. Word-oriented editors have cropped, reduced, enlarged, or eliminated illustrations for considerations of space rather than the intended impact of the communication."† It is up to the artist to demonstrate that illustration is an increasingly important part of scientific communication. There is a great difference between pretty pictures and an informative illustration. The medical illustrator must present solutions. As Demarest states, he or she must "illuminate areas that words cannot reach." It is the medical illustrator's responsibility to articulate, clarify, and simplify the author's words to a degree of immediate comprehension.

Photography vs illustration

Who needs an illustrator when photography can do so much? Medical photography has made tremendous strides in the past fifty years and there is no denying its value. The arts of illustration and photography should work hand in hand. A camera can make a cell stand still and pose; but that camera, no matter how refined and sophisticated, records only what it sees. An illustrator can eliminate the unnecessary, superimpose a diagram,

---

*Cullen, T. S.: Max Brodel, 1870-1941, Director of the first department of art as applied to medicine in the world, Bulletin of the Medical Library Association **33:**27, 1945.
†Netter, F. Cited in Mellori, B.: Frank Netter, dean of American medical illustrators, Visual Medicine **1:**38, 1966.
‡Lieberman, J.: AV communication, the constant renewal, Journal of the Association of Medical Illustrators **18:**5, 1967.

*Osburn, W. A.: Editorial, Journal of the Association of Medical Illustrators **16:**17, 1965.
†Demarest, R. J.: Publisher's comment, Journal of Biocommunications, vol. 5, 1978.

or reduce to a diagram. The illustrator can cut windows to the inner reaches of the anatomy. He or she can cross-section the body and still keep the patient alive!

Training

In order to know what to expect of medical illustrators it might help to understand what goes into their training. Aside from training in artistic crafts, they have enrolled in a medical illustration department in a medical center. They concentrate on the study of human anatomy. They dissect, drawing as they do so, every layer of tissue, every nerve, artery, vein, muscle and organ, learning the functions and the "feel" of them all. Illustrators devote perhaps three times the time a medical student does to gross anatomy. Histology, embryology, and comparative anatomy are also included in their studies. Their libraries are amply filled with illustrated reference books in these fields. They have knowledge of graphic, plastic, and photo reproduction processes. They have observed and sketched countless surgical procedures and autopsies and can communicate the "feel" in their work. They can transform words into pictures that demonstrate visually what the author is saying. The illustrator articulates and clarifies to the common denominator of sight.

COST

The cost of medical illustration varies in different parts of the country. In medical illustration the aphorisms, "time is money" and "you get what you pay for" are apropos. If you employ an artist who is not a trained medical illustrator, you pay the price of inexperience. So your niece is "artistic"? Forget it. Unless you have someone already trained in medical vocabulary, operating room procedures, and anatomy, you are putting an unnecessary, time-consuming, and trying burden on yourself and the artist. Get a qualified person. Have an understanding with the artist about the cost at the outset. It could be an hourly rate, and total cost would depend upon the number of conferences, number of hours in the operating room, travel expenses, and cost of materials. On the other hand, the artist may give you a total charge in advance. Extras add up. The better prepared you are in advance, the less cost in money and time there will be for you both.

The artist can tell you what type of illustrations you will need for your particular situation and the relative costs of reproduction. For clarity in reproduction, basic black and white is best. Color is exciting, but unless it is for slides the reproduction costs are high and publishers will print color plates only if color is a significant factor. The simple outline drawing is more effective and frequently more eloquent than the elaborate one. It is truer, bolder, costs less to produce, and is less likely to be distorted in the printing process.

FINDING A MEDICAL ILLUSTRATOR

Besides letting "your fingers do the walking" in the Yellow Pages, look for a medical illustrator the way you would for any other professional. Ask your colleagues, study published medical journal articles, or write the nearest medical center. Most medical schools have a list; also the Association of Medical Illustrators has a directory with names of qualified illustrators in the country. Look at samples of several illustrators' work and make your choice. You are fortunate if your clinic or medical school has an artist on its staff.

WORKING WITH AN ILLUSTRATOR

If you know in advance of an operation that you will want the services of an artist, call him or her for a conference about the upcoming case. Infect the artist with your enthusiasm and reasons for recording the procedure. He or she is by nature a questioning, curious, and inventive person. Arm yourself with X-rays and a description of the expected procedure. Even your own sketches, as crude as you may think they are, will reveal much. The artist will work from a format of normal to pathologic or injured to the corrected or reconstructed results. If you will tell the artist in advance the anatomic areas involved and the proposed operative procedure, he or she can do some preliminary study, and this research will enhance your understanding of one another. The artist will be able to enter the operating room fortified by study and make sketches as you proceed, following your commentary and direction. Do not be dismayed at the sketches that are "dashed off." The illustrator is simply recording pertinent details for his or her own memory and record. You will usually need three conferences with the artist—one before surgery and two afterward: first to view the preliminary sketches for corrections and additions, followed by evaluation of the finished drawings.

Often you become aware of the need for an artist after the fact. (If only I had known . . .) In this instance provide the artist with an operative report, X-ray films, your own sketches, and other reference material you may have. He or she can work from these materials after you describe your findings and operative procedure. The artist will then provide you with preliminary drawings in which the unnecessary has been eliminated and procedures have been diagrammed for simplicity and clarity. From these you can suggest additional details or changes and assist the artist with legends and labels.

SUMMARY

Your paper puts your reputation on the line. For a professional job, you must call a professional to help you. Work with the artist and know and appreciate his or her contribution.

CHAPTER 16

Medical illustration techniques

Denis C. Lee

Illustrations for plastic surgeons may vary greatly from complex surgical drawings to simple cartoons. A medical illustrator must decide which technique will best represent the procedure to be illustrated.

Because of the expense of printing, most illustrations are done in pen and ink. This medium is fast and reproduces well. However, if the original drawing is not sent to the publisher, the results, usually a copy from a photograph, may be unsatisfactory.

Fig. 16-1 shows three different types of tube skin grafts. These are represented by simple line drawings of the grafts without detracting from the basic idea by placing each graft on a patient. A little humor is added to stress the caterpillar type of movement of the skin graft.

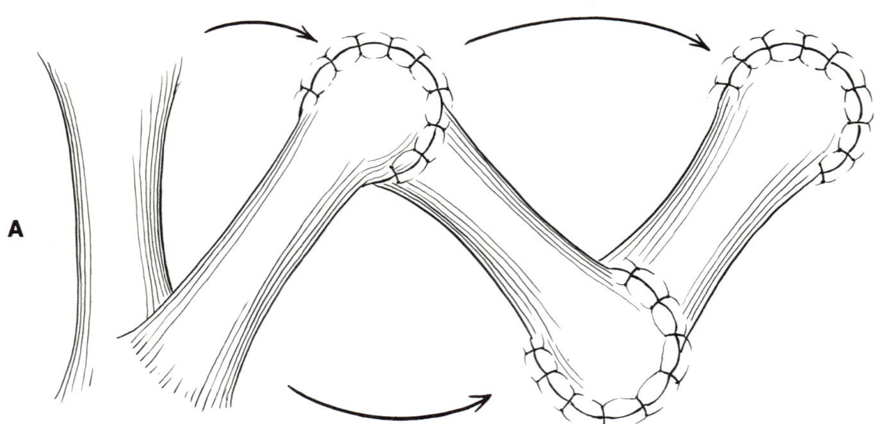

Fig. 16-1. From Grabb, W.C., and Myers, M.B.: Skin flaps, Boston, 1975, Little, Brown & Co. Reproduced with permission.

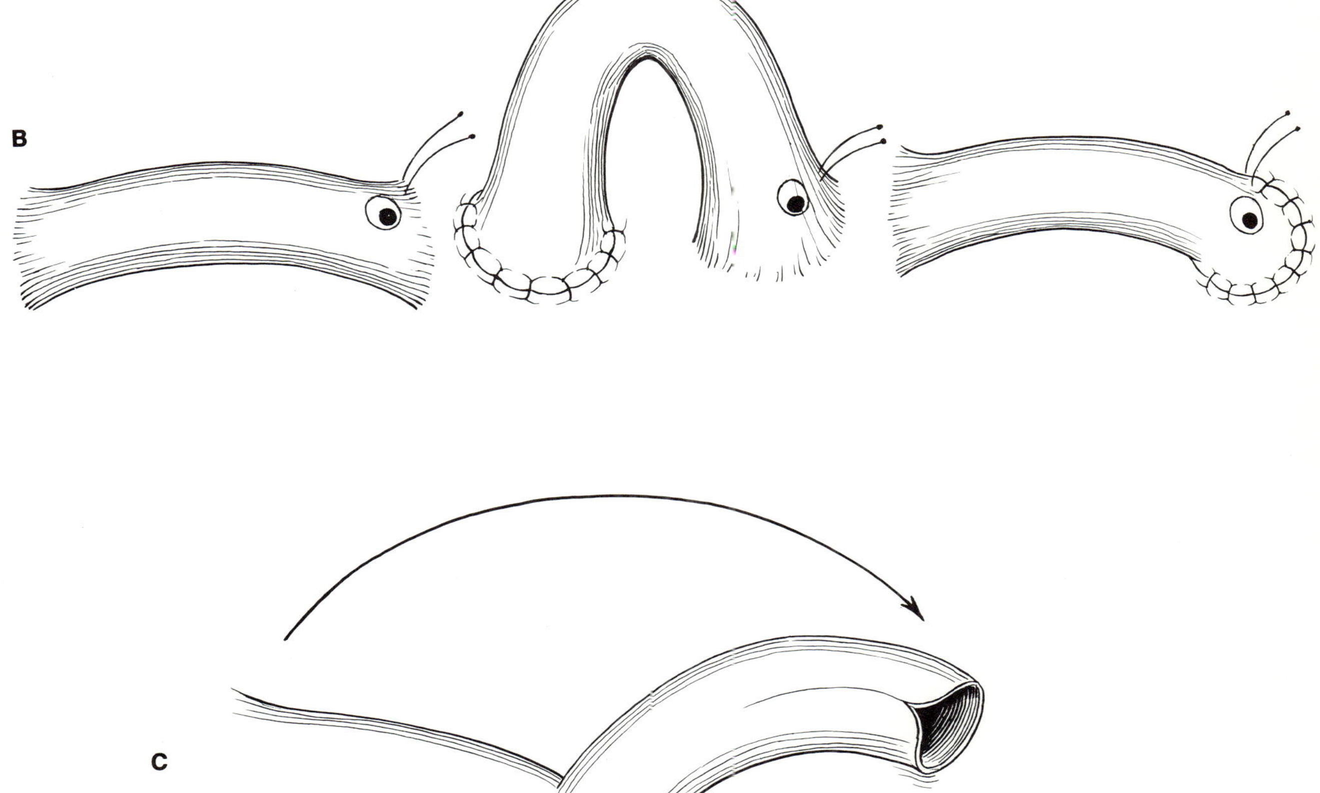

Fig. 16-1, cont'd.

Illustrating surgery of the hand is a real challenge; the hand is one of the most difficult parts of the body to draw. A simple outline of the hand with emphasis on the surgical area is most effective. Excessive shading of the hand would merely detract from the center of interest (Fig. 16-2). A little stippling illustrates the affected area and a dotted line, the extent of the incision. A foreshortened view is difficult to draw but makes the drawing more interesting and affords the most effective view of the important area between the fingers.

When surgery of the fingertip is involved it would be distracting to show the rest of the hand (Fig. 16-3). Simple cross-sections are used to illustrate correct and incorrect techniques.

In Figs. 16-4 and 16-5 illustrations of the entire hand were required to illustrate incision lines. Instead of trying to show all of the incisions on one hand, simple outlines of the dorsal and palmer views plus insets of fingers provide a view of all areas of the hand. It would be superfluous and confusing to place the same incisions on each finger or to illustrate incorrect and correct incisions on one hand.

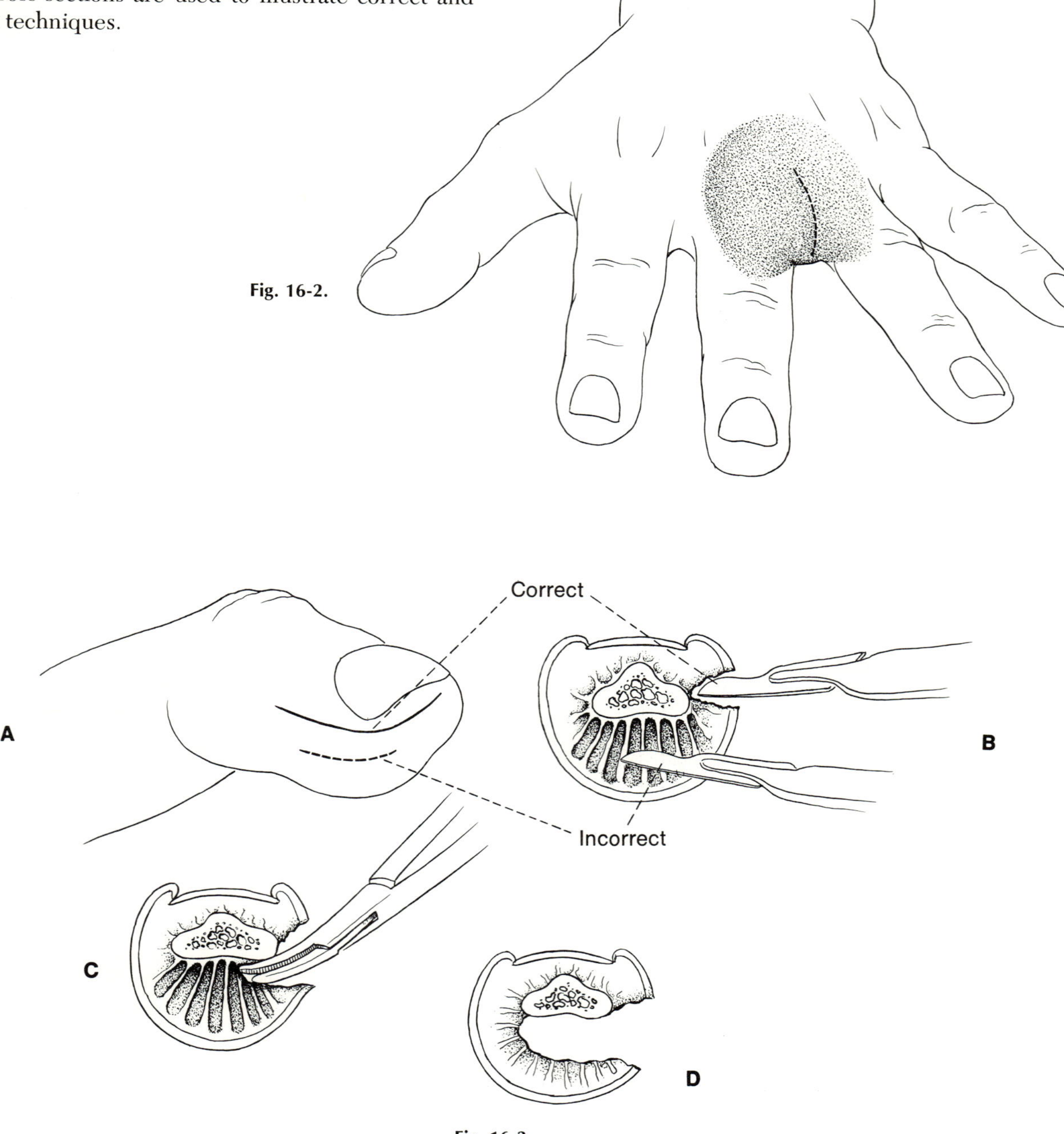

Fig. 16-2.

Fig. 16-3.

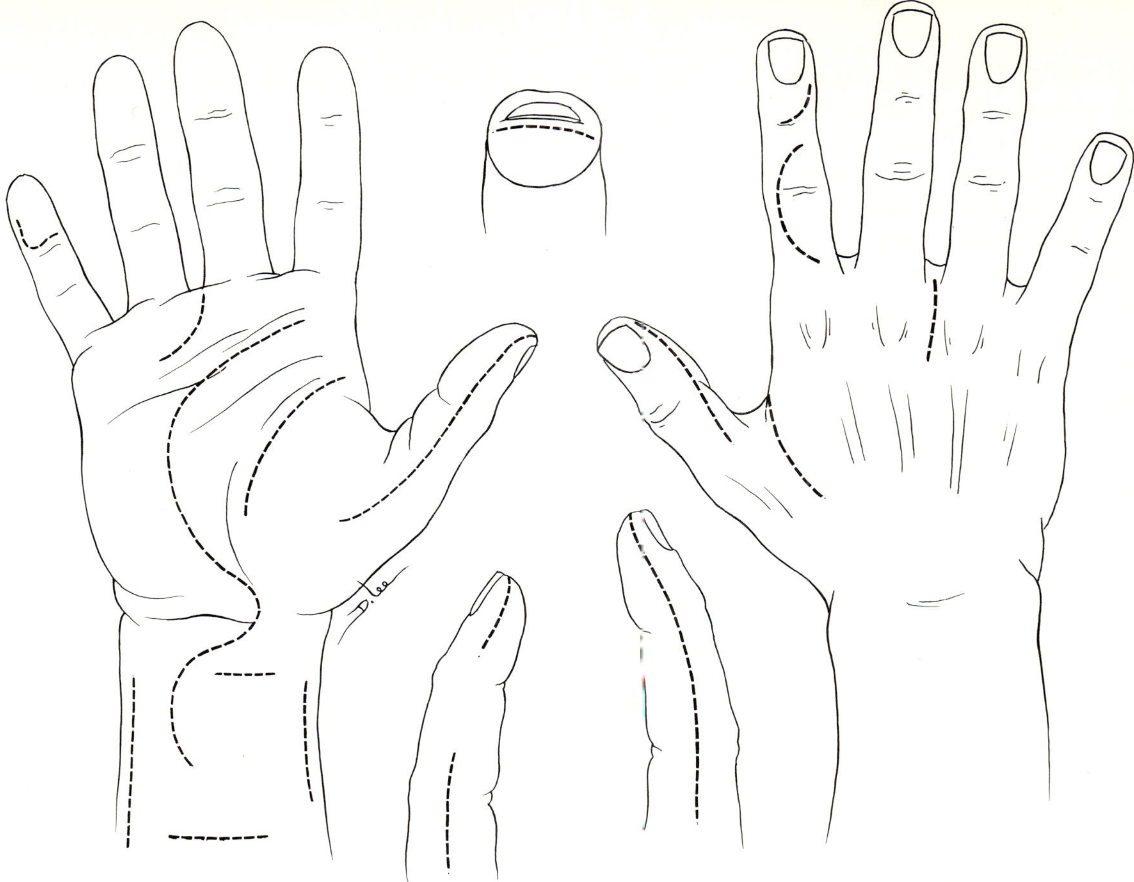

Correct incisions

Fig. 16-4.

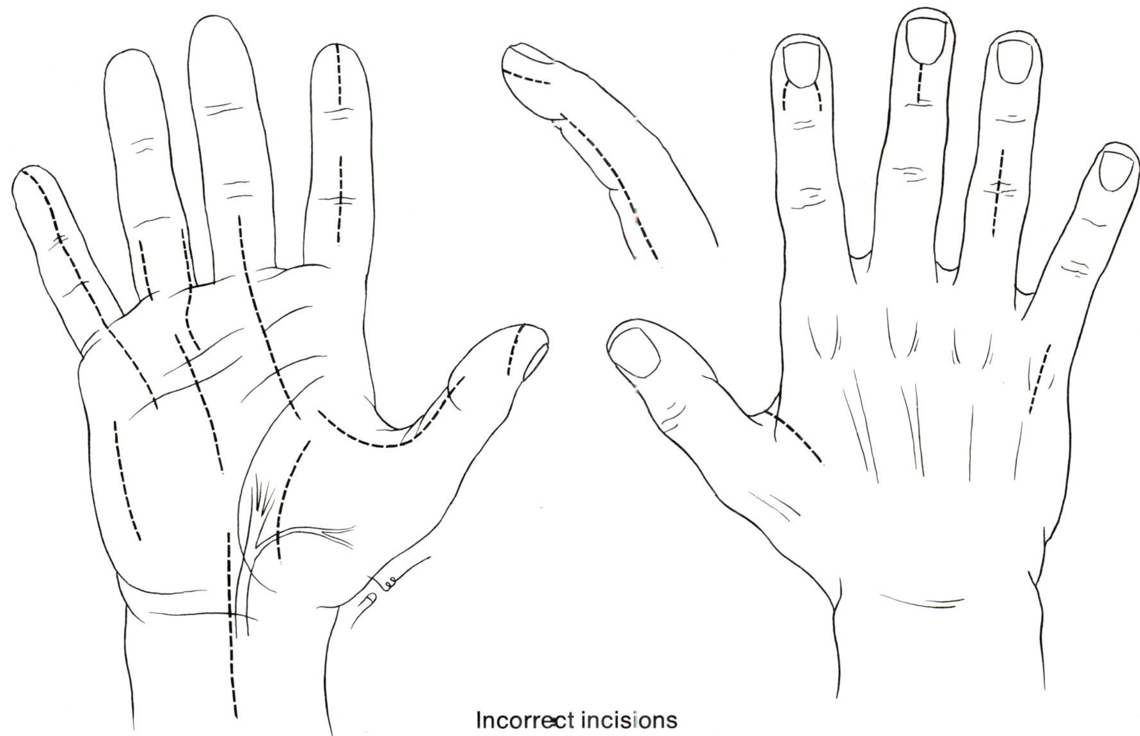

Incorrect incisions

Fig. 16-5.

Figs. 16-6 to 16-8 illustrate a more involved pen-and-ink technique depicting procedures for skin flaps to larger areas of the body. Here again only the important areas of this procedure are shaded so that the viewer's eye focuses on the important part of the drawing and is not distracted by the figures themselves.

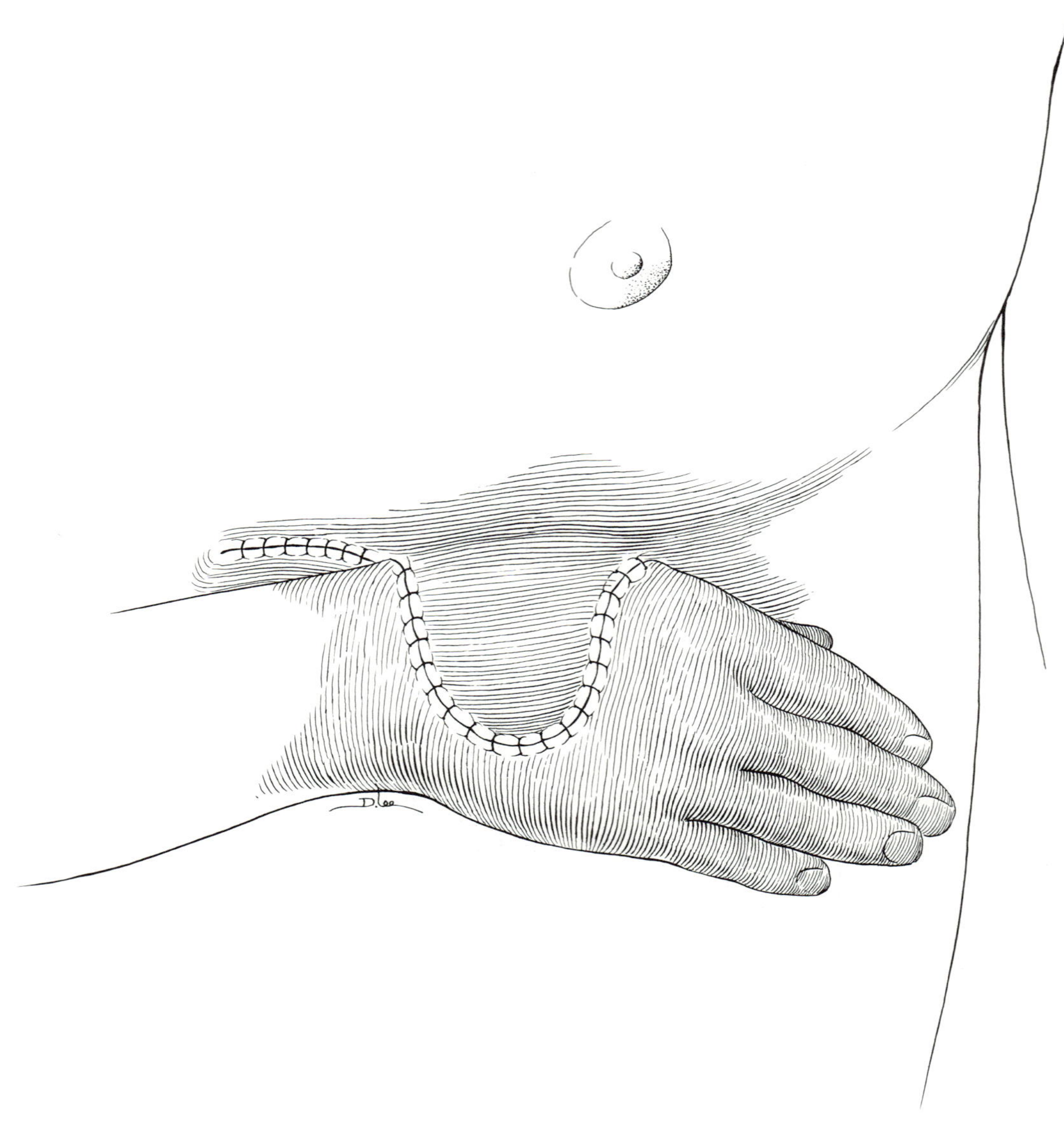

Fig. 16-6. From Grabb, W.C., and Myers, M.B.: Skin flaps, Boston, 1975, Little, Brown & Co. Reproduced with permission.

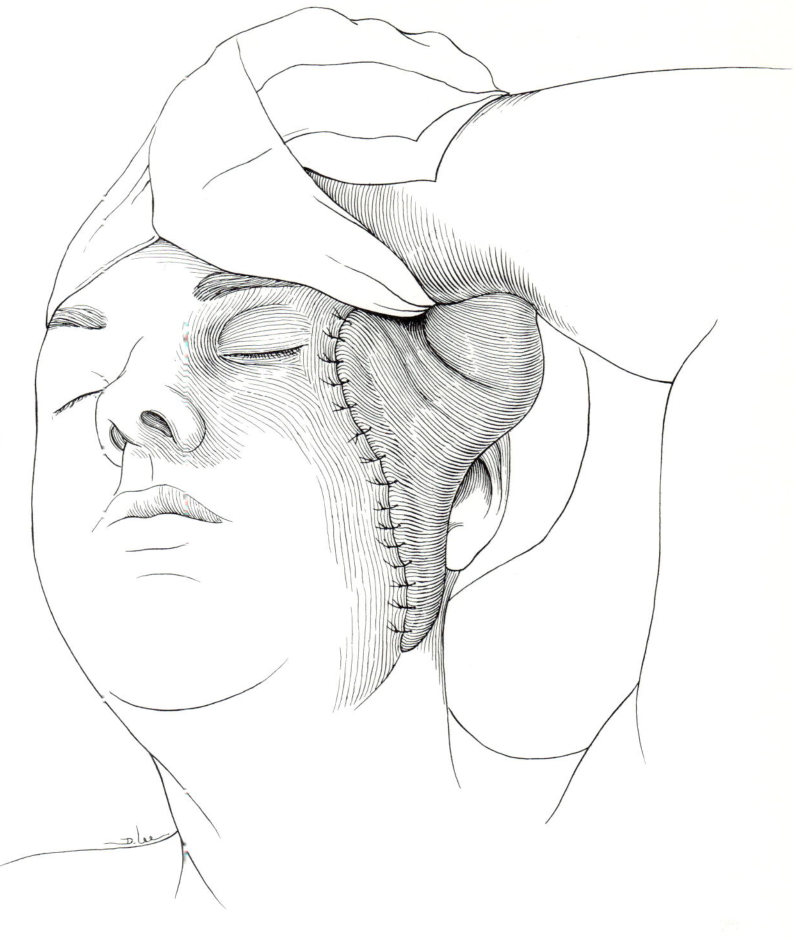

Fig. 16-7. From Grabb, W.C., and Myers, M.B.: Skin flaps, Boston, 1975, Little, Brown & Co. Reproduced with permission.

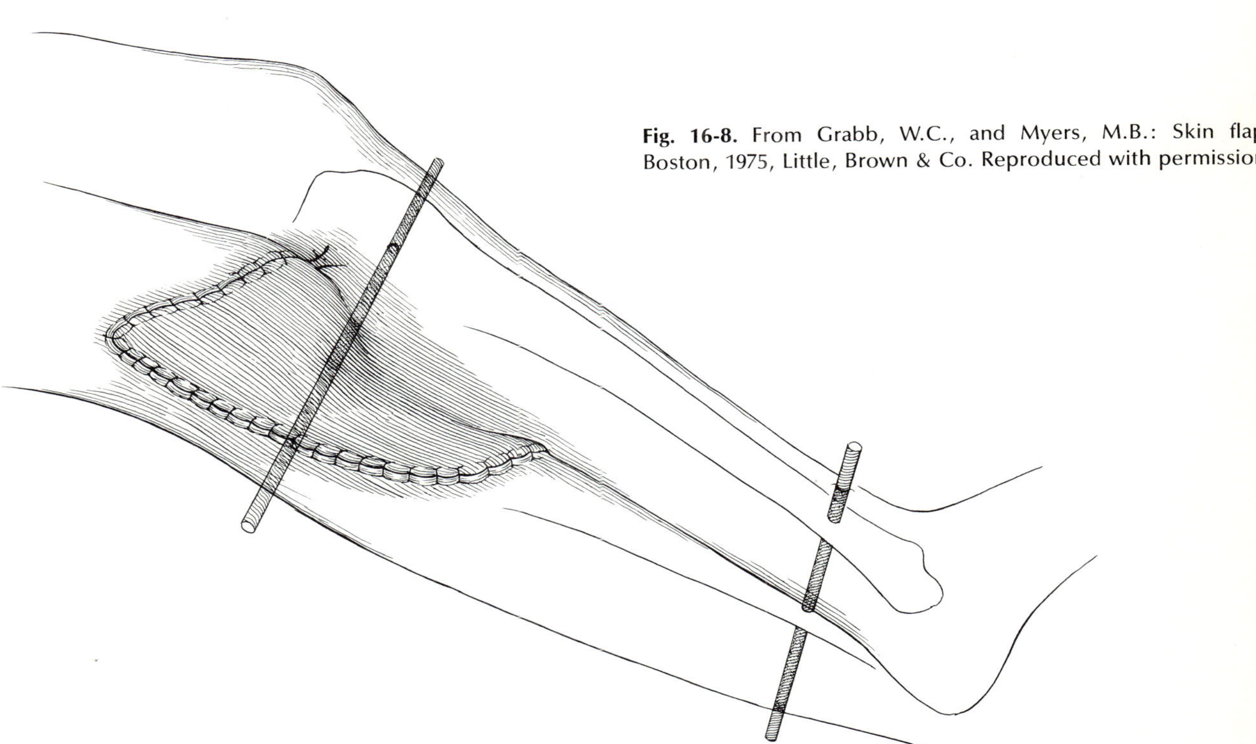

Fig. 16-8. From Grabb, W.C., and Myers, M.B.: Skin flaps, Boston, 1975, Little, Brown & Co. Reproduced with permission.

Illustrating plastic surgery procedures involving the head may become confusing if the illustration is not objective. Figs. 16-9 to 16-11 illustrate clearly and simply a facelift procedure. In Fig. 16-9, tone is used to illustrate the area of the scalp to be excised. The hair line is only lightly suggested for orientation. Drawing more hair on the head would only be distracting and serve no pur-

pose. Simple arrows are used to illustrate the extent of undermining involved in this procedure. Fig. 16-10 illustrates an important step in the dissection of the scalp. Only the important structures are emphasized. Fig. 16-11 illustrates the closure of the incision and the type of suturing involved.

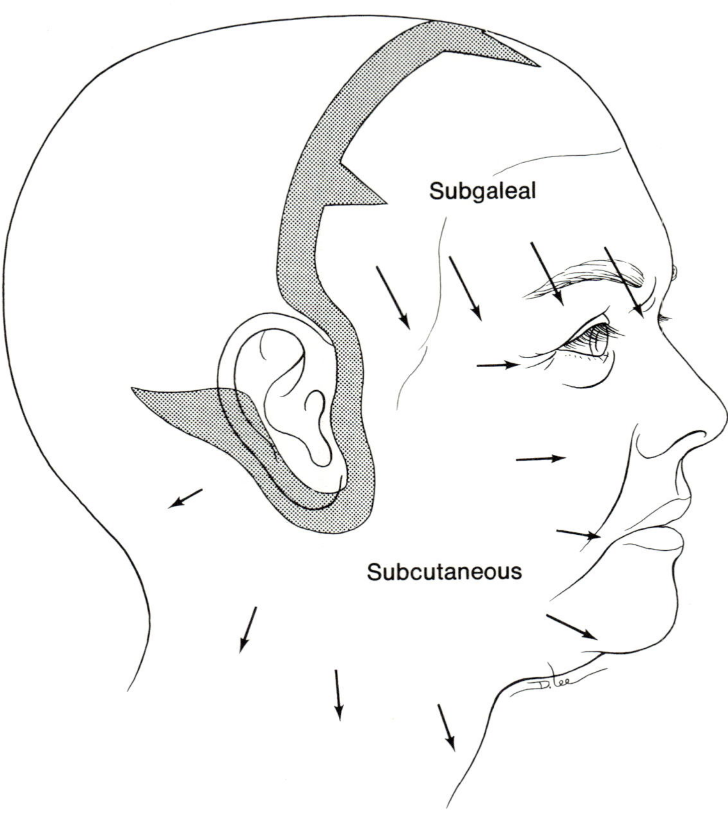

Fig. 16-9.

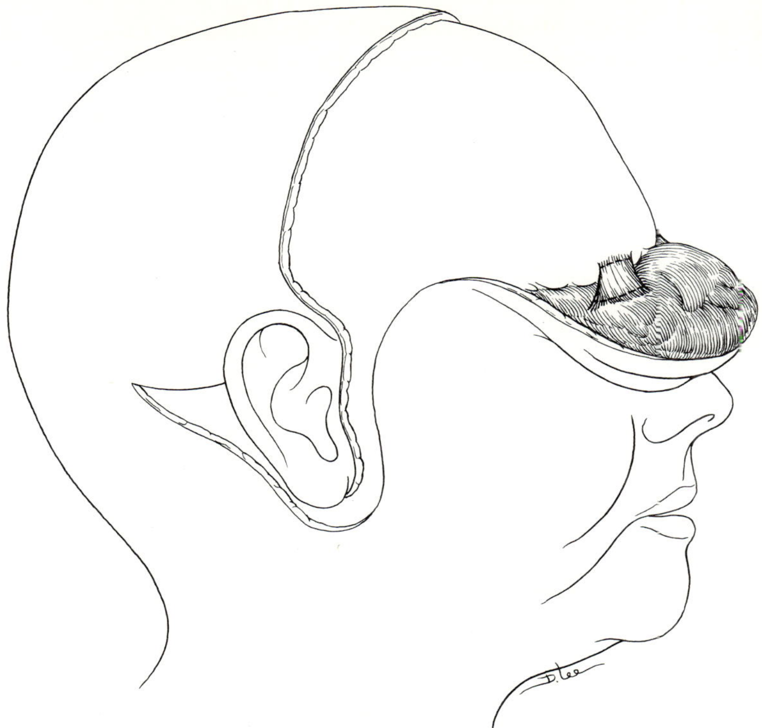

Fig. 16-10.

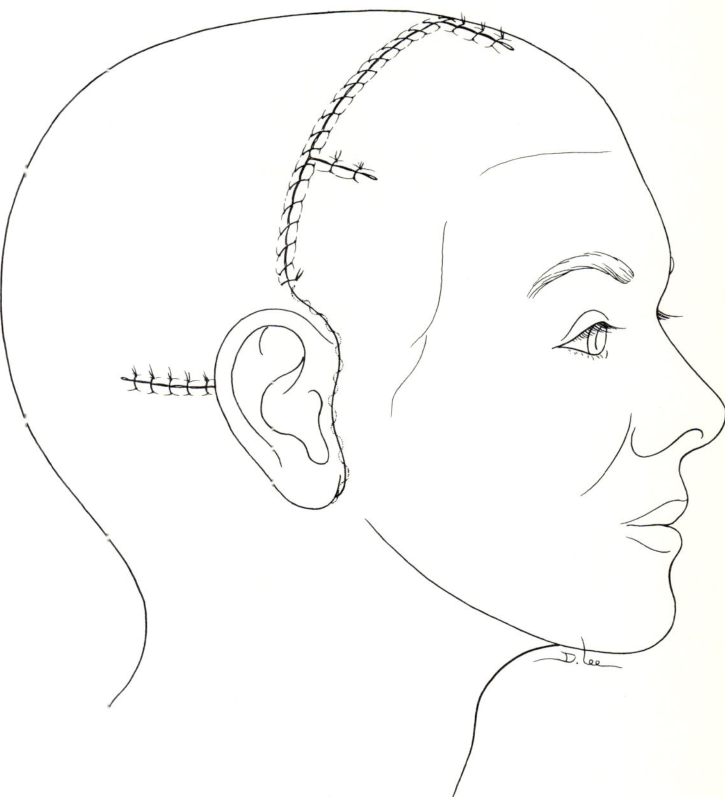

Fig. 16-11.

Fig. 16-12 is a more detailed drawing with emphasis on the areas of the face involved in surgery. The portion of the nose used for the skin flap is important. The second step illustrates the closure and how the scar is hidden in the natural lines of the face. The total procedure is placed on one plate.

Fig. 16-12, *C*, is a simple illustration for surgery of the lacrimal duct. The entire operation is shown in one step by ghosting in the duct and tubing.

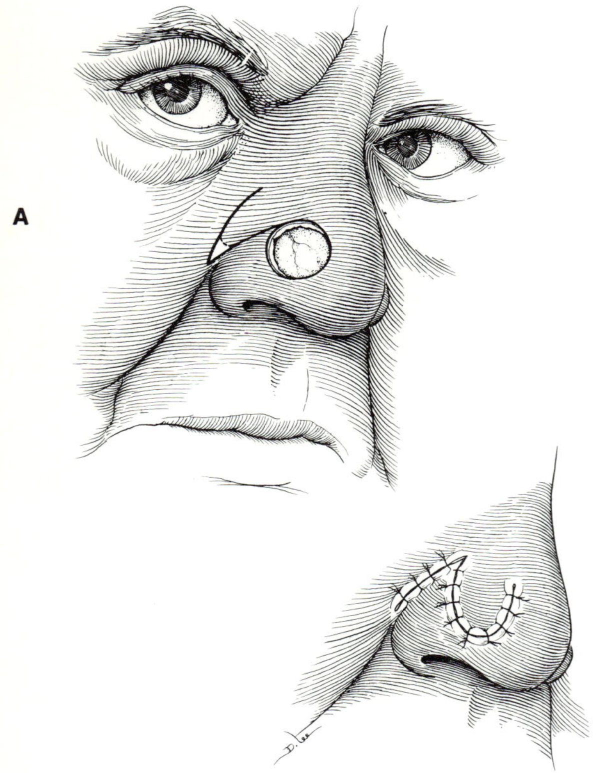

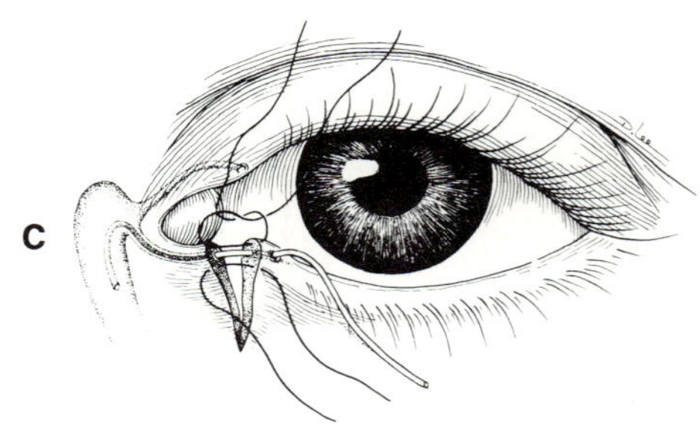

Fig. 16-12.

Surgery of the cleft lip may often be confusing. Fig. 16-13 illustrates one way of clearly depicting the procedure with the use of more shading and black areas for depth. In this technique the important areas are left white so that the sutures may be easily seen.

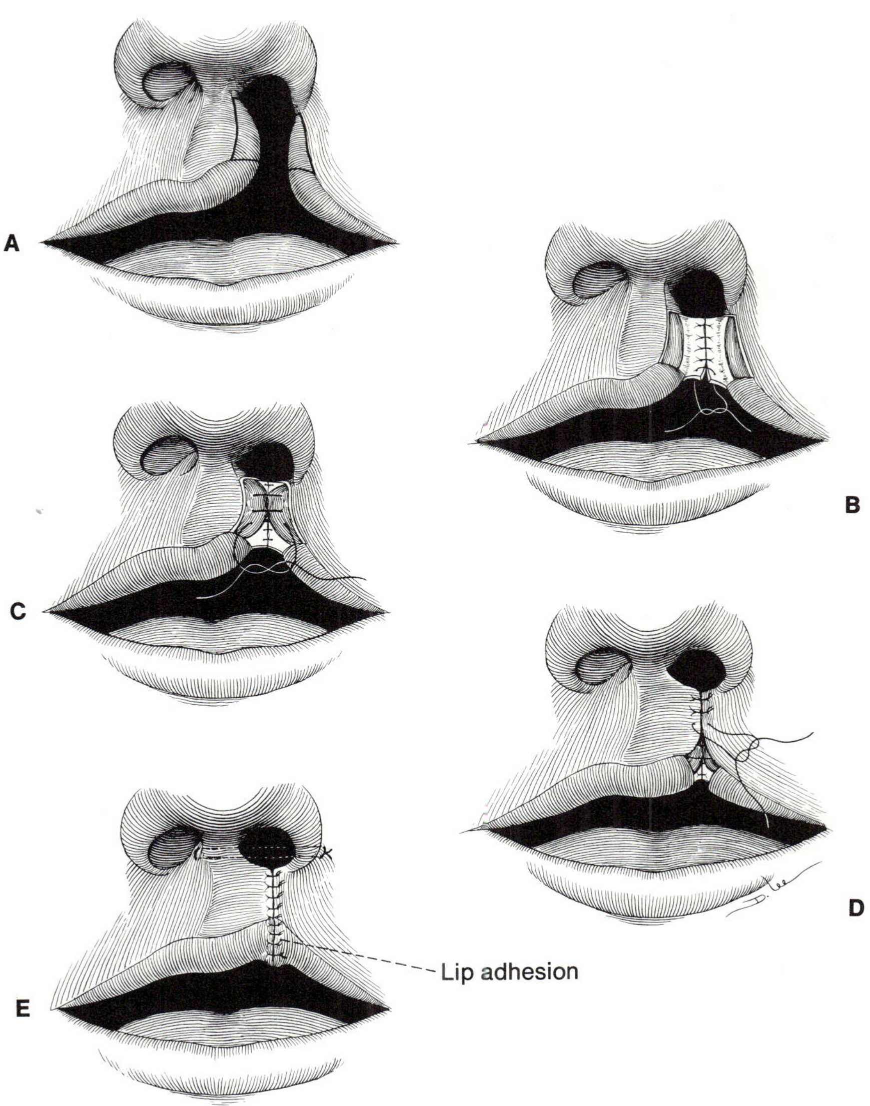

Fig. 16-13.

When the complex area of the mouth and throat are illustrated, simplicity is again most effective. In Fig. 16-14 a cross-section is added for better orientation to the procedure.

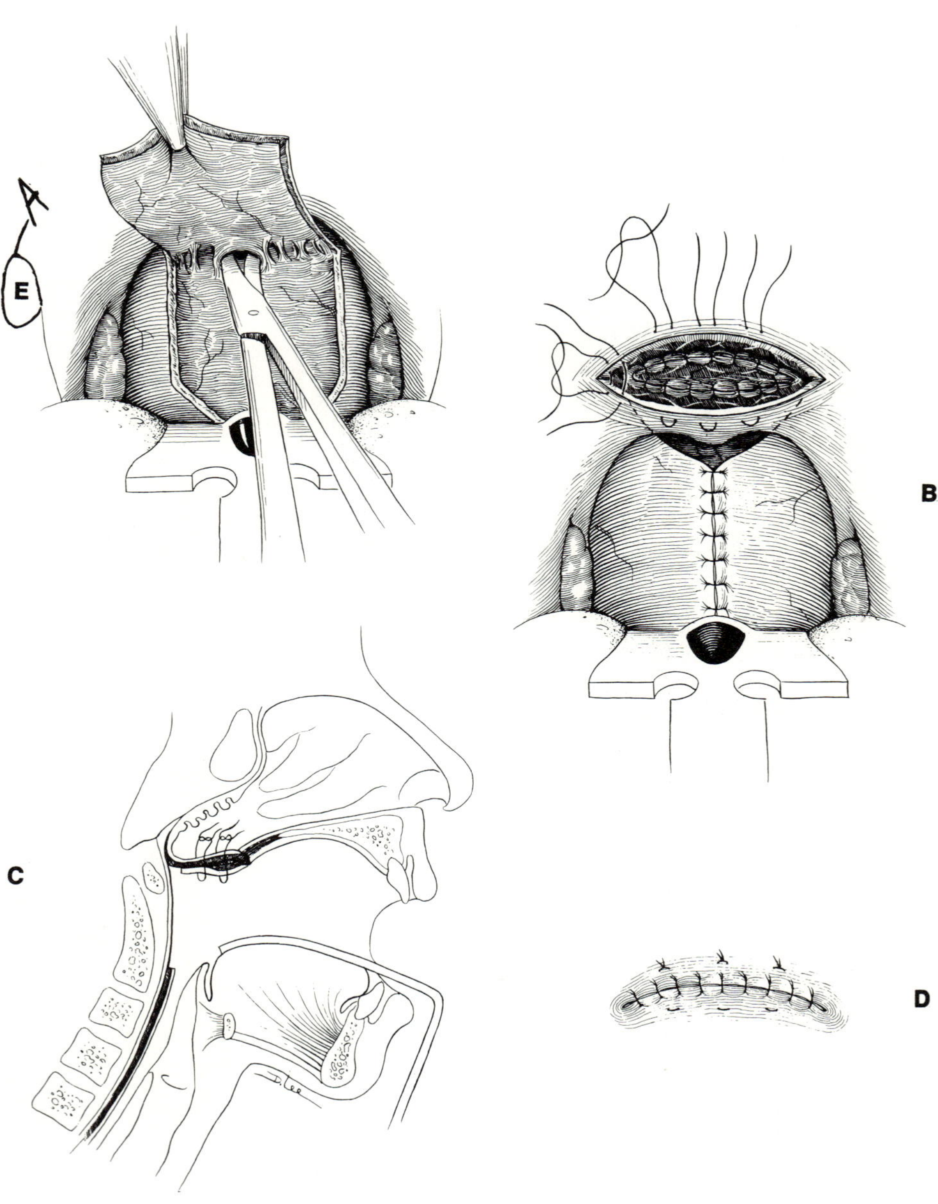

Fig. 16-14.

Fractures of the jaw are more clearly illustrated in cross-section (Fig. 16-15) or by simple drawings of the skull (Fig. 16-16).

Anatomy of specific areas of the skull can be illustrated effectively with the use of line and shading (Fig. 16-17).

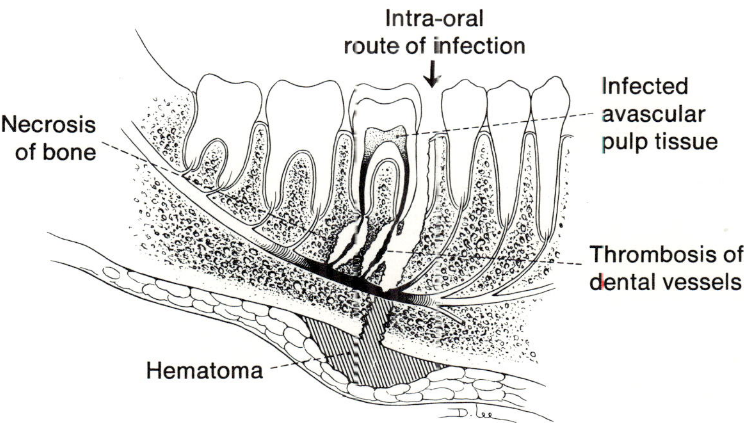

Fig. 16-15. From Goldwyn, R.M., editor: The unfavorable result in plastic surgery, Boston, 1972, Little, Brown & Co. Reproduced with permission.

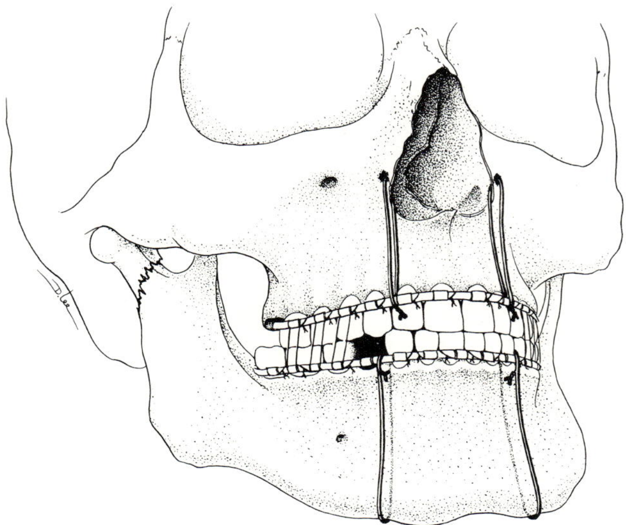

Fig. 16-16.

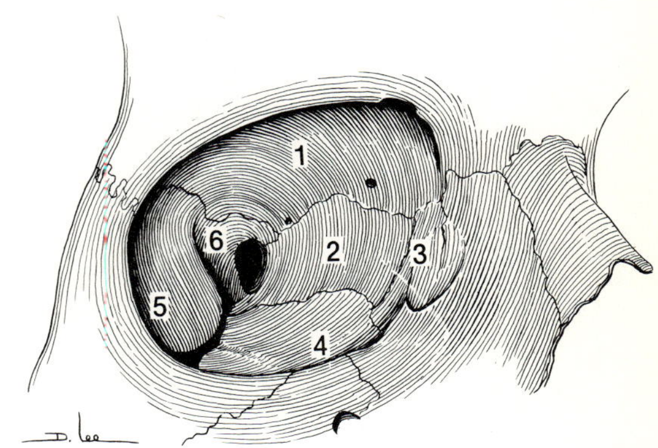

Fig. 16-17.

When complex surgical procedures involving the skull are illustrated, again simplicity is the secret. A small drawing of the patient's head with incision lines quickly orients the reader. Line drawings of the skull in various positions are used to show locations for bone incisions. Depicting tissue over bone would only add confusion to this type of procedure (Figs. 16-18 to 16-20).

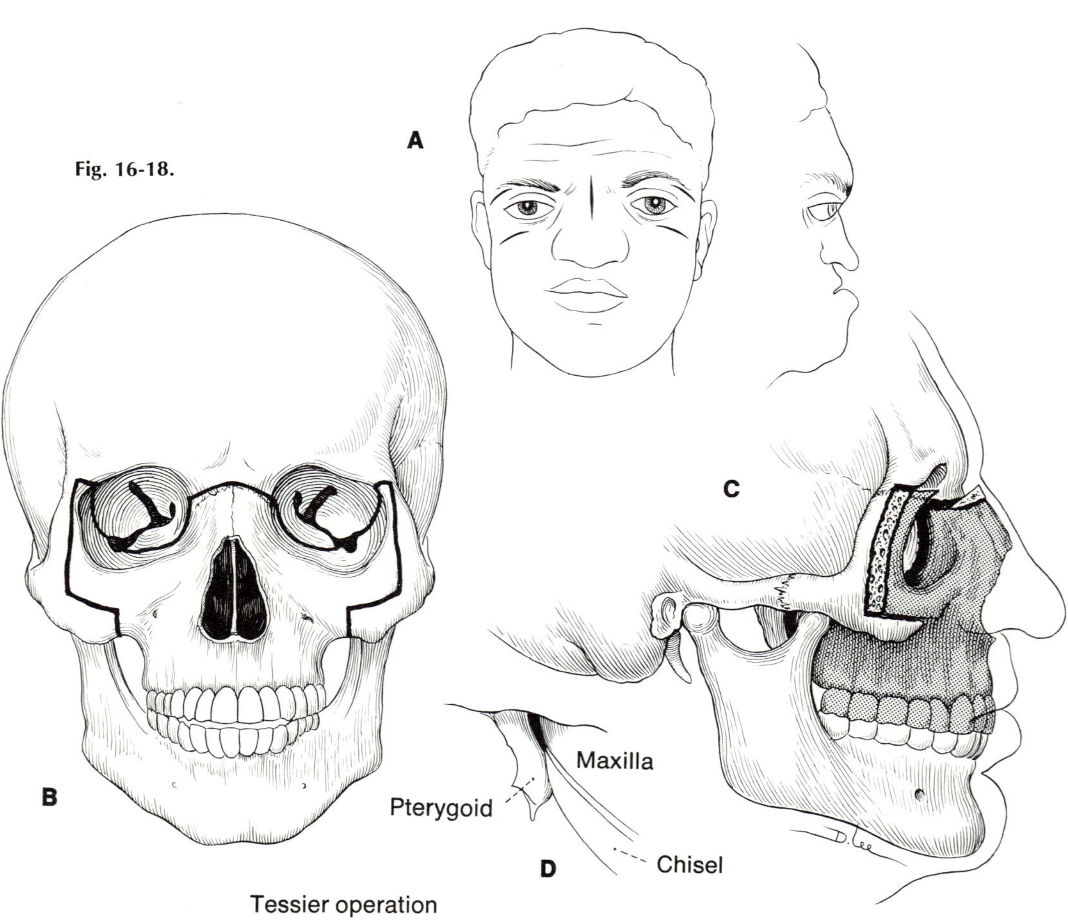

Fig. 16-18.

Tessier operation

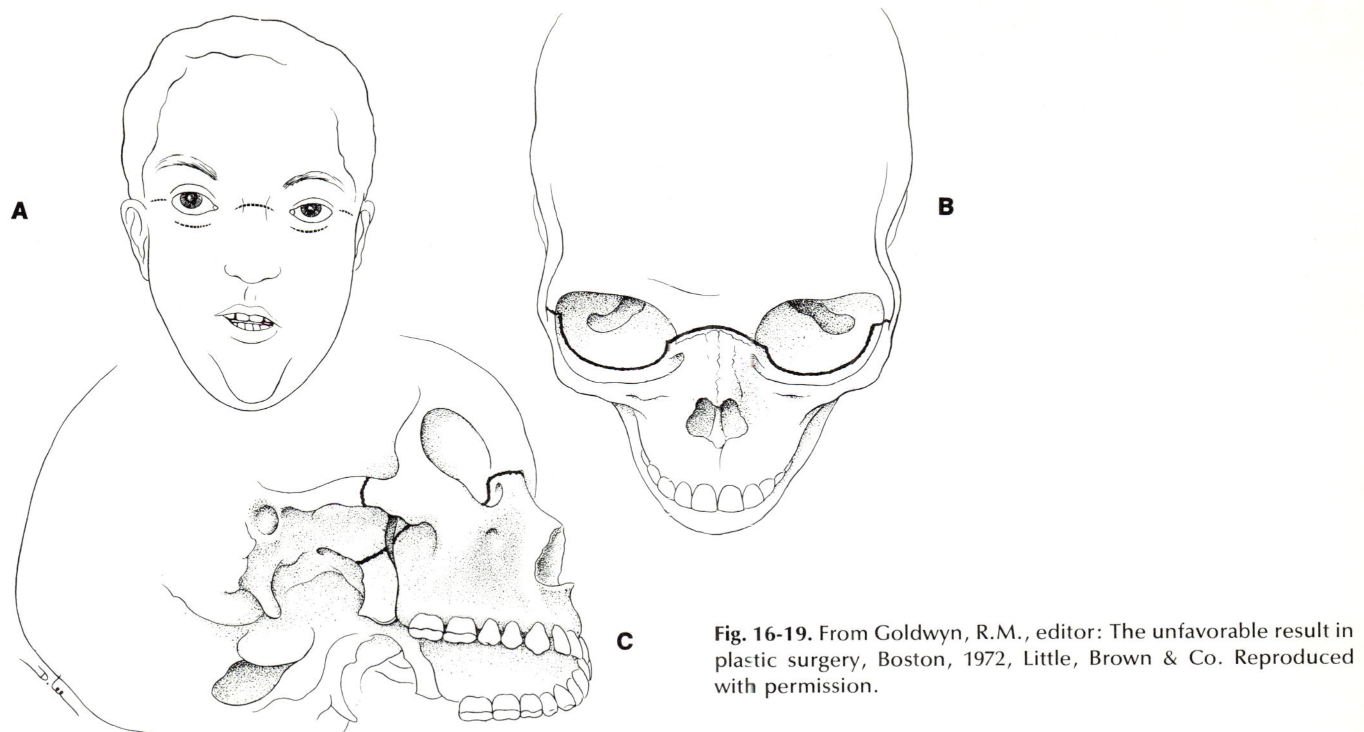

Fig. 16-19. From Goldwyn, R.M., editor: The unfavorable result in plastic surgery, Boston, 1972, Little, Brown & Co. Reproduced with permission.

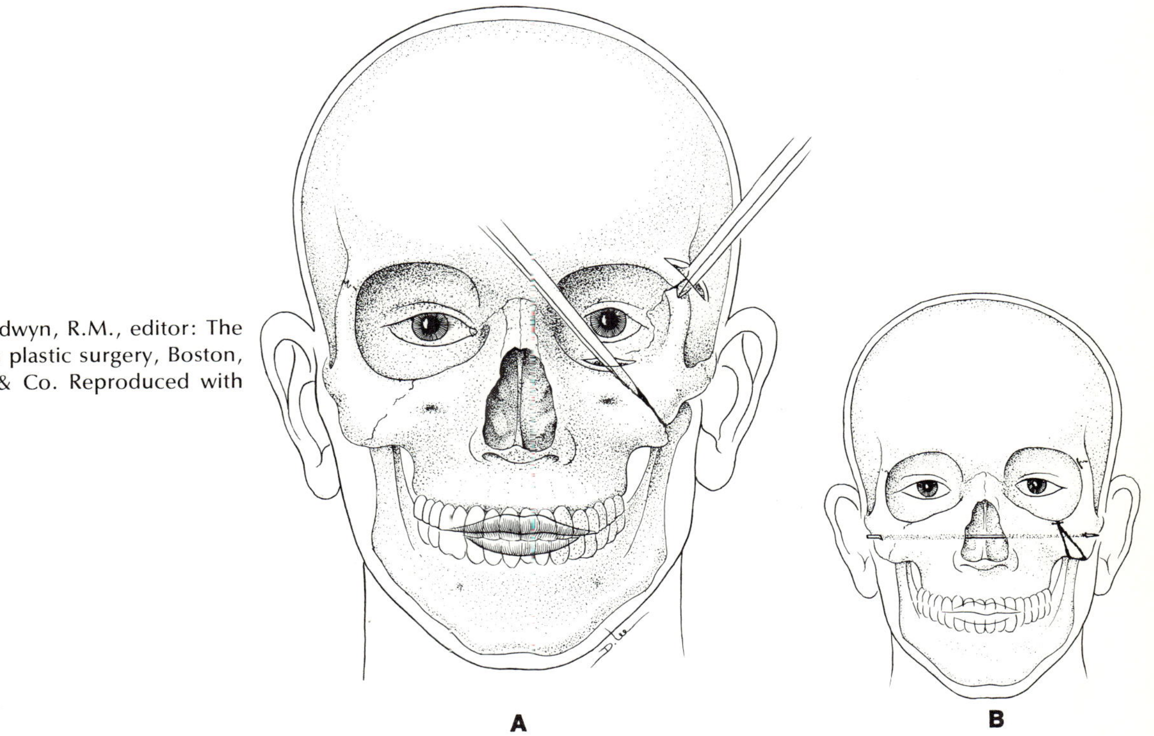

Fig. 16-20. From Goldwyn, R.M., editor: The unfavorable result in plastic surgery, Boston, 1972, Little, Brown & Co. Reproduced with permission.

Fig. 16-21, *A*, is a complex illustration of the head demonstrating the use and design of a particular type of mouth gag. Shading is used to illustrate depth of the mouth and throat.

Fig. 16-21, *B*, illustrates the use of carbon dust on halftone to demonstrate anesthesia of the face and ghosting of important nerves and vessels. This technique usually involves more time for completion and does not reproduce as well as pen and ink; however, when handled well and used for certain surgical procedures it provides a more esthetic quality to the illustration.

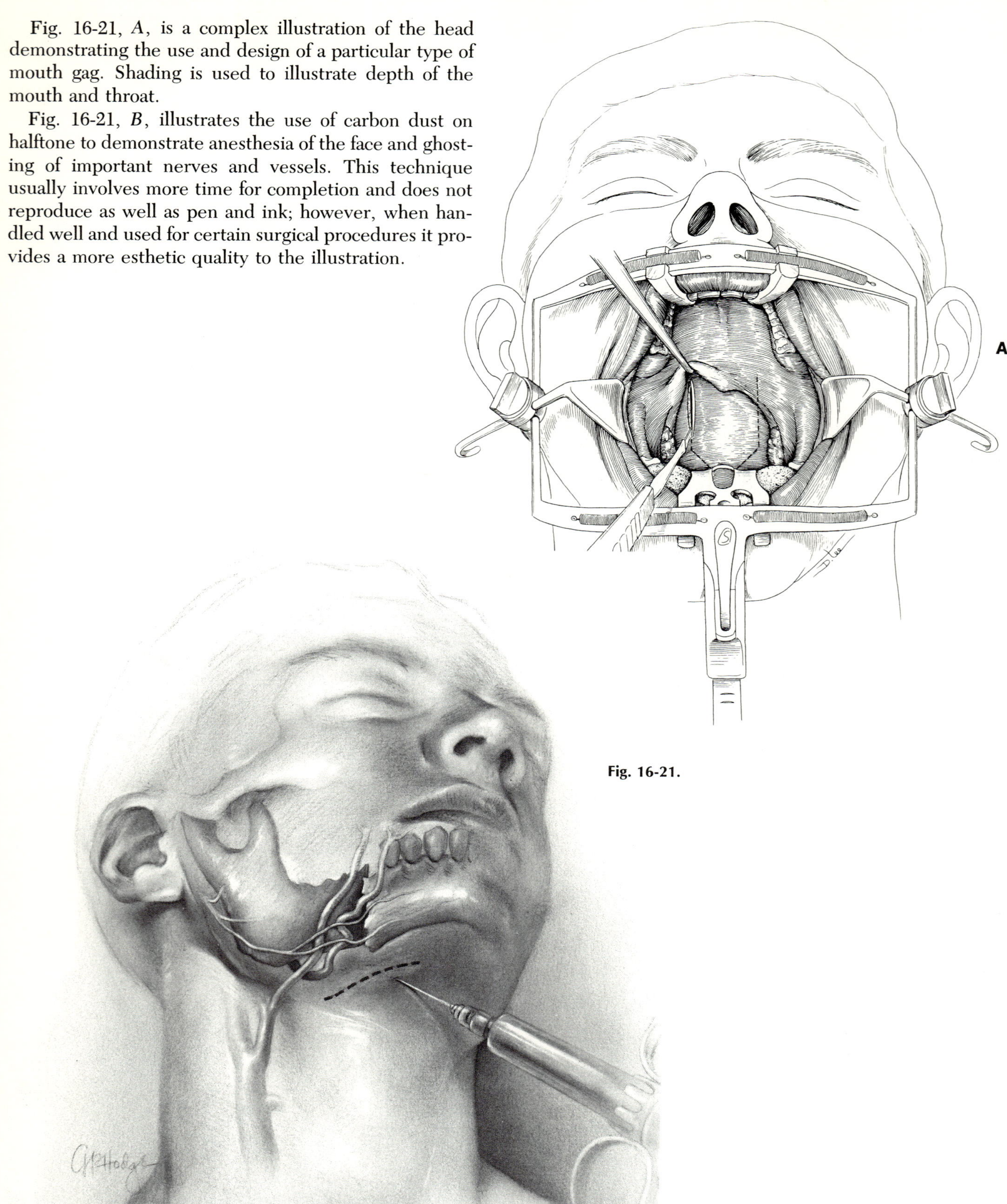

Fig. 16-21.

Illustrating plastic surgery of the breast often requires a variety of techniques. Incision, drains, and other illustrations of this type are most effective on simple line drawings (Figs. 16-22 to 16-24). More extensive pro-

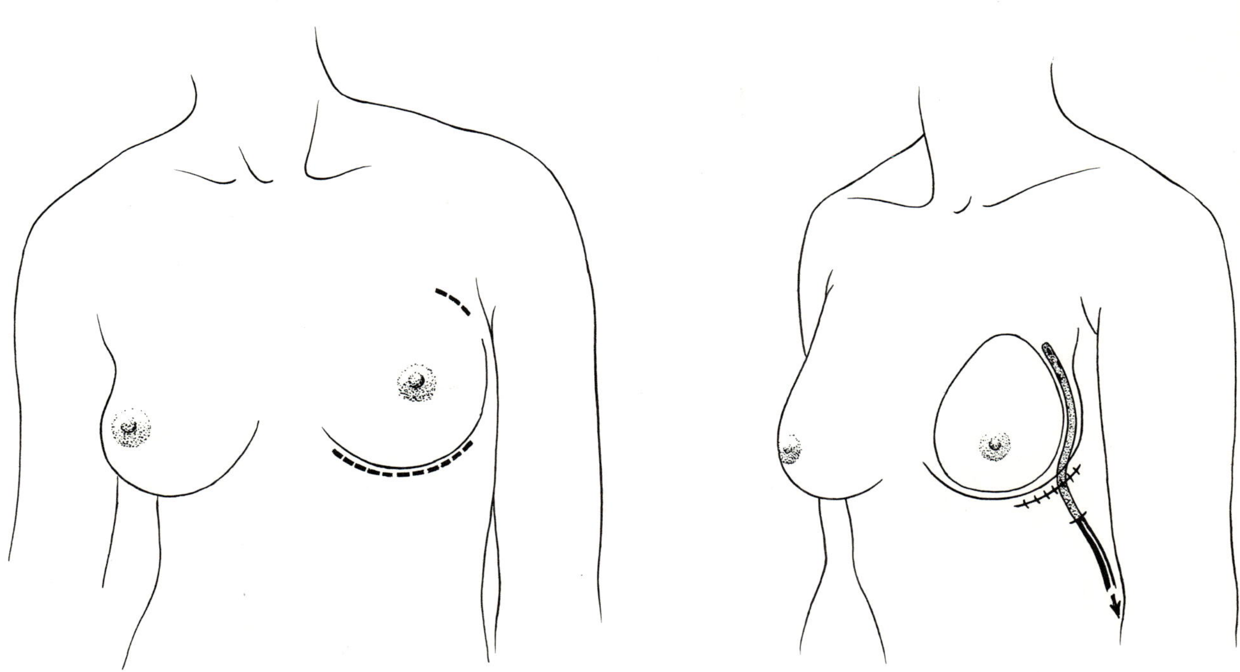

Fig. 16-22.

Fig. 16-23.

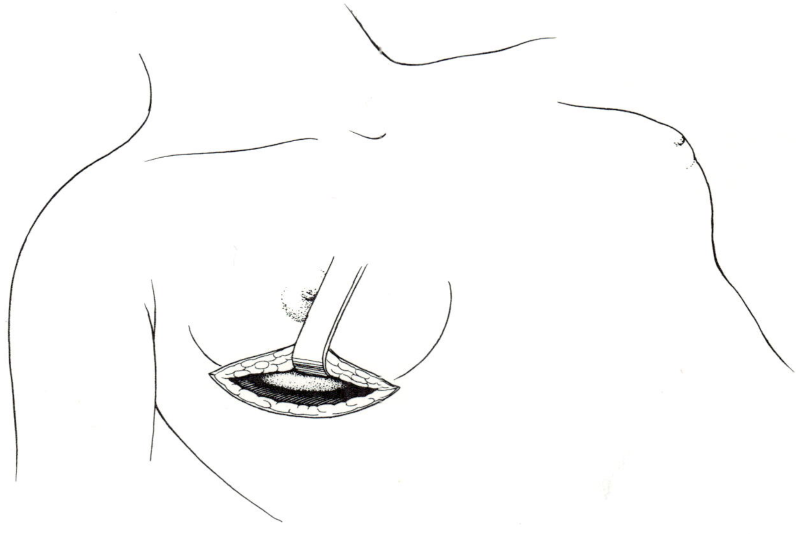

Fig. 16-24.

cedures are often best illustrated by shaded areas (Fig. 16-25) and by ghosting in instruments (Fig. 16-26). Fig. 16-27 illustrates the use of a new instrument, which is ghosted under the skin. A more shaded drawing illustrates the incision and position of the hand. A cross-section, Fig. 16-28 illustrates the depth and tissue separated by the instrument.

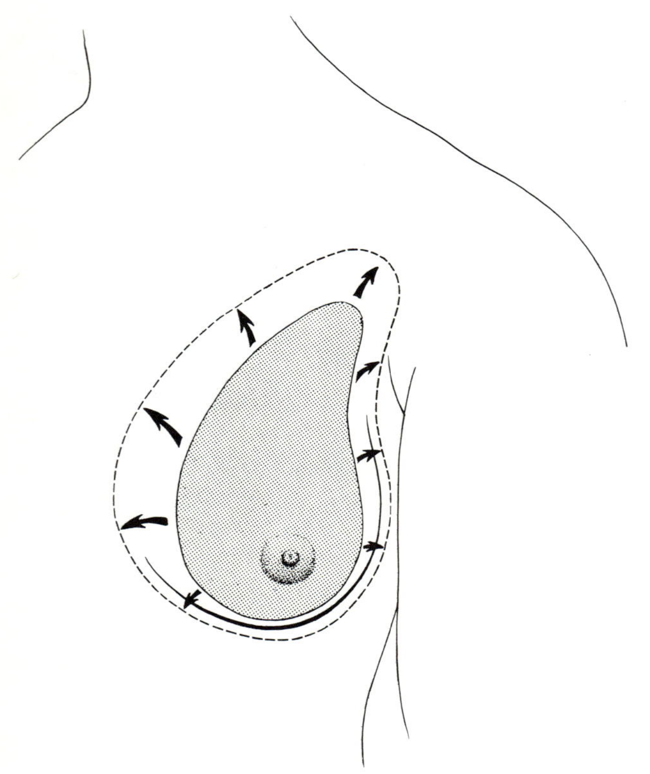

Fig. 16-25.

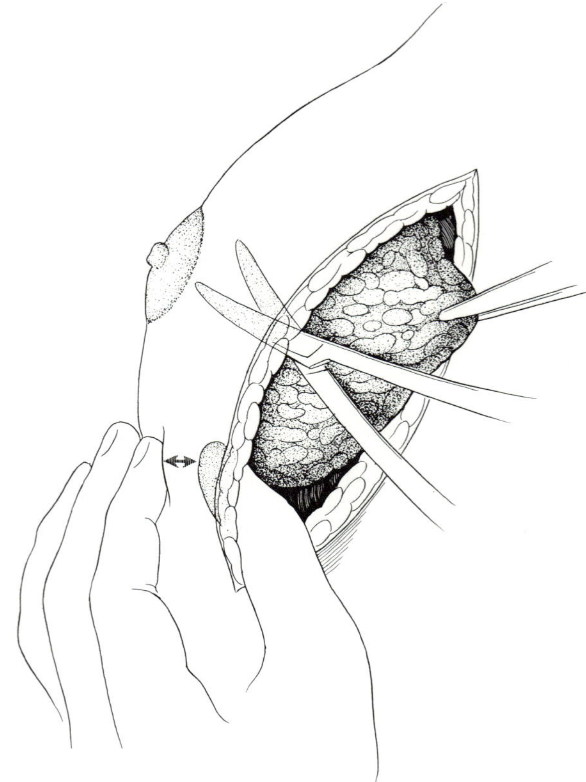

Fig. 16-26.

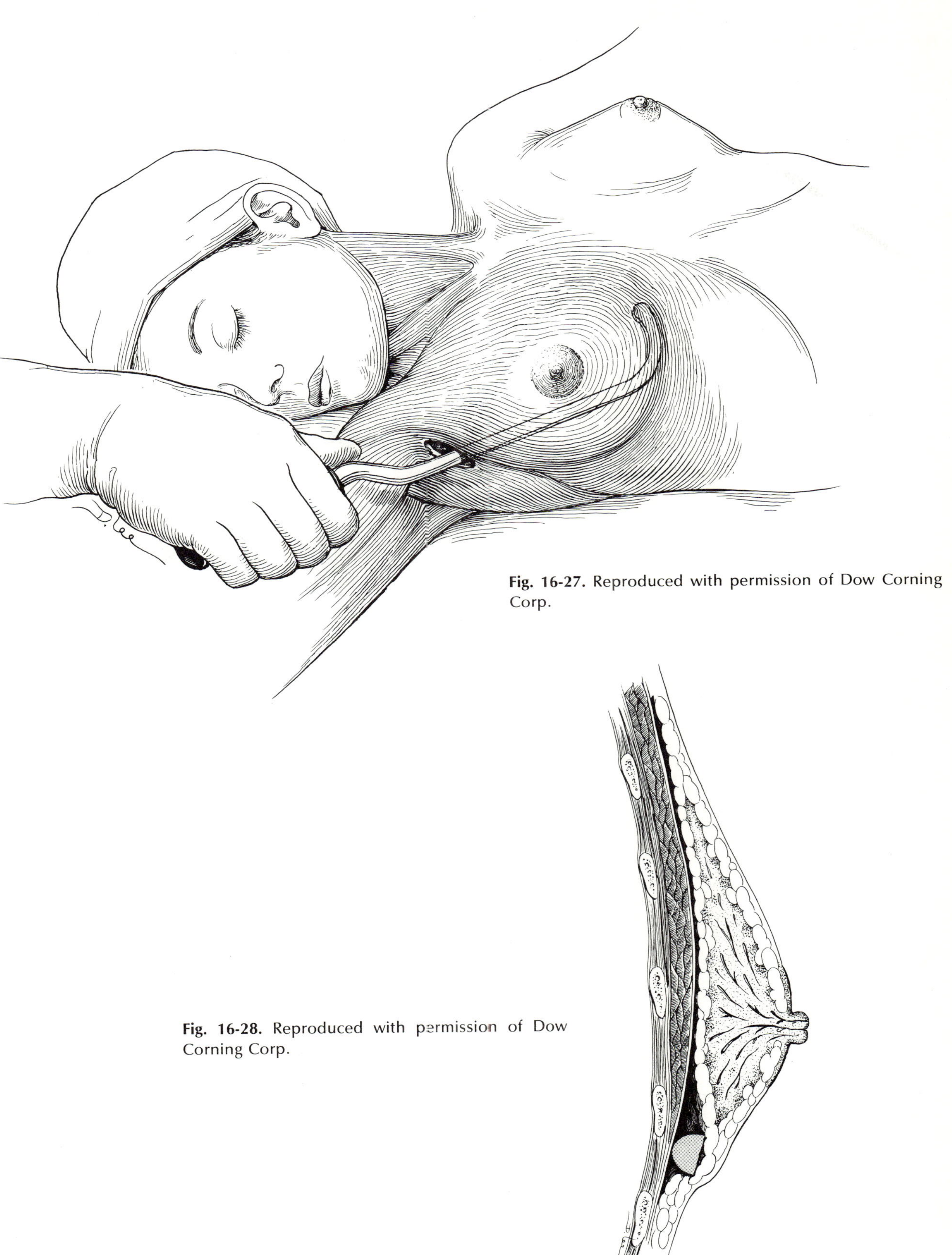

Fig. 16-27. Reproduced with permission of Dow Corning Corp.

Fig. 16-28. Reproduced with permission of Dow Corning Corp.

In Fig. 16-29 the area of the chest undermined for insertion of a breast implant is illustrated with the use of shading. Skin and muscle incisions are indicated with dotted lines. The blood supply to this area is also shown. This illustration shows everything the surgeon considers important—yet is accomplished by a simple drawing.

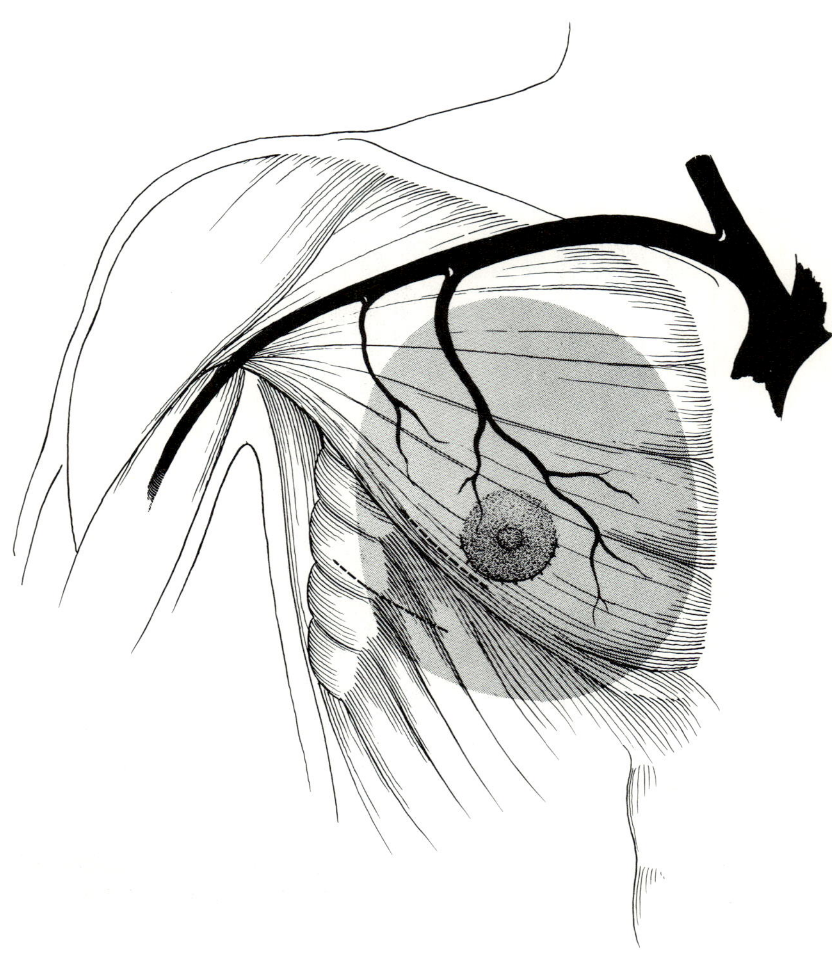

Fig. 16-29.

Complex surgical procedures may involve several important steps. Figs. 16-30 and 16-31 illustrate an involved technique for breast reduction. These plates include simple diagrams, cross-sections, ghosting, and detailed anatomy.

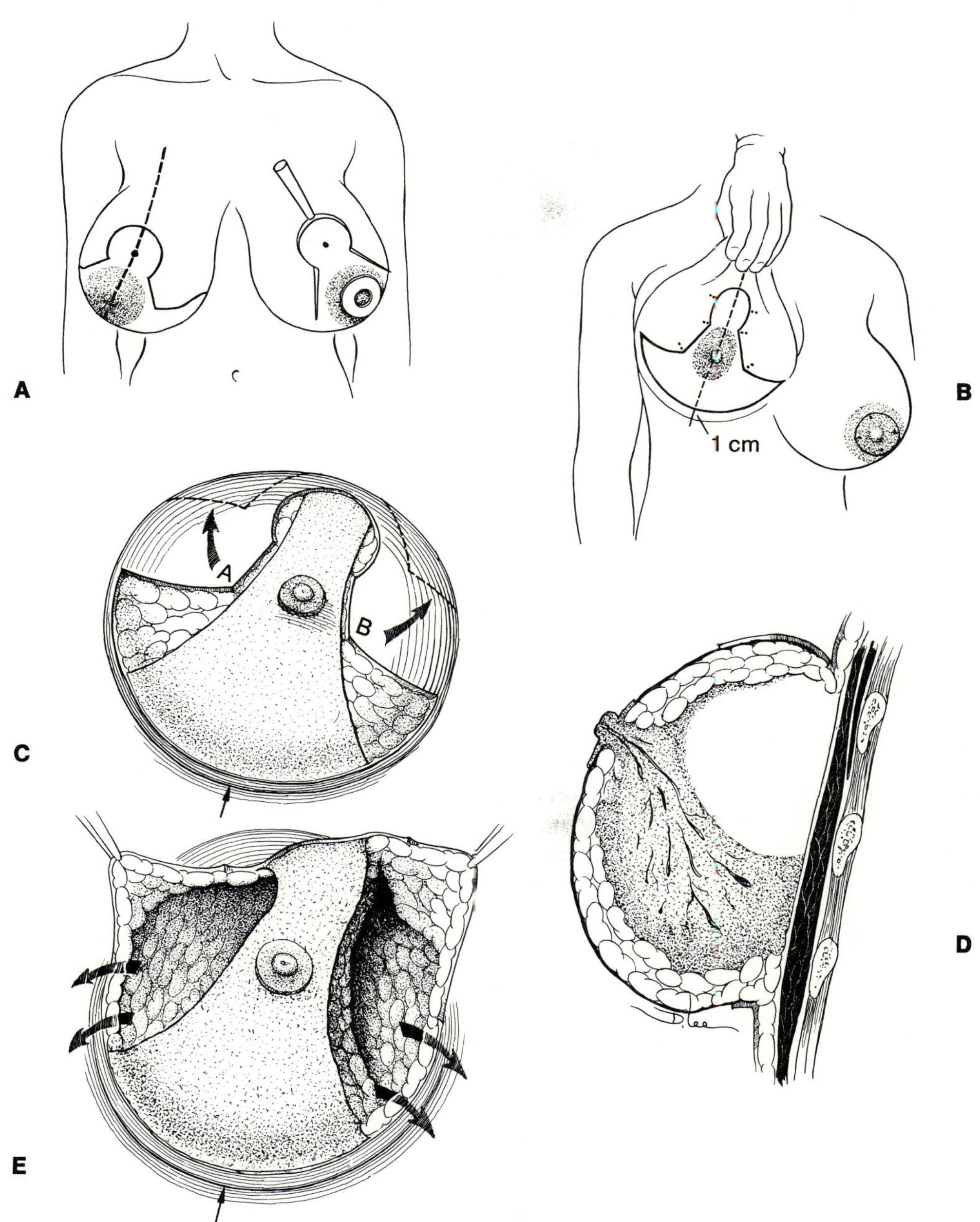

Fig. 16-30.

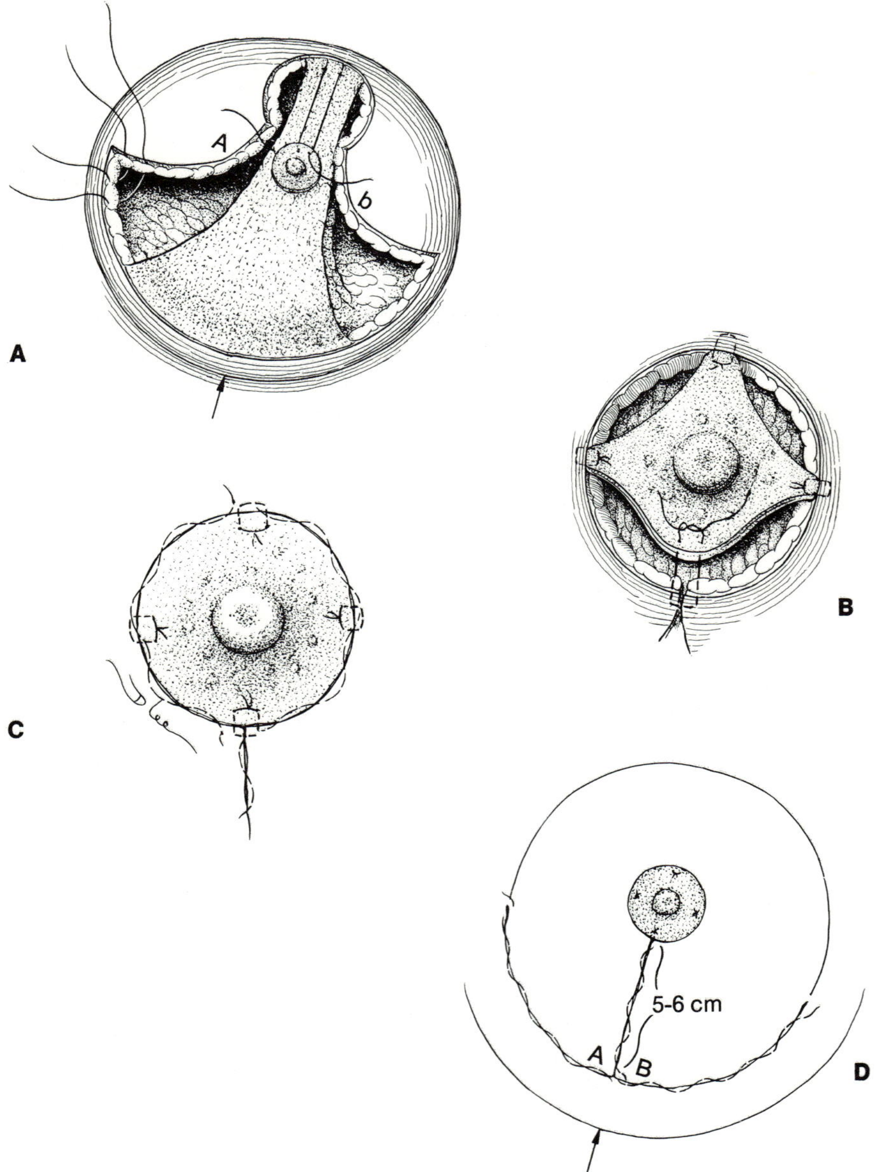

Fig. 16-31.

CHAPTER 17

Copying and special photographic techniques

Sheldon Phillips

How can I improve my lecture slides? How can I make my visuals look more professional? These are questions frequently asked of me when I attend trade shows, medical meetings, and other professional conventions. In this chapter I will offer suggestions for strengthening your teaching skills and making better use of slides. Most of these techniques are inexpensive, require a minimum of time and talent, and use materials that are readily available.

Professional meetings, conferences, and lectures are typical situations in which visuals can be used to inform the audience. Slides are versatile and can be used not only in large lecture halls but also in small group meetings or individual learning situations. Packaged slide programs are an effective means of informing patients about their diagnosis and treatment. Slides can also be used to communicate with people outside the hospital, such as business and community leaders. In all these areas, the use of visuals adds four strengths to your communications.

1. Slides hold the attention of your audience.
2. Visuals help to clarify information. Difficult subjects can become interesting and more easily understood.
3. Visuals provide a common starting point for you and all members of your audience. The same word often means different things to different people. The visual leaves no doubt about what you have in mind.
4. Visuals can overcome time and space limitations and provide experiences otherwise impossible or impractical to communicate.

LEGIBILITY

If your slides are to be effective you must be certain that the audience can read the information projected on the screen (see also Chapter 13 and Appendix C-11). You must, therefore, evaluate the legibility of your slides and prepare your artwork for maximal legibility. A practical rule for legibility is: If you can read the print on your slides with the unaided eye, it will project well and be read by the audience (Fig. 17-1). Often a slide will contain so much information that it is impossible for the audience to determine what is important (Fig. 17-2). It is better to extract the pertinent data, type or letter it, and copy this as a slide (Fig. 17-3).

When making slides containing text, give some thought to the style of type you use. Block letters are more legible than those in script or other decorative styles (Fig. 17-4 and Appendix C-1).

If you must use an existing drawing for illustration that is "busy" or has distracting elements in it, try using color to outline or emphasize the important parts.

To summarize legibility requirements:

1. Keep your material big and simple.
2. Use legible typefaces and open spacing; stay away from decorative faces.
3. Highlight your data in some way to emphasize the important points.

EQUIPMENT

If you want to make good slides or visuals, you must have proper equipment to photograph your artwork.

The 35 mm single lens reflex camera allows you to view the area that will be photographed directly through

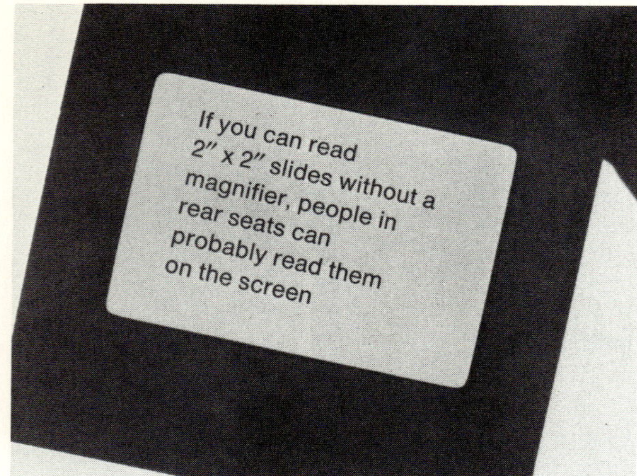

Fig. 17-1.

Table 3—Age-at-Appearance Percentiles for Major Postnatal Ossification Centers (in Years)

Ossification Center	Boys 5th	Boys 50th	Boys 95th	Girls 5th	Girls 50th	Girls 95th
1. Head of humerus	—	.03	.32	—	.03	.30
2. Proximal epiphysis of tibia	—	.04	.10	—	.01	.04
3. Coracoid process of scapula	—	.04	.36	—	.03	.42
4. Cuboid of tarsus	—	.07	.30	—	.05	.16
5. Capitate of carpus	—	.25	.60	—	.15	.56
6. Hamate of carpus	.03	.31	.82	—	.18	.59
7. Capitulum of humerus	.06	.33	1.07	.05	.26	.77
8. Head of femur	.06	.35	.64	.04	.33	.62
9. Third cuneiform of tarsus	.05	.46	1.58	—	.23	1.23
10. Greater tubercle of humerus	.25	.83	2.33	.20	.51	1.14
11. Primary center, middle segment of 5th toe	—	1.04	3.81	—	.74	2.08
12. Distal epiphysis of radius	.53	1.10	2.30	.38	.82	1.70
13. Epiphysis, distal segment of 1st toe	.71	1.21	2.10	.39	.78	1.68
14. Epiphysis, middle segment of 4th toe	.40	1.21	2.88	.40	.92	3.00
15. Epiphysis, proximal segment of 3d finger	.77	1.37	2.15	.41	.85	1.61
16. Epiphysis, middle segment of 3d toe	.41	1.40	4.27	.21	1.02	2.47
17. Epiphysis, proximal segment of 2d finger	.78	1.41	2.17	.40	.87	1.64
18. Epiphysis, proximal segment of 4th finger	.80	1.49	2.40	.41	.90	1.66
19. Epiphysis, distal segment of 1st finger	.75	1.51	2.70	.42	.99	1.73
20. Epiphysis, proximal segment of 3d toe	.90	1.58	2.52	.51	1.05	1.88
21. Epiphysis of 2d metacarpal	.93	1.61	2.82	.64	1.09	1.69
22. Epiphysis, proximal segment of 4th toe	.95	1.64	2.65	.61	1.24	2.06
23. Epiphysis, proximal segment of 2d toe	.97	1.74	2.65	.63	1.19	2.05
24. Epiphysis of 3d metacarpal	.95	1.79	3.01	.65	1.13	1.94
25. Epiphysis, proximal segment of 5th finger	1.00	1.85	2.82	.65	1.19	2.07
26. Epiphysis, middle segment of 3d finger	1.01	1.97	3.31	.63	1.28	2.36
27. Epiphysis of 4th metacarpal	1.09	2.03	3.60	.75	1.29	2.17
28. Epiphysis, middle segment of 2d toe	.89	2.04	4.05	.49	1.18	2.24
29. Epiphysis, middle segment of 4th finger	1.00	2.05	3.24	.63	1.24	2.43
30. Epiphysis of 5th metacarpal	1.27	2.17	3.82	.86	1.37	2.35
31. First cuneiform of tarsus	.89	2.17	3.77	.50	1.43	2.82
32. Epiphysis of 1st metatarsal	1.39	2.18	3.12	.96	1.58	2.23
33. Epiphysis, middle segment of 2d finger	1.30	2.19	3.31	.67	1.36	2.54
34. Epiphysis, proximal segment of 1st toe	1.45	2.35	3.31	.89	1.55	2.47
35. Epiphysis, distal segment of 3d finger	1.31	2.41	3.72	.72	1.46	2.69
36. Triquetral of carpus	.49	2.43	5.47	.29	1.70	3.73
37. Epiphysis, distal segment of 4th finger	1.37	2.44	3.73	.73	1.52	2.82
38. Epiphysis, proximal segment of 5th toe	1.53	2.45	3.65	.97	1.73	2.67
39. Epiphysis of 1st metacarpal	1.45	2.59	4.32	.92	1.60	2.67
40. Second cuneiform of tarsus	1.19	2.65	4.21	.81	1.80	3.00
41. Epiphysis of 2d metatarsal	1.93	2.86	4.33	1.22	2.14	3.43
42. Greater trochanter of femur	1.92	2.96	4.35	.96	1.85	3.03
43. Epiphysis, proximal segment of 1st finger	1.84	3.00	4.57	.93	1.71	2.84
44. Navicular of tarsus	1.12	3.02	5.40	.77	1.94	3.58
45. Epiphysis, distal segment of 2d finger	1.80	3.17	4.97	1.06	2.50	3.29
46. Epiphysis, distal segment of 5th finger	2.06	3.29	4.98	1.01	1.96	3.45
47. Epiphysis, middle segment of 5th finger	1.94	3.40	5.84	.88	1.97	3.54
48. Proximal epiphysis of fibula	1.86	3.47	5.24	1.33	2.61	3.92
49. Epiphysis of 3d metatarsal	2.33	3.48	5.00	1.42	2.48	3.68
50. Epiphysis, distal segment of 5th toe	2.34	3.94	6.30	1.17	2.31	4.07
51. Patella of knee	2.55	4.00	5.96	1.47	2.48	4.01
52. Epiphysis of 4th metatarsal	2.92	4.02	5.74	1.77	2.84	4.05
53. Lunate of carpus	1.53	4.07	6.77	1.08	2.62	5.65
54. Epiphysis, distal segment of 3d toe	2.99	4.36	6.19	1.37	2.73	4.11

Fig. 17-2.

Ossification Center	Boys 5th	Boys 50th	Boys 95th
Primary center, middle segment of 5th toe	—	1.04	3.81
Epiphysis, middle segment of 4th toe	.40	1.21	2.88
Epiphysis, middle segment of 3rd toe	.41	1.40	4.27
Epiphysis, middle segment of 2d toe	.89	2.04	4.05
Epiphysis, proximal segment of 1st toe	1.45	2.35	3.31

Fig. 17-3.

Table 1—Indications for Sialography

Recurrent pain or swelling in parotid or submandibular region

Palpation of mass in salivary region

Dryness of mouth and eyes of obscure origin

Table 1 — Indications for Sialography

Recurrent pain or swelling in parotid or submandibular region

Palpation of mass in salivary region

Dryness of mouth and eyes of obscure origin

Fig. 17-4.

the picture-taking lens. This feature is particularly important when you are doing copy work at close distances. A simple camera with adjustable shutter speed and f stops and that accepts interchangeable lenses is quite acceptable. Close-up lenses may be added to the normal camera lens for close copy work. A macro lens may be a wise investment. While such a lens is expensive, it is capable of focusing over a wide range, including down to a few inches, without the use of attachments.

A copy stand provides a handy platform for photographing charts and artwork. Copy lights can be balanced and left in position so that you get the same results each time (Fig. 17-5). The lights should be placed at a 45-degree angle to the copy (Fig. 17-6). Overlapping the lights avoids creating a central hot spot that could result in glare or uneven illumination. An easy way to check for even lighting is to place a pencil on the copy surface, then adjust the lights so that the shadows on either side of the pencil are equal in density (Fig. 17-7).

Before you begin shooting, make sure the camera is level. You can determine this by either "eyeballing" it or using an inexpensive bubble level that can be purchased at a hardware store. Some copy work requires long exposure times. A flexible cable release will prevent your hand from shaking the camera during time exposures. Another handy piece of equipment is a baffle board constructed of black cardboard (Fig. 17-8). This is attached to the camera with either a retainer ring or lens hood and cuts down on reflections produced by shiny surfaces.

Polarization of copy lights will help to further elimi-

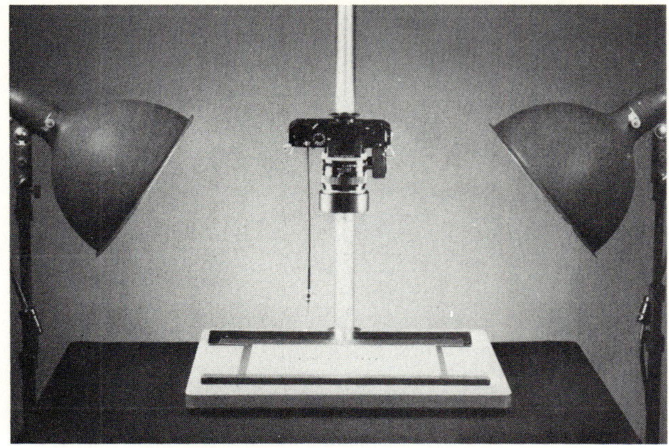

Fig. 17-5.

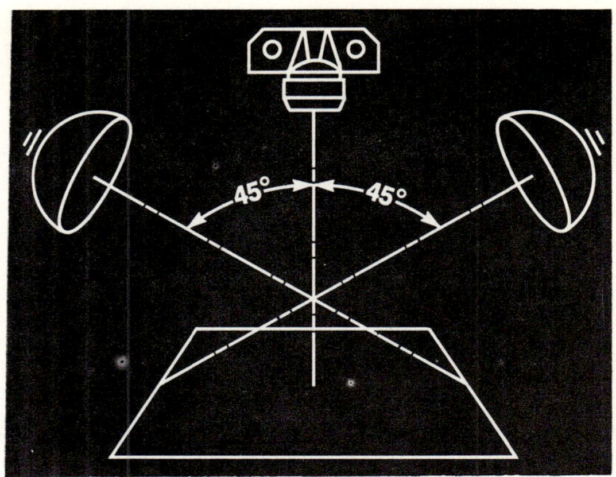

Fig. 17-6.

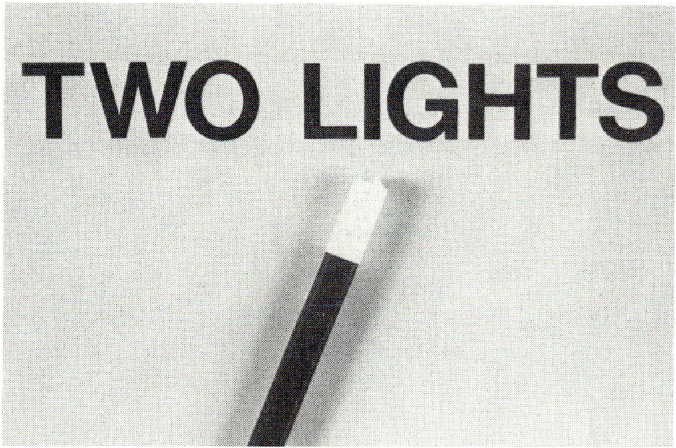

Fig. 17-7.

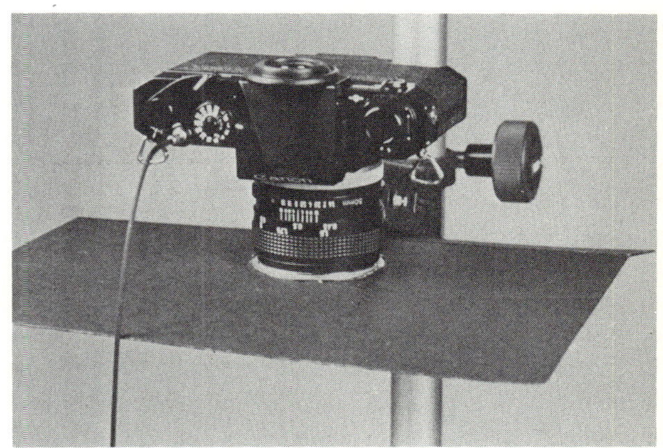

Fig. 17-8.

nate glare. Place a polarizing filter over each light and a complimentary polarizing filter over the camera lens to filter the light reflected from the artwork. Even without a glare problem, copying under polarized light produces brighter colors and deeper color saturation.

Determining the correct exposure is a key to the successful use of any film. You can use an empirical approach by making a series of test exposures, evaluating the results, and finding that combination of shutter speed and aperture that gives the best exposure. Or, you can use a separate hand-held exposure meter, which will give precise exposure indication for any type of reflection artwork or radiograph. Finally, you can use the through-the-lens meter in a 35 mm single lens reflex camera. If this type meter is used, you will still need to make some test exposures, since these are not always accurate when copying radiographs or other transparent materials. They are, however, accurate when copying reflection artwork. Regardless of which type meter you use, the exposure readings should be taken from a gray card, such as the Kodak Neutral Test Card (Fig. 17-9).

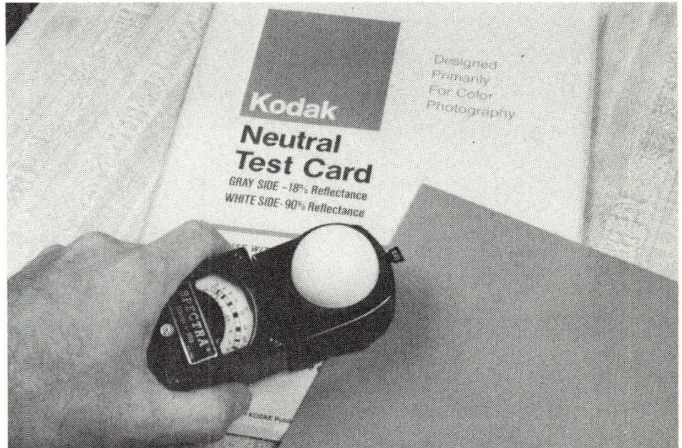

Fig. 17-9.

Place the card over your artwork with the copy lights on and determine correct exposure with whichever type meter you are using. Be certain that the exposure meter is not reading any area outside the gray card. Even after determining proper exposure by this method, you should "bracket" the indicated exposure by shooting additional exposures of 1 or ½ f stop over and under that recommended. A better copy may occasionally result when the film is slightly over- or underexposed.

FILM

There are two types of film: negative and reversal (see also Appendix C-2). Reversal film produces a correct reading image polarity relative to the original. This process is accomplished in a one-step development operation. The reversal films with which most people are familiar are those that produce color transparencies such as Kodachrome or Ektachrome. Negative films, as the name implies, are those in which the image polarity is reversed from the original; thus dark colors appear light and light ones dark.

Black and white reversal films

There are two black-and-white reversal films you may find useful. The first is Kodak Rapid Processing Copy Film. It is available in 36 exposure rolls and is excellent for reproducing wide density ranges of the type found in medical radiographs. Other continuous tone orignals, such as electron micrographs, also reproduce well on Rapid Processing Copy Film.

The second black-and-white reversal film is Kodak Precision Line Film, LPD-4. It is faster and has a higher contrast and density than Rapid Processing Copy Film. It is well suited to produce reversal images of typewriter copy, line drawings, or oscilloscope tracings.

Color reversal films

Although many color reversal films are available, perhaps the most versatile are Kodak Ektachrome films. They have a wide range of uses from color copying to documenting surgical procedures to comparison views of patients before and after treatment. They are available in several film speeds and in daylight and tungsten illumination types. The daylight type is used for natural illumination and electronic flash, while tungsten is used for artificial light, copying, or photomicrography.

ARTWORK TECHNIQUES

The necessary materials for producing artwork are easy to use and are available in photo, stationery, or art supply stores.

Lettering can do much to make your slides look more professional. Many varieties of typefaces and symbols are available in dry transfer lettering (Fig. 17-10). It is easy to use; simply position the letter or symbol you wish to transfer, and rub with a pencil, ballpoint pen, or burnishing tool. Lift the carrier sheet and the characters will be transferred to the artwork (Fig. 17-11). Mechanical devices are also available to produce lettering for artwork. The Varityper "Headliner" machine (Fig. 17-12)

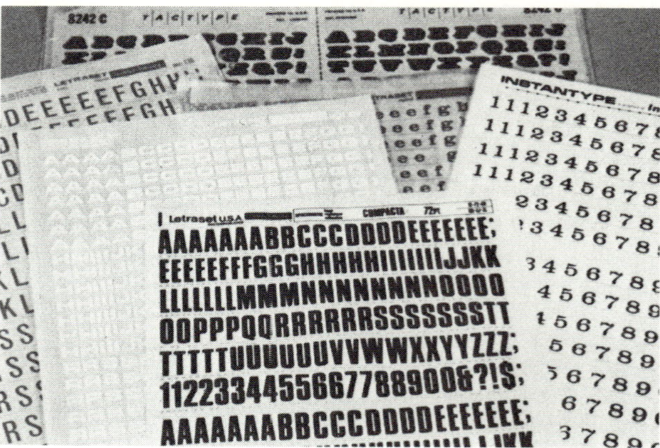

Fig. 17-10.

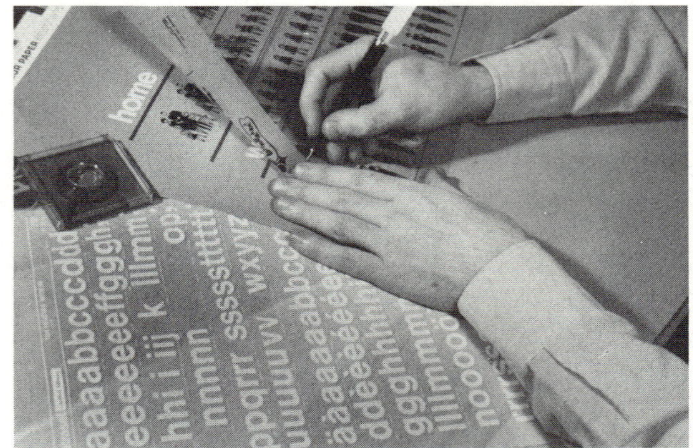

Fig. 17-11.

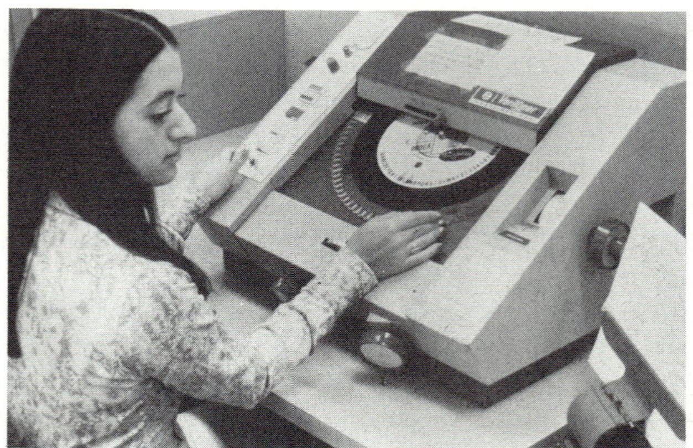

Fig. 17-12.

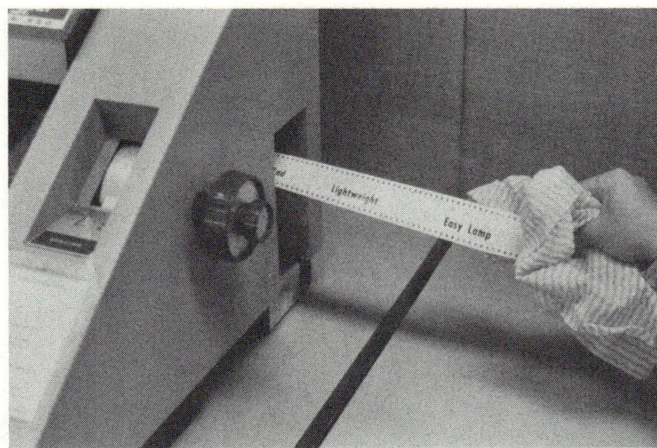

Fig. 17-13.

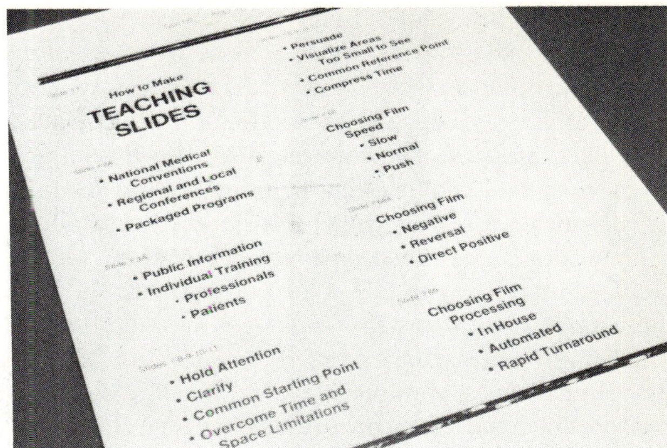

Fig. 17-14.

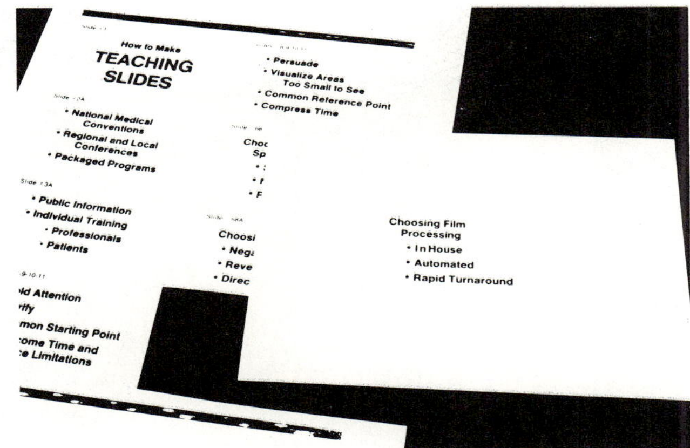

Fig. 17-15.

Fig. 17-16.

uses disks that, when rotated to the proper letter, print the character on photographic film or paper (Fig. 17-13). The finished print is pasted on a layout sheet and shot as a slide. Another method of obtaining fairly inexpensive titles is to "gang" or batch title requirements and have a printer pull a single typesheet for you (Fig. 17-14). Each title is then cut apart and photographed to create the individual slides (Fig. 17-15).

Do not overlook the typewriter as a titling tool. Typing should be done with a carbon, rather than cloth, ribbon for clear, sharp letters (Fig. 17-16). If you must use a typewriter with a cloth ribbon, place a sheet of carbon paper, carbon side up, behind your typing sheet. The additional build-up of carbon on the back of the impression will minimize some of the raggedness caused by the pattern of the cloth ribbon.

An easy way to make typed titles is to position, directly behind the paper you intend to type on, a paper on which a 2 × 3 inch rectangle is drawn. This is the format of the 35 mm film frame. It will give an approximation of what your finished title will look like.

COPYING ARTWORK

Many titles and much artwork can be photographed effectively with high-contrast black-and-white film. Kodalith film is one type that gives a negative image of the original copy. It has a low film speed, thus you must use a longer exposure than with most other black-and-white film. It is opaque; you cannot see light through it when properly exposed. This film is available only in 100 foot rolls and must be spooled into usable 35 mm cassette lengths. Since it is not overly sensitive to red light, it can be loaded and developed under limited red safelight conditions. After processing, the film can be cut, mounted, and used as a slide.

Kodalith slides can be dyed to produce a more pleasing appearance or to emphasize a particular point. It is best to dye on the emulsion side, although it is possible to dye on the base side. If you want an especially vivid color, dye both sides of the film. Use a water-soluble dye. We have found Dr. Phillip Martin's water-soluble colors to be practical. Simple food coloring dye, which can be purchased at the supermarket, also does a good job, although the color range is limited. Pens made especially for coloring overhead transparencies produce a heavy coating of transparent dye, but they tend to streak. Another way to add color to a Kodalith slide is to sandwich it together with a color gel in a slide mount. Transparent colored tapes can be applied to a Kodalith slide, but if this technique is used, the slide should be copied, since the tapes on the original may loosen because of heat and jam the projector.

Kodalith slides can be used effectively for a technique called "progressive disclosure." If you have a series of points to make, disclose them one at a time rather than all at once, which may tend to distract your audience (Figs. 17-17 to 17-21). This type slide can be made in several ways. One technique is to shoot a series of exposures of the full copy, dye the film, then use black tape to mask off the unwanted material. As suggested with colored tapes, copy the masked slides rather than projecting the originals. The same result may be obtained when copying the original artwork by covering unwanted material with a white paper. Another effective technique is to dye the information line a light color, or leave it white, and dye the other lines a darker contrasting or harmonizing color.

You can enliven a piece of black-and-white copy by covering it with a color gel and photographing it on color film. The same effect can be obtained by copying it with a colored filter over the camera lens. Another technique for adding color is to start with a black-and-white photograph, add color with dyes or felt-tip pens, and copy this on color film. To emphasize a specific area of a photograph, start with a color print, trace the important parts on layout paper, then copy the two as a comparison slide (Fig. 17-22).

Another method of adding color to black-and-white artwork is to use color overlay film. This is transparent, has an adhesive backing, and is available in a wide range of colors. After the sheet is adhered to the original artwork, use an artist's knife to remove color from any areas you wish to emphasize (Fig. 17-23) or leave color on only the area of emphasis (Fig. 17-24).

Illustrations can also be used to enhance slides. To use these you do not have to be an artist or order expensive artwork. Simply consult books of line engravings, which are available in libraries, bookstores, or art supply stores (Fig. 17-25). An effective slide can be made by photographing and enlarging an illustration, placing a sheet of color gel or overlay film over it, and adding an appropriate title (Fig. 17-26).

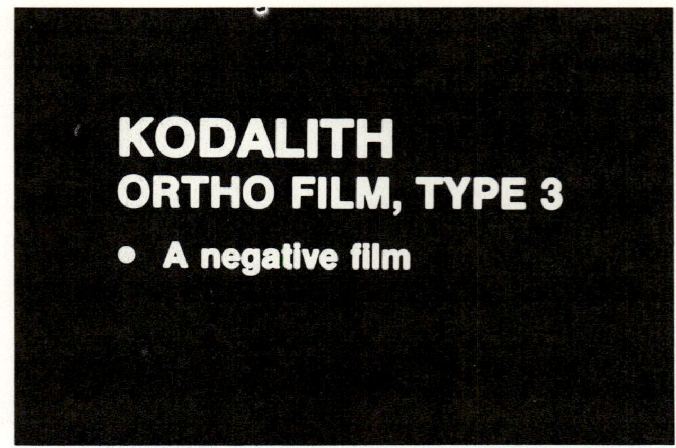

Fig. 17-17.

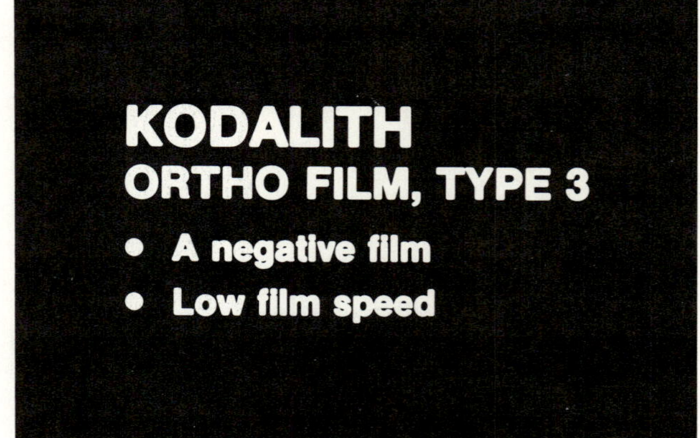

Fig. 17-18.

Fig. 17-19.

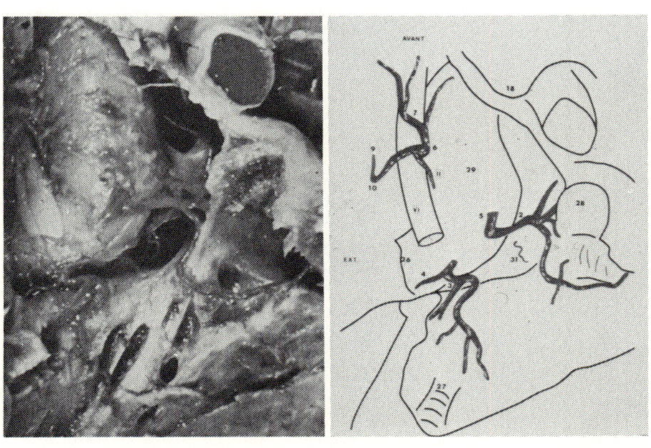

Fig. 17-20.

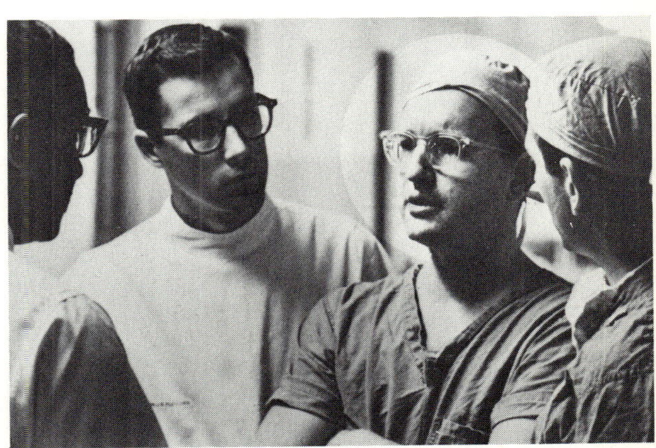

Fig. 17-21.

Fig. 17-22.

Fig. 17-23.

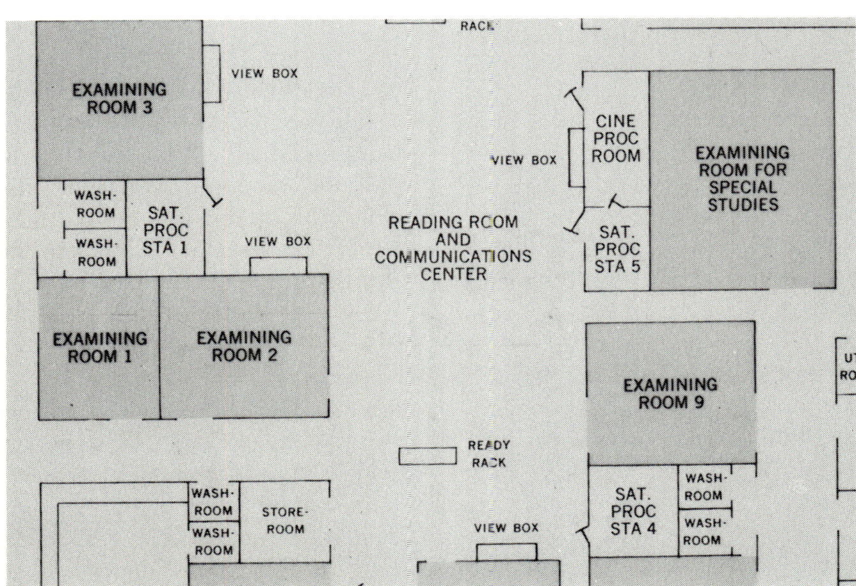

Fig. 17-24.

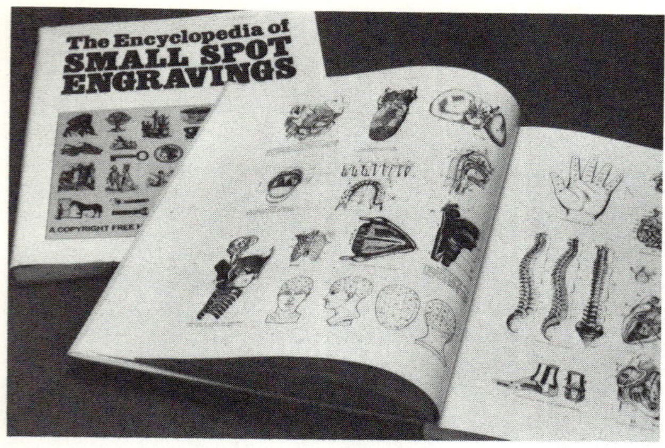

Fig. 17-25.

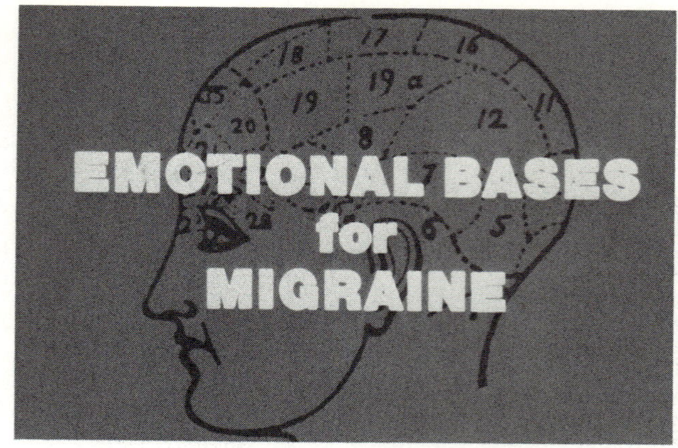

Fig. 17-26.

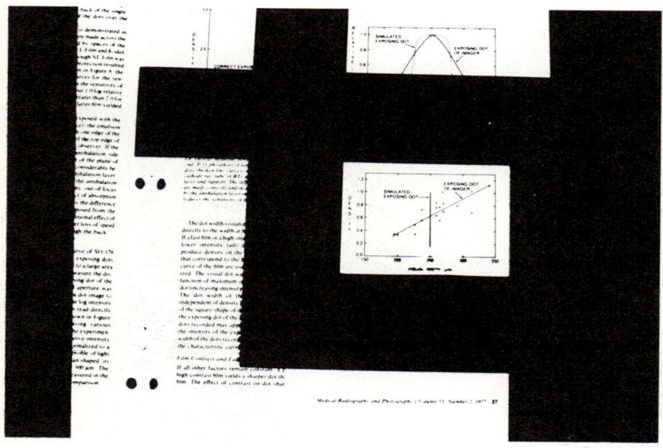

Fig. 17-27.

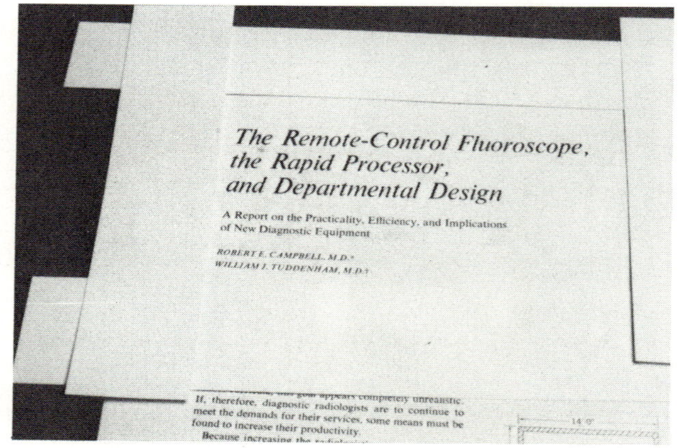

Fig. 17-28.

SPECIAL COPYING TECHNIQUES

All of the techniques mentioned thus far involve photocopying in one form or another. While camera, lighting, and exposure have been discussed, other specialized techniques may prove helpful.

If you have a lot of book copying to do, a book holder is a worthwhile investment. It holds the pages open and flat. Black-masking Ls are a simple way to delete extraneous material (Fig. 17-27). It is not always necessary to go to the trouble of making a title; these may be copied directly from journal articles. If you are copying with Kodalith film, use white masks to eliminate unwanted detail (Fig. 17-28).

OPTICAL TITLING

Once you get into production of your own teaching slides, you may want to experiment with double-exposed titles. These are referred to as "optical titles." Start with a color slide that you want to use as a background and a black-and-white Kodalith title slide. Using a light box or a slide copying device, first make a copy exposure of the background slide; then without advancing the film, expose (or "double expose") the title slide. The order in which this is done is not important; the result will be the same. The resultant slide has white or clear letters "burned through" the background image (Fig. 17-29).

Slide duplicating units vary from the professional, which cost from $500 to $600 (Fig. 17-30), to the light box (Fig. 17-31) to a variety of less expensive devices (Fig. 17-32). The difference in cost is a measure of the unit's ability to change focal length. The more expensive devices permit zooming in to enlarge sections of a slide.

Slide duplicating requires a low-contrast film emulsion. We recommend Kodak Ektachrome Slide Duplicating Film 5071. If you copy slides with a camera original film, you get a build-up of contrast which, in most cases, is undesirable.

When making optical titles, avoid background slides

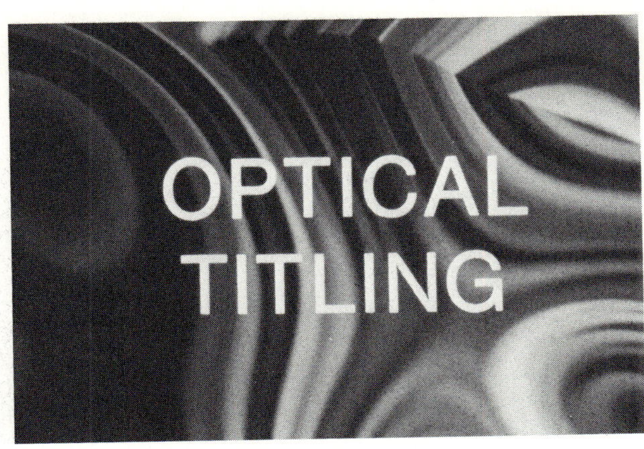

Fig. 17-29.

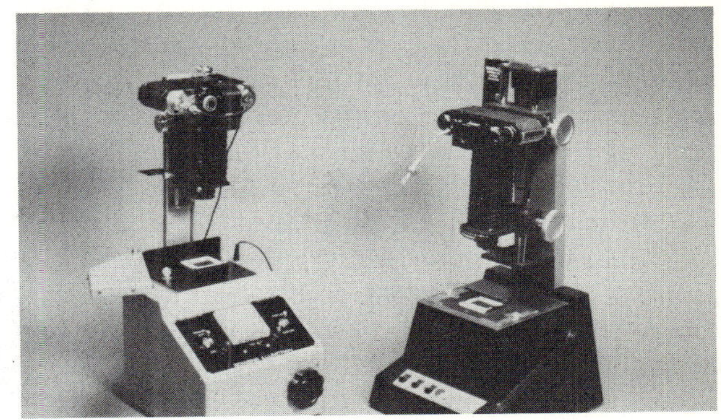

Fig. 17-30.

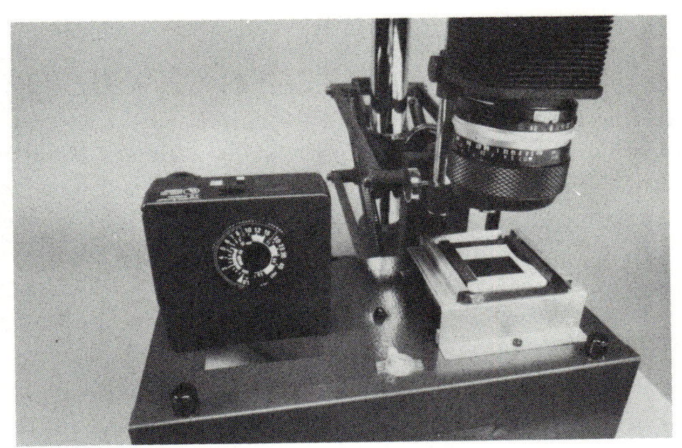

Fig. 17-31.

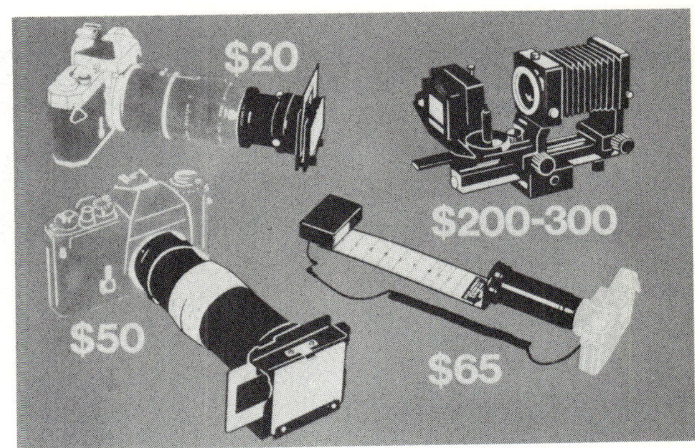

Fig. 17-32.

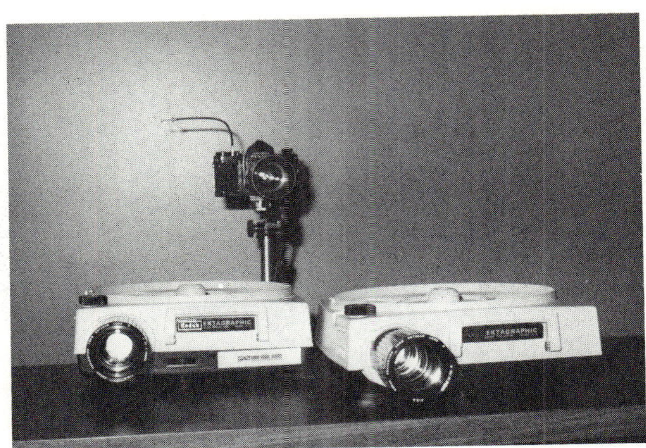

Fig. 17-33.

that conflict with the title being "burned in." Select backgrounds that offer the greatest contrast and visibility to your titles. As you look for background slides to add to your files, consider these possibilities: if you have a few exposures left at the end of a roll, finish if off with filters over the lens to darken the scene. Other methods are to copy extra slides using dark filters or to use colored gels over existing scenes.

It is possible to make optical title slides without investing in special equipment. Just set up two projectors, each projecting one of the two slides you wish to combine, put your camera between them, and photograph the composite image on the screen (Fig. 17-33). Use a zoom telephoto lens on the camera because you want to get as far away from the screen as possible to minimize image distortion. Read the light intensity directly off the wall, but to be on the safe side, take a wide range of bracketed exposures.

Title slides can also be created by sandwiching a color slide or gel with a Kodalith slide, either positive or negative. The resultant "sandwich" can be mounted in a single mount for projection, or better, copied onto color film.

REVERSE TEXT SLIDES

We have discussed the creation of black-and-white slides using Kodalith. Attractive reverse text slides may also be made in color, using Kodak Vericolor Slide film and color filters. This technique involves a bit of color physics.

As you know, additive color is made up of the primaries—red, blue, and green. Subtractive colors are the minus ones: yellow, cyan, and magenta. If you work with a subtractive color to get, for example, a blue background, you must shoot your copy through a yellow filter (yellow being minus blue). When this technique is used, the Vericolor Slide film is developed in a negative process (C-41). This allows you to obtain clear letters on a colored background.

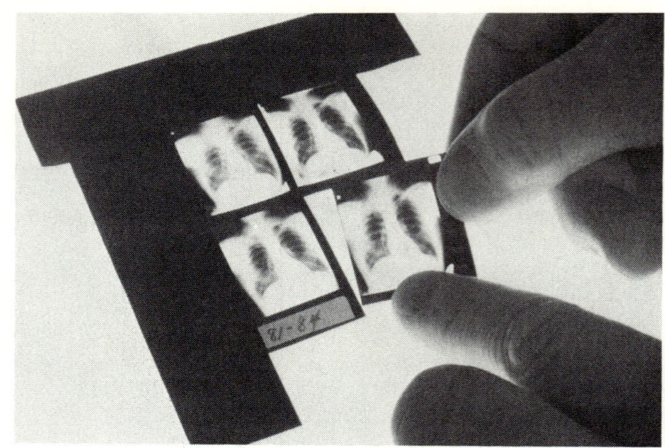

Fig. 17-34.

MASKING

You may want to display more than one image at a time. Masks and multiple frame mounts are a helpful way of doing this. Many shapes of ready-made mounts are available. Some can be used directly with a film frame; others require that you cut up your images to fit in the respective areas. Also many cardboard insert masks are available. These are usually added to the film frame and sandwiched in a glass mount. Still another way to produce multiple images is to assemble several photographs or images, tape them together, and copy the resultant layout (Fig. 17-34).

SUMMARY

It does not require a lot of effort to improve the quality of teaching slides. Using techniques outlined in this chapter can be a rewarding communication experience. A number of Kodak publications are listed in the Bibliography that cover these and other techniques in detail. A final word of advice is to try these techniques and become familiar with them. By so doing you will significantly improve the quality of your teaching slides.

CHAPTER 18

Office sketching

Melvin Spira, M.D.

The ability to draw can be learned and developed with practice. It can be effectively employed in the office practice of a plastic surgeon, both as a method for teaching patients so that they can give "informed consent" and as an adjunct in the planning of surgery. A brief drawing demonstrating the form to be achieved, where scars are to be placed, and/or the mechanics of an operation will reinforce the most specific of nonvisual discussions. In addition to its primary purpose, sketching can be utilized as an operating room aid in the orientation of pathologic specimens and to enhance the recording of surgical procedures, particularly those involving flap reconstructions in complicated deformities. While artists may not be plastic surgeons, plastic surgeons are frequently artistic and must utilize methods and techniques similar to those employed by artists in the conceptualization of both the desired postoperative result and the technique to be used in achieving it. In addition, sketching can serve as a practice builder and subtle reinforcement of a good patient-physician relationship. Finally, drawing can also be a pleasurable avocation.

I begin my drawing course by asking students to make, in addition to a straight line, a series of simple geometric forms, including circles, squares, and rectangles in rapid succession. Then, beginning with parts of the face such as the ear and nose, they are shown how to put them together and form a face (Figs. 18-1 to 18-6).

Text continued on p. 137.

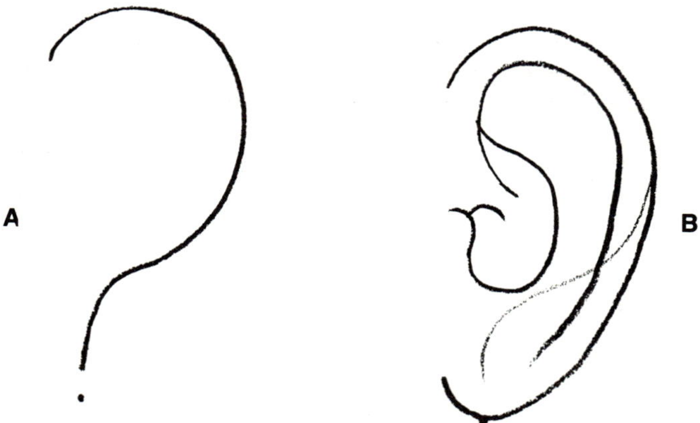

Fig. 18-1. Ear. A "question mark" is made first **(A)**, followed by the outlining of the helix and antihelix lobe and tragus **(B)**. Note that the root of the helix extends into the concha and that the ear is angulated about 30 degrees.

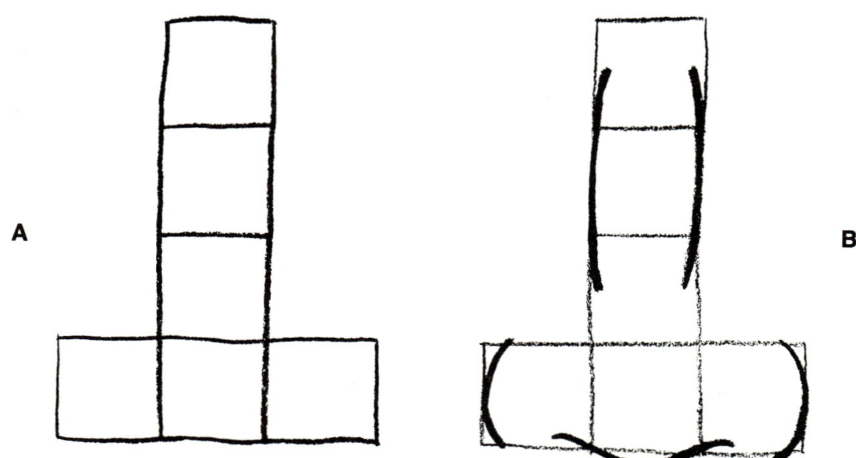

Fig. 18-2. Nose, front view. **A,** "Building blocks" of four squares in the vertical dimension and three in the horizontal. **B,** The base of the nostrils are rounded off and the tip borders are outlined, with the final form. Primary error involves inadequate width-to-length ratio.

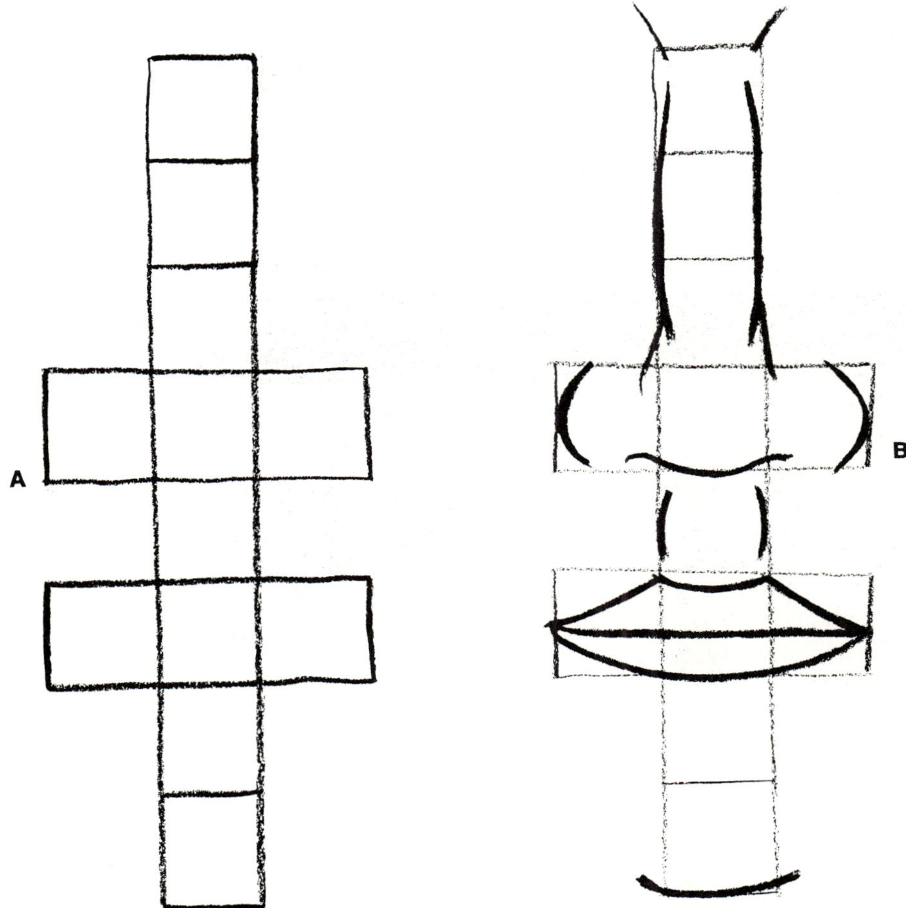

Fig. 18-3. Mid lower face, front view. The "building blocks" are seen in **A,** composed of eight vertical squares, with the lateral squares added for the base of the nose, as well as for the lips. **B,** The proportions for the nose, upper and lower lips, and chin are seen in final form. Note that the same proportions are maintained in both the front and lateral view. Compare this with Figs. 18-4 to 18-6.

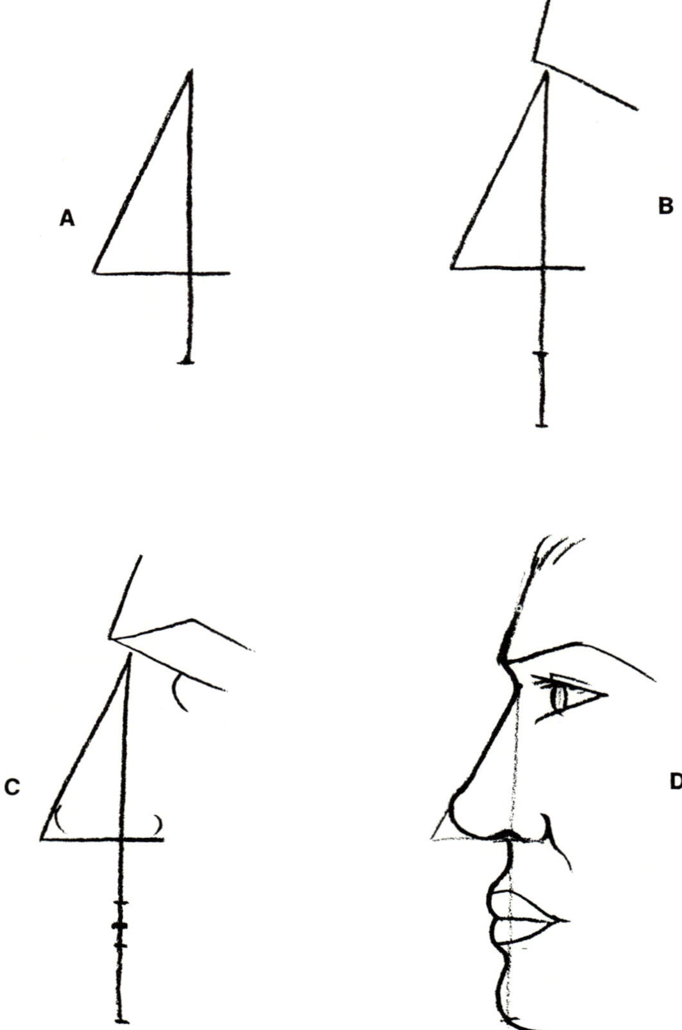

Fig. 18-4. Anterior facial profile. Begun by drawing a 4, as seen in **A. B,** The vertical limb is doubled, and the forehead and brow are added. **C,** The 4 is then shortened, the lip levels are added, being approximately half the vertical dimension of the chin. **D,** Final configuration. Note that the base of the nose lies just anterior to the vertical plane dropped down from the cornea which, in turn, lies just anterior to the commissure of the mouth.

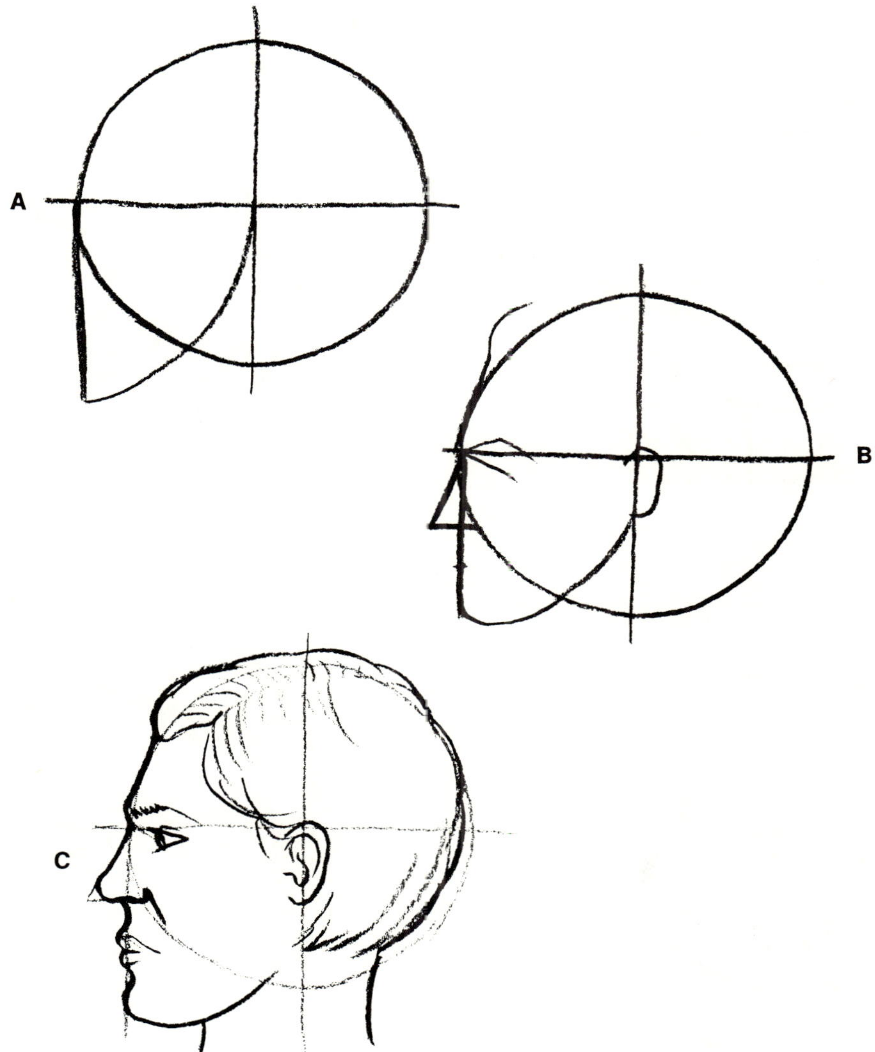

Fig. 18-5. Full head and neck, lateral view. **A,** A circle is drawn first, together with a "quarter pie." **B,** the basic 4, as seen in Fig. 18-4, is drawn in, together with the portions for the upper and lower lip and chin. The ear is located in back of, or posterior to, the center of the circle. **C,** The addition of the lips, alar base, and eyes, as well as filling in the nose, employing the technique as described above, completes the picture profile of the head and neck.

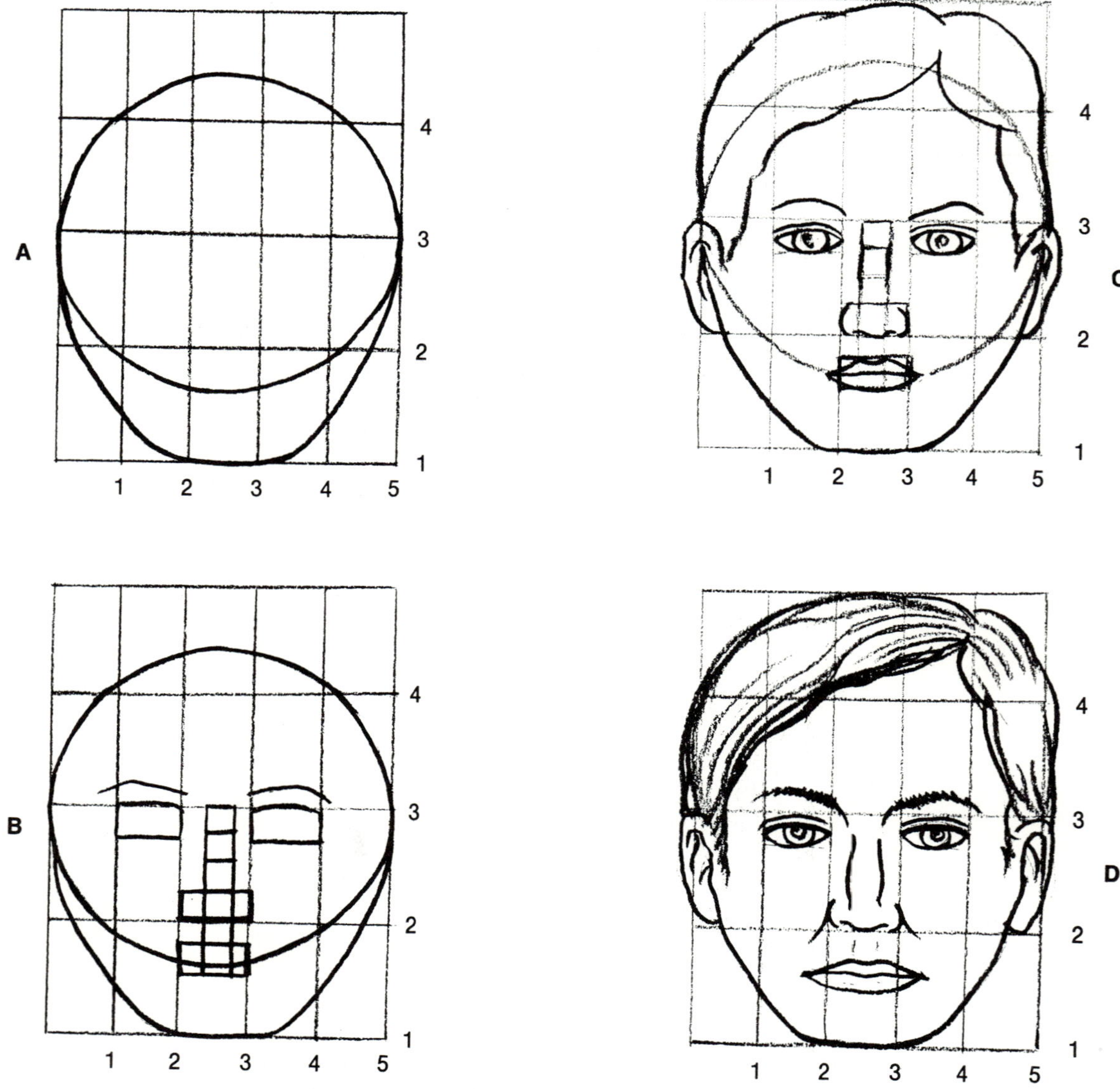

Fig. 18-6. The head, frontal view. **A,** A circle is drawn first with the "pie," the additional inferior dimension for the chin and jaw line. The circle is then divided into five segments vertically and four segments horizontally, with the proportions seen in **B. C,** The general features are filled in. **D,** The final drawing.

A specific example of what sketching can accomplish is its utilization in rhinoplasty. At the first office visit the patient's profile is sketched directly on the examining table disposable paper. What can be accomplished by removal of the hump, overall reduction in size of the nose, elevation of the tip, or some other procedure can be rapidly and graphically explained (Fig. 18-7). The advantage of a chin implant to augment mental contour for a hypoplastic chin can be convincingly demonstrated. Specific methods for similarly demonstrating and determining such diverse procedures as rhytidectomy, reduction and augmentation mammoplasty, and excision of a skin cancer are seen in Figs. 18-8 to 18-11. Typical instances in which sketching is useful in the hospital are described in Figs. 18-12 and 18-13.

Text continued on p. 143.

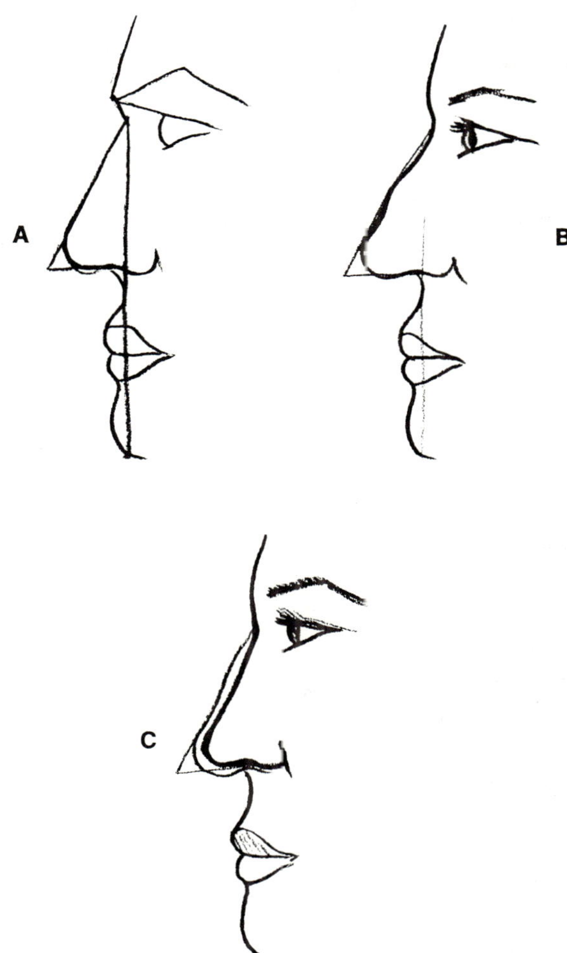

Fig. 18-7. Drawing the rhinoplasty candidate. **A,** We see the 4 again with the vertical limb extension above and below the 4 to simulate the brow and chin area, as seen in Fig. 18-4. **B,** The typical patient with a hump nose deformity, coupled with a lack of chin protrusion. **C,** The surgical goal following rhinoplasty and chin augmentation.

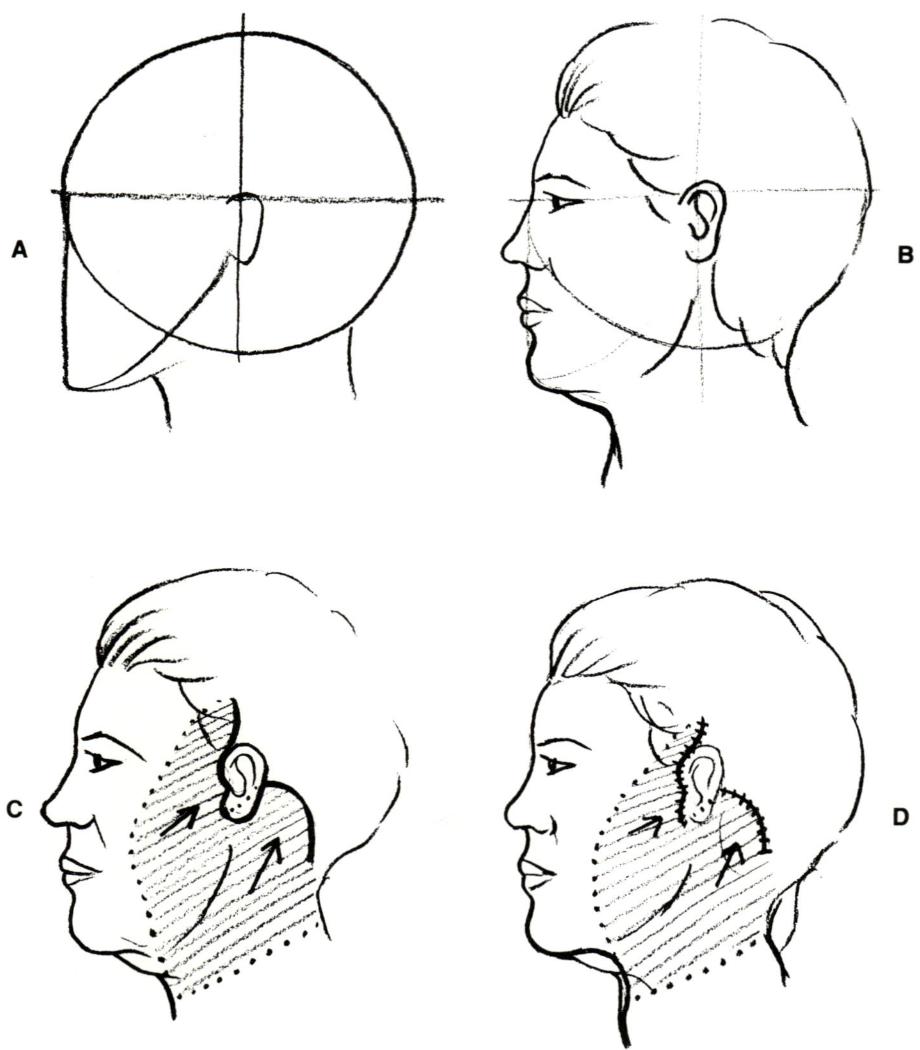

Fig. 18-8. Giving the patient informed consent for the cervicofacial rhytidectomy. **A** and **B,** The initial drawing is developed. **C,** The area of undermining required in order to accomplish the lift and outlining of the permanent scars together with direction of pull. **D,** The resulting improvement in contour.

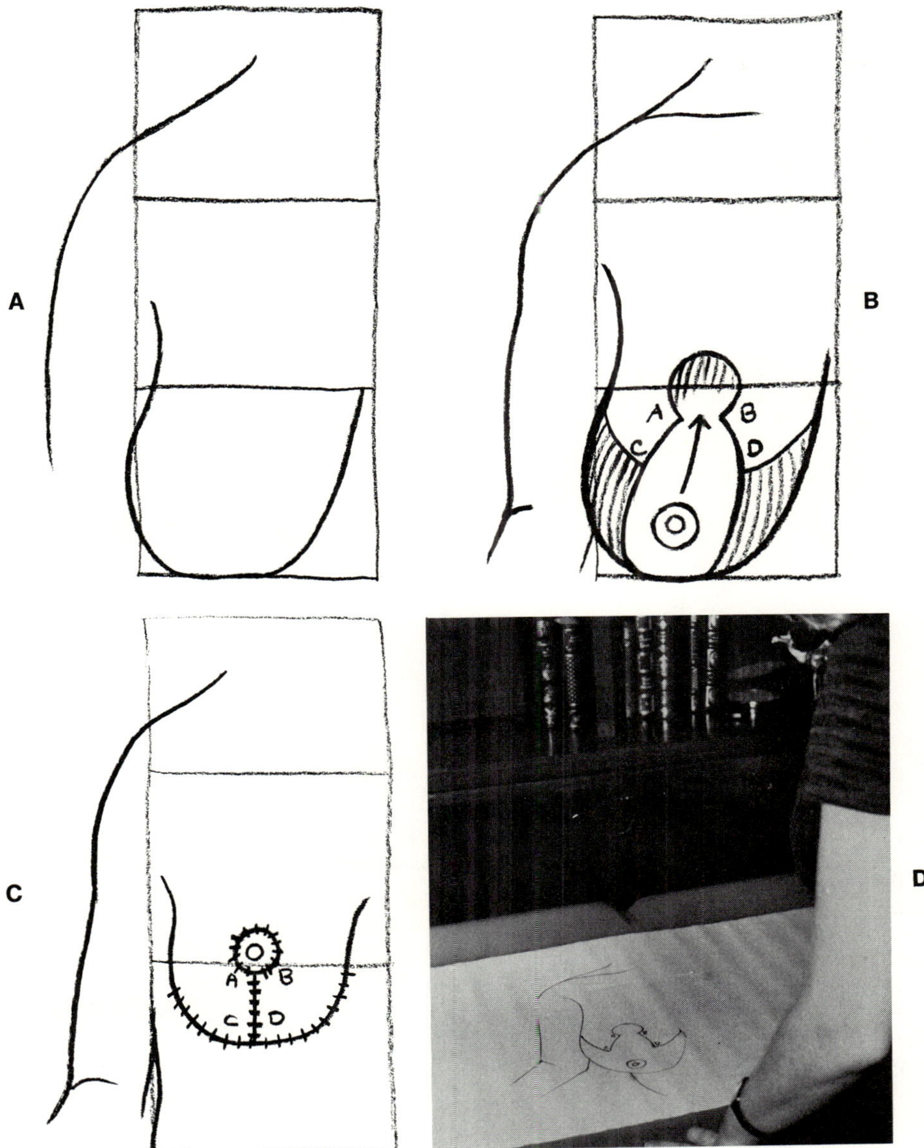

Fig. 18-9. Preoperative discussion of the reduction mammoplasty. **A,** Three squares are made to proportion the initial frontal view in the vertical plane. **B,** Flaps are outlined so as to demonstrate the incisions and general technique for breast reduction. The flap corners are lettered and the amount of tissue to be resected is seen as shaded. The elevation of the nipple on the dermal pedicle to a more superior position is described. **C,** The projected new configuration is drawn, side by side with the old. In explaining the technique, the patient is told that point A goes to point B, point C goes to point D, etc. In **D,** The examining table disposable paper is used for drawing paper.

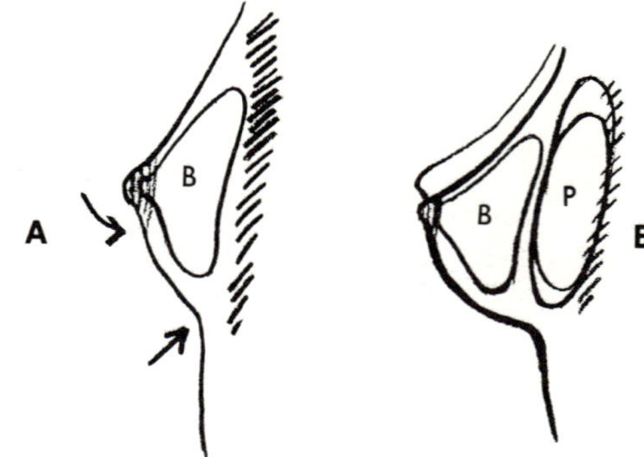

Fig. 18-10. Discussing the augmentation mammoplasty. **A,** An outline is drawn with the relationship of the breast tissue *(B)* to the underlying muscle. **B,** The routes of entry to develop a space between the breast tissue and muscle and the placement of the implant in the "pocket," *P.*

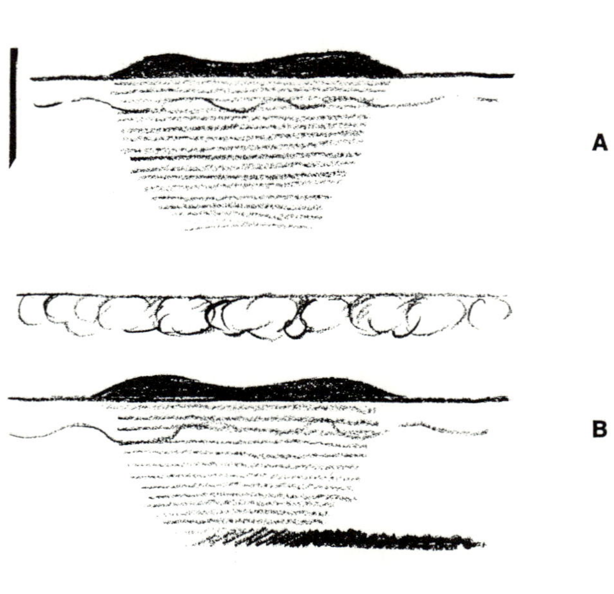

Fig. 18-11. Discussing the surgical excision of a basal cell carcinoma. **A,** The usual lesion is seen in cross-section. **B,** A possible lateral extension in the dermis. **C,** The usual resection *(1),* as visualized by the external lesions, and the need for taking an additional section *(2)* can be discussed. Following a frozen section that demonstrates "tumor at the margins," the patient better understands the occasional need for a much larger resection of skin and a more complicated reconstruction than what would normally be required by the size of the external lesion on the skin.

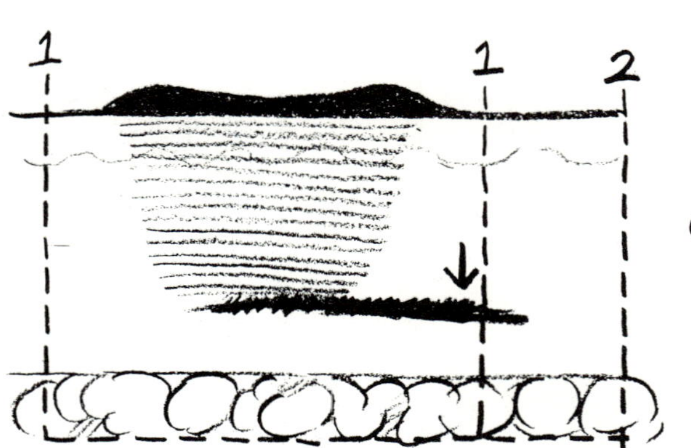

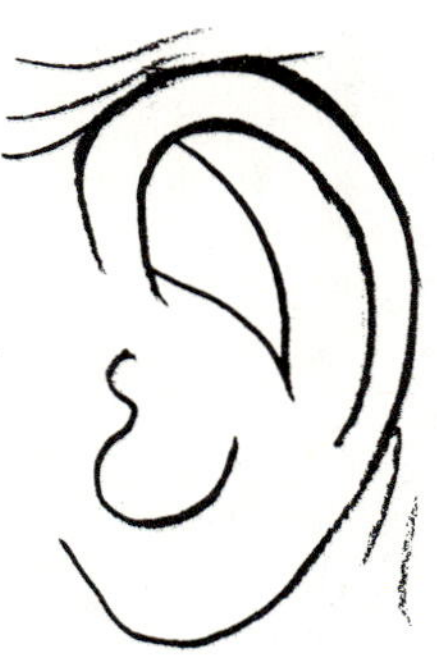

Fig. 18-12. A lifesize sketch made in the operating room will serve as a base on which the specimen is taken to the pathologist so that rapid identification of the location and orientation of the lesion is possible.

Fig. 18-13. A quick sketch in the emergency room saves the time required for lengthy written descriptions and supplement the dictated note.

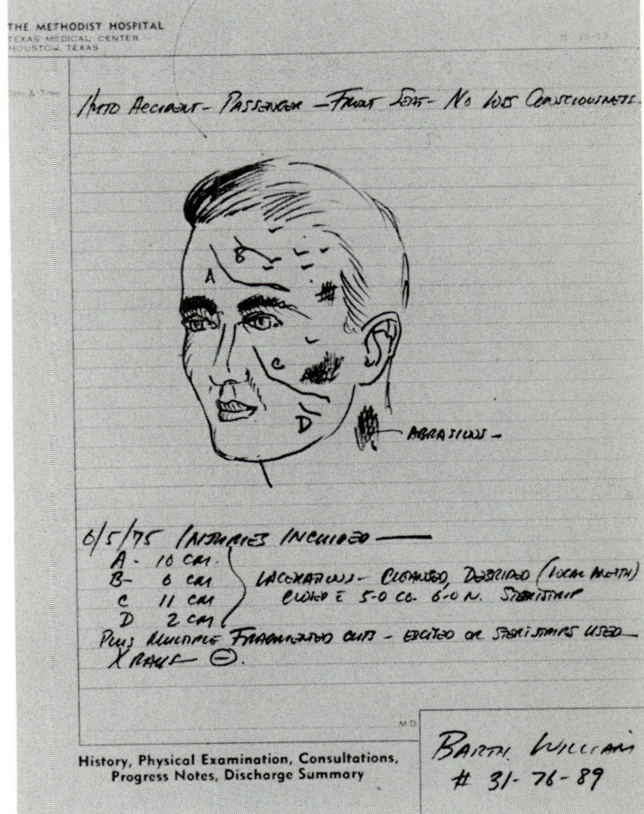

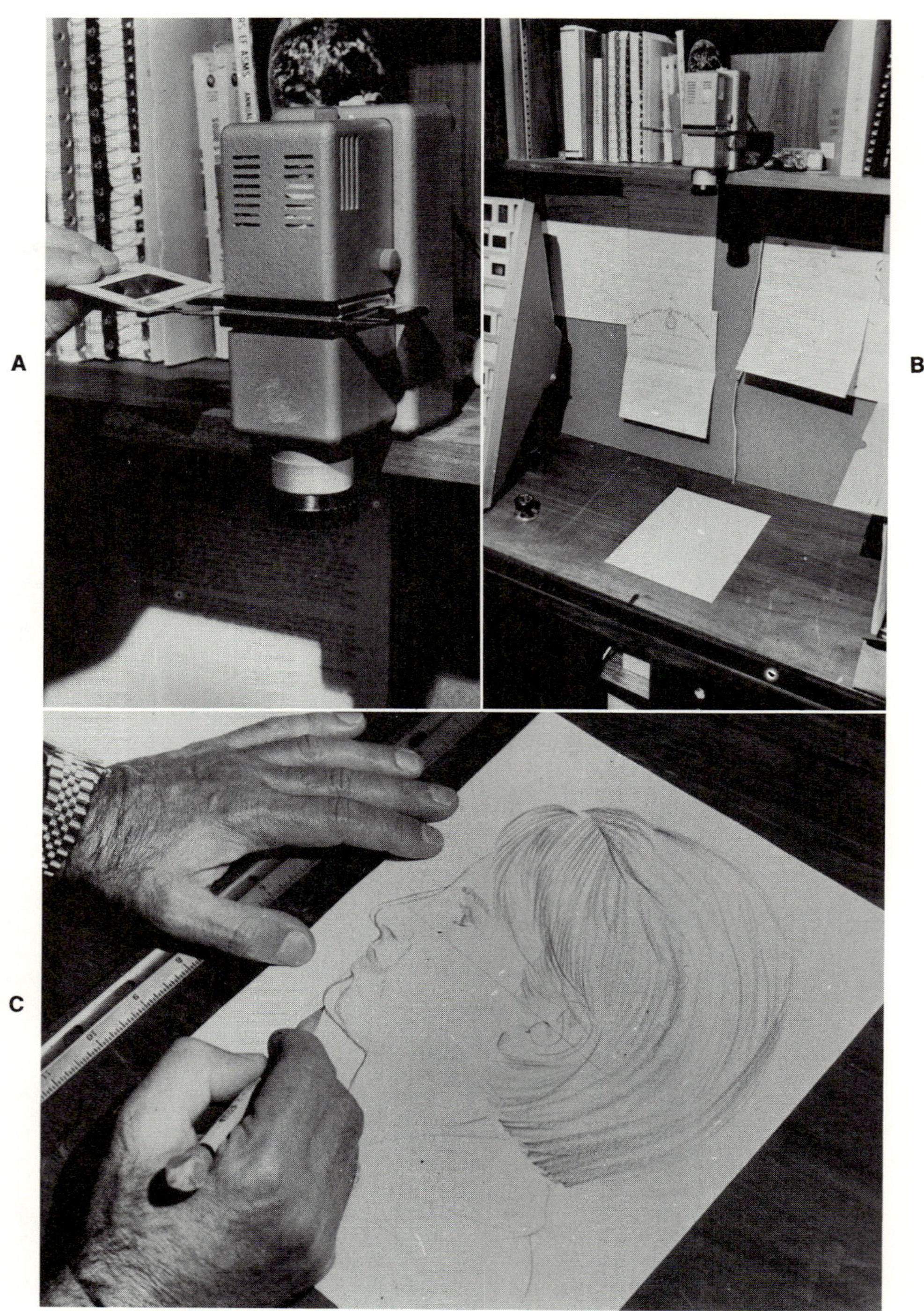

Fig. 18-14. Using a small 35 mm projector **(A)**, mounted so as to project a lifesize image from a color slide **(B)**, will enable the surgeon to make a sketch to exact proportions **(C)**. See text.

In certain cases planning the procedure involves making a tracing from a Kodachrome 2 × 2 inch slide transparency, the enlargement being lifesize. For this purpose an inexpensive short focal length lens projector is used (Fig. 18-14). Such procedures as the specific amount of "hump" to be removed or the amount of caudal septum to be excised to elevate the tip can be determined in millimeters by such preoperative planning. The sketches are then utilized in the operating room as a direct aid in executing the operative procedure. Finally, by comparing the preoperative sketches of the patient with the final clinical result, one can discern discrepancies in the preoperative plan versus the procedure actually performed to hopefully improve the results of future similar operations.

The ability to draw can be taught and learned just as can playing the piano or violin. All of us are not Van Cliburns but many of us can play the piano, and the ability to do so comes through hard work and practice. I was once told by a successful commercial artist that if you make ten drawings a day of any subject from life you will develop enough ability at the end of one year to take a position in a commercial art house, and I believe it.

Practice perception of correction proportions and perspectives, add a pencil, pad, and some pastime, and you will develop a talent that will satisfy you beyond belief!

To assist those interested in pursuing this concept further, *Drawing the Head and Hands* by Andrew Loomis is highly recommended.

CHAPTER 19

Medical photography

Robert C. Reeder, M.D.

"A picture is worth a thousand words." That phrase is so often used that it has become a cliche; yet nowhere is it more appropriate than when describing clinical photography. No matter how articulate he or she may be, it is a rare physician who can verbally describe as concisely or accurately the appearance of an unusual or abnormal condition as can a single well-done clinical photograph.

Photographic equipment is like an artist's materials; the results produced depend upon the skill with which each is used. There is no mystique about the skills or equipment necessary to produce good clinical photographs. All that is needed is a relatively simple combination of camera, lens, and light source; and attention to some basics of composition, background, and standardization of views.

EQUIPMENT

A bewildering variety of photographic equipment is available. Thumb through any camera magazine or catalog and you will be assailed with the virtues and capabilities of the many products. Reading about automatic exposure, shutter-preferred versus aperture-preferred exposure, center-weighted metering, the various camera sizes available, and the number of accessories available can make one thoroughly confused and wishing for the return of the simple "box Brownie." No wonder so many are confused about the selection of suitable equipment for clinical use.

A system for clinical photography need not be complex. All you need is a simple but adequate camera, the proper lens or lenses, and an appropriate light source. The system for clinical photography should be just that; it should not be used for family photographs or for recording your vacation to the beach. If it is used for clinical work only, a very simple system will suffice and you need not worry about expensive options that expand the potential of the camera, but at the same time make its use more complicated. Try to select a system that is reliable, gives reproducible results, and can be used by even the most inexperienced of your office or operating room staff with a minimum of instruction.

Camera

35 mm single lens reflex. The best camera for clinical photography is the 35 mm single lens reflex (Fig. 19-1). With this type of camera you view and focus through the lens that is used to take the picture. By means of a mirror and prism the exact image to be photographed is shown on the viewing screen. This eliminates problems with parallax and allows critical focusing and framing of the subject. Since the viewing system uses the camera lens, this type camera works equally well with all lenses.

If you are going to use the camera for clinical photography only, you do not need one that has through-the-lens exposure metering or automatic exposure features. Most, if not all, clinical photographs are taken with an electronic flash, which requires the use of only one shutter speed (X synchronization). If you do chose a camera with automatic exposure, however, be sure that it has provision for setting exposure manually.

The clinical camera should accept interchangeable lenses. There are several different types of lens mounts used on these cameras (breech lock, bayonnet, screw mount, etc.). Be sure that the camera you choose uses a system compatible with a variety of accessory lenses. If you already own several lenses, choose a camera that will accept them.

Many cameras offer an automatic winder as a accessory. These are relatively inexpensive and eliminate the need to refocus and recompose the picture between exposures.

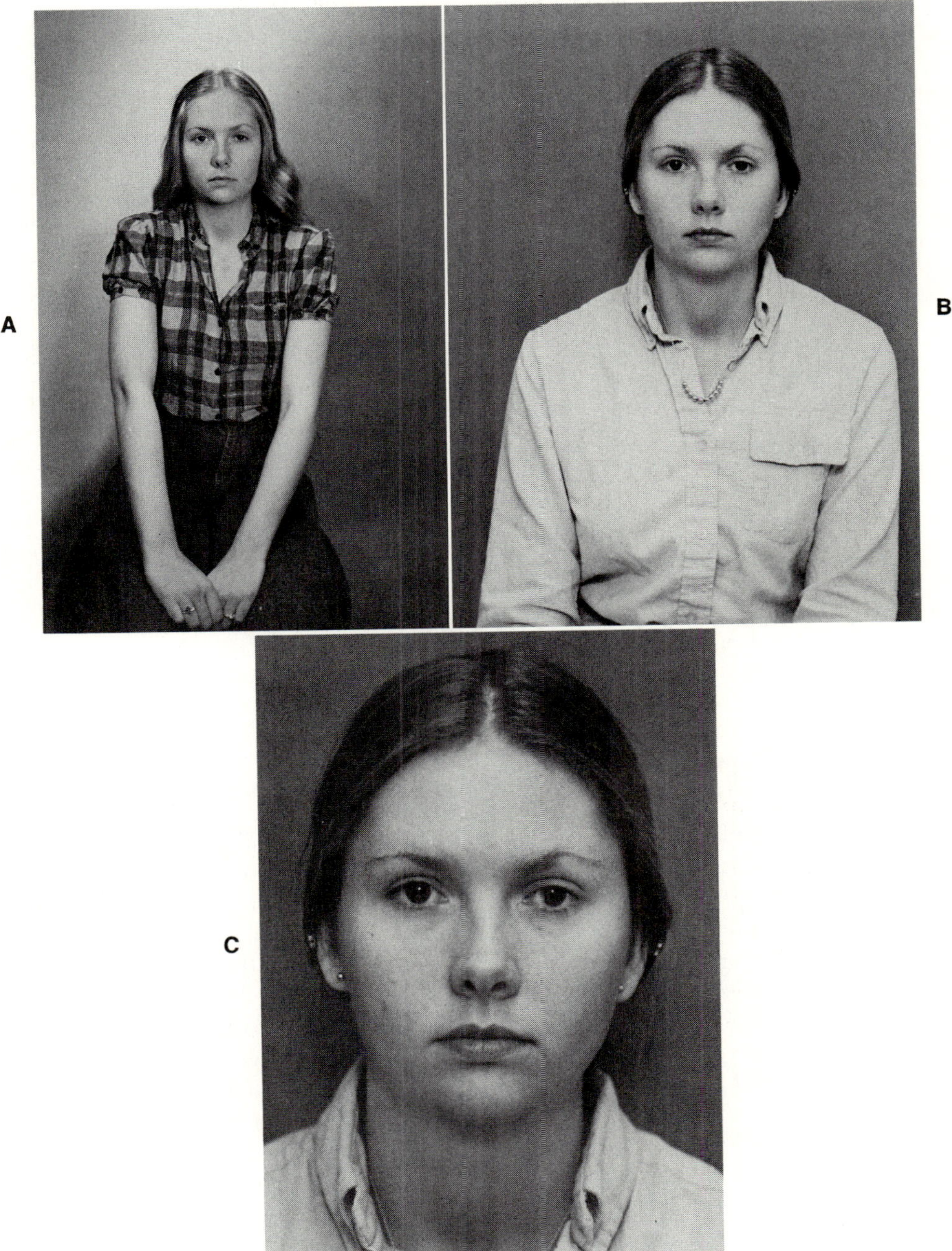

Fig. 19-4. Selection of proper lens to record normal perspective. All of these photographs were taken from a distance of 4 feet. **A** was taken with a 28 mm lens, **B** with a 50 mm lens, and **C** with a 100 mm lens. Note that the one taken with the 100 mm lens fills the frame and records perspective accurately. If the camera is moved closer to the subject to fill the frame with the image projected by the other lenses, distortion may occur (see Fig. 19-6).

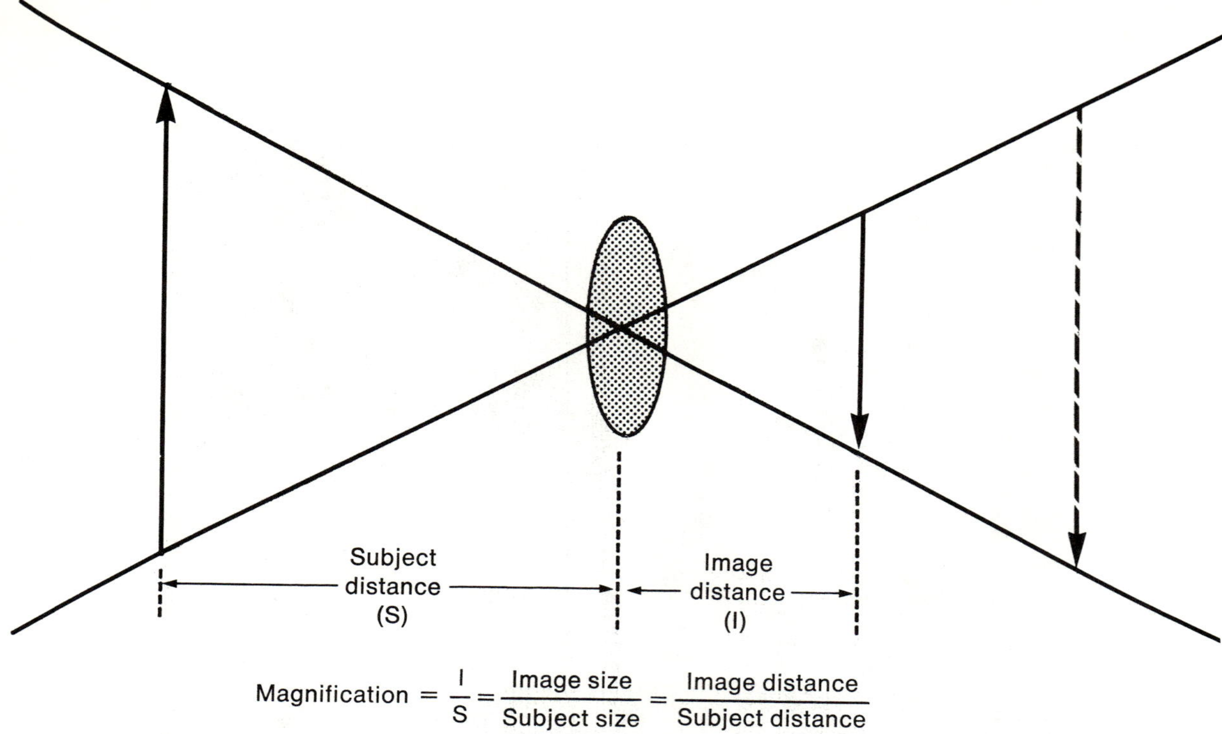

Fig. 19-5. Magnification is a function of the ratio of image distance to subject distance. When these distances are equal the magnification is 1:1 or life size. (Redrawn from Shipman, C.: How to select and use canon SLR cameras.)

lens is moved farther from the film plane, then magnification will be increased. This can be expressed as a formula: $M = I/S$ where M = magnification, I = image size or image distance from the lens, and S = subject size or subject distance from the lens. Therefore, to increase magnification we must either move the lens closer to the subject or increase the lens-to-film distance. We must be aware, however, that if the lens is moved closer to the subject, we may encounter a phenomenon known as "foreshortening" in which objects closer to the lens are magnified, thus introducing distortion into the resultant photograph (Fig. 19-6).

The selection of a proper lens, therefore, requires that it have an appropriate angle of view and that its focal length is such that it permits photographs to be taken at a distance that will fill the film frame but not introduce distortion of perspective.

Lenses are marked with f stops. This is an expression of the ratio between the focal length of the lens and the diameter of the diaphragm opening of that lens. The f stop determines the amount of light that will reach the film by varying the diameter of the diaphragm opening. For example, a 50 mm lens set at f8 will have an aperture diameter of 6.25 mm (50/8 = 6.25). Conversely, a 50 mm lens set at f16 will have an effective aperture of

3.125 (50/16 = 3.125). We can see, therefore, that since the number assigned the f stop is a reciprocal of the diameter, the larger the f stop number, the smaller the diameter of the diaphragm opening. Obviously, the smaller the opening, the less light will reach the film.

There are formulas that help to determine correct exposure. Changing the f stop changes the amount of light that will reach the film. The amount of light transmitted is doubled or halved by each "stop" change; f8 allows twice the light to pass as does f11. Changing the shutter speed has a similar effect; 1/50 second allows twice as much light to reach the film as does 1/100 second. Therefore, if you wish to retain the same exposure but want to increase the size of the aperture one stop, you must reduce the shutter speed by one increment to compensate. For example, if the correct exposure is f:8 at 1/100 second and you wish to change the lens opening to f:11, you must change the shutter speed to 1/50 second to compensate for the lessened amount of light reaching the film if exposure is to remain constant.

Depth of field is defined as the zone of apparent sharpness that exists in front of and behind the point of critical focus. This can be affected by several factors, the most important of which are the focal length of the lens and the aperture of the diaphragm. The shorter the focal

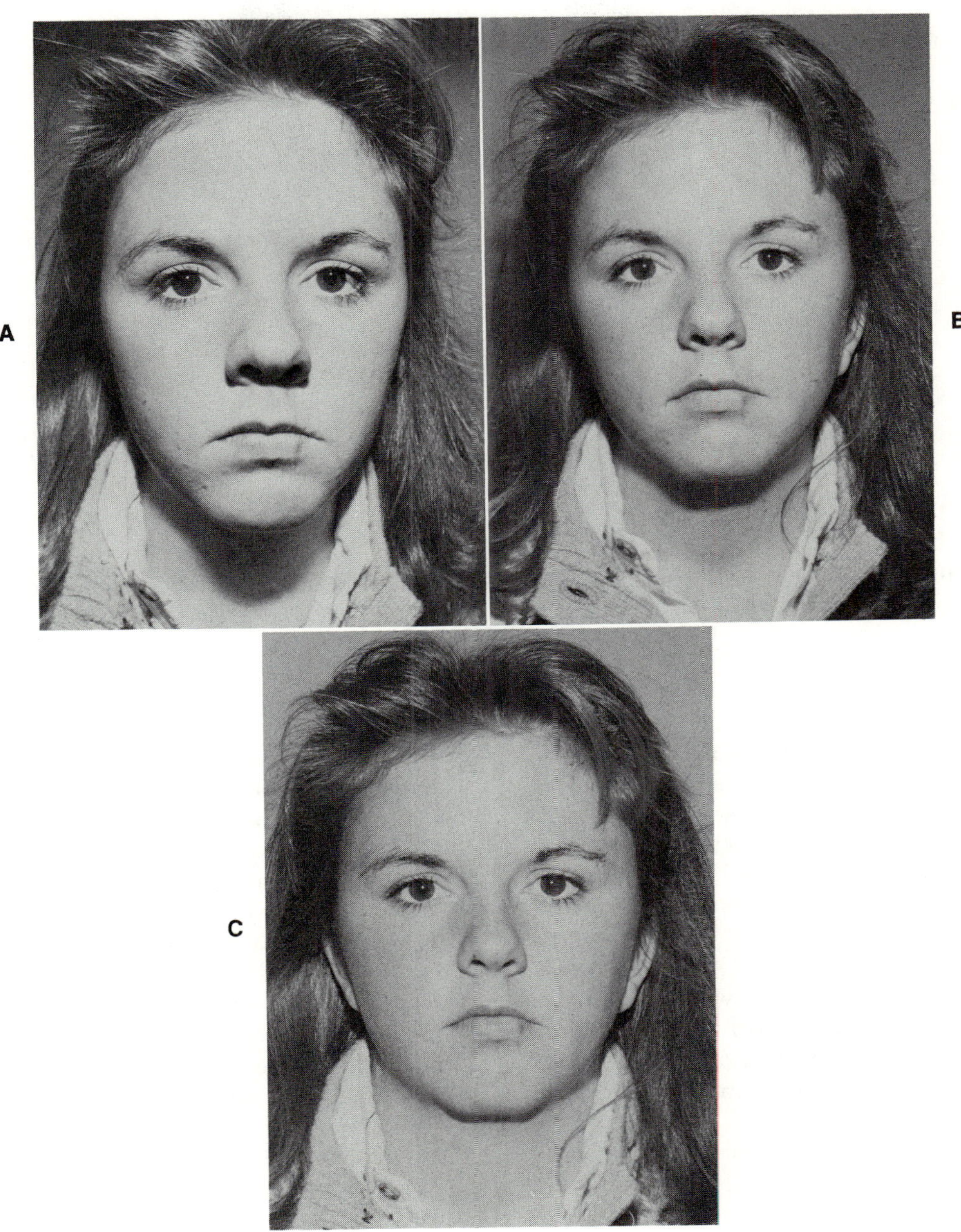

Fig. 19-6. Distortion produced by foreshortening. These photographs were taken from a distance that would allow the image to fill the film frame. The shorter the focal length of the lens used, the closer the camera must be to the subject in order to fill the frame. **A** was taken with a 28 mm lens, **B** with a 50 mm lens, and **C** with a 100 mm lens. Note that when the camera is moved closer to the subject, objects in the foreground are magnified, producing distortion. Note also that the 100 mm lens yields the most normal perspective.

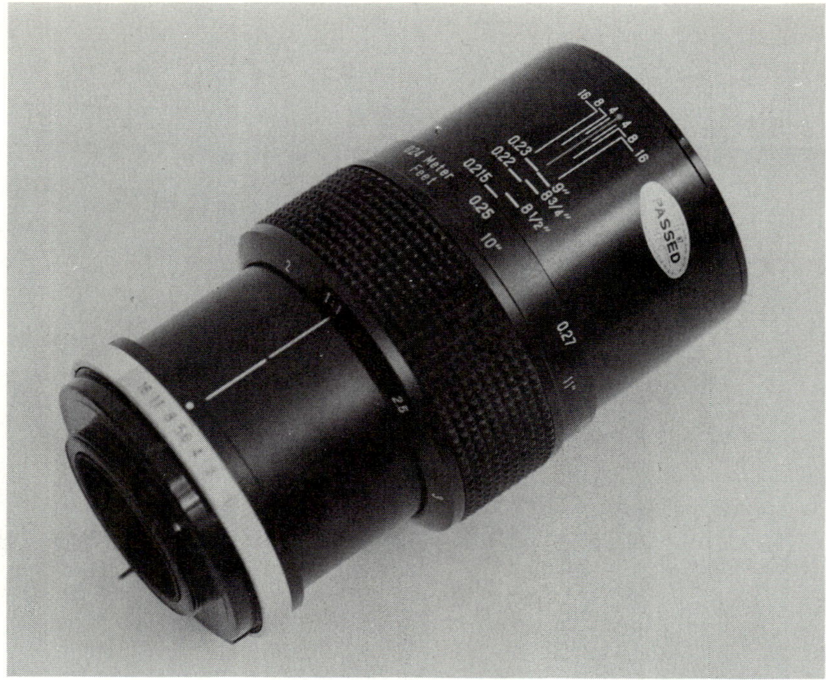

Fig. 19-7. Macro lens. A true macro lens is capable of life size, or 1:1 reproduction ratio, as shown here by the markings on the lens barrel. When used for other than close ups, it acts as a normal lens of the designated focal length.

length of a lens, the greater the depth of field. Similarly, the longer the focal length, the less the depth of field. Changing the aperture of a lens affects both exposure and depth of field. The smaller the aperture, the greater the depth of field; but this is accomplished by a corresponding reduction in the amount of light transmitted to the film.

A number of options are available to produce the proper magnification and angle of view for good clinical photographs. Remember that the goal is to fill the frame of the photograph without distortion of the subject and to devise a system that will give reproducible results each time.

Macro lenses (Fig. 19-7). A macro lens, by definition, is capable of producing an image on the film equal to or larger than life size. This is usually expressed as 1:1 or 1× reproduction. While a macro lens has this capability, it will also act as a lens of the designated focal length when used in other than the macro function. Thus a 100 mm macro lens not only can focus closely enough to yield a one-to-one reproduction ratio, but also is a medium telephoto lens otherwise. This, then, permits this type lens to record normal perspective of a face, and at the same time allows it to accurately record, life-size, a small lesion.

Zoom lenses (Fig. 19-8). A zoom lens allows, within certain limits, the focal length to be varied. This gives the photographer a continuously variable focal length within the design limits of the lens. It allows changes in framing and composition without varying the camera to subject distance. In theory, at least, it should replace several single focal length lenses but this is not done without some compromise in speed and simplicity of operation.

The average zoom lens is heavier and bulkier than a fixed focal length lens. Its design is such that the maximal aperture is less than that of a single focal length lens. Also, unless you are careful to set the focal length at precisely the same mark when taking pre- and postoperative or comparison photographs, you may introduce variables in composition and perspective that make the photographs invalid or deceptive.

Many zoom lenses are referred to as "macro zoom." This is a misnomer, since most of them have a maximal reproduction ratio from 1:2 to 1:6; not the 1:1 of a true macro lens. These lenses, then, should be called "close focusing" rather than "macro." The limitations in maximal reproduction ratio may negate the advantages of variable focal length for clinical photography.

Accessories for close-up photography

Close-up lenses. Close-up lenses (Fig. 19-9) provide the simplest and least expensive way to take close-up photographs with a normal focus lens. These are simple magnifying lenses that attach to the front of the camera lens and make it possible to focus on subjects nearer the cam-

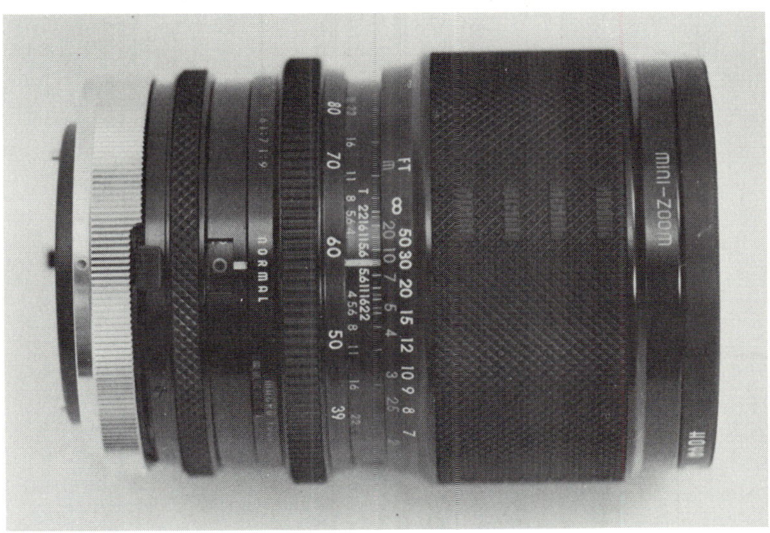

Fig. 19-8. Zoom lens. The focal length of this lens can be varied from 39 mm to 80 mm. It is advertised as a macro lens, but the maximal reproduction ratio is only ⌐:3.5; therefore, it should be called a close focusing, rather than a macro lens.

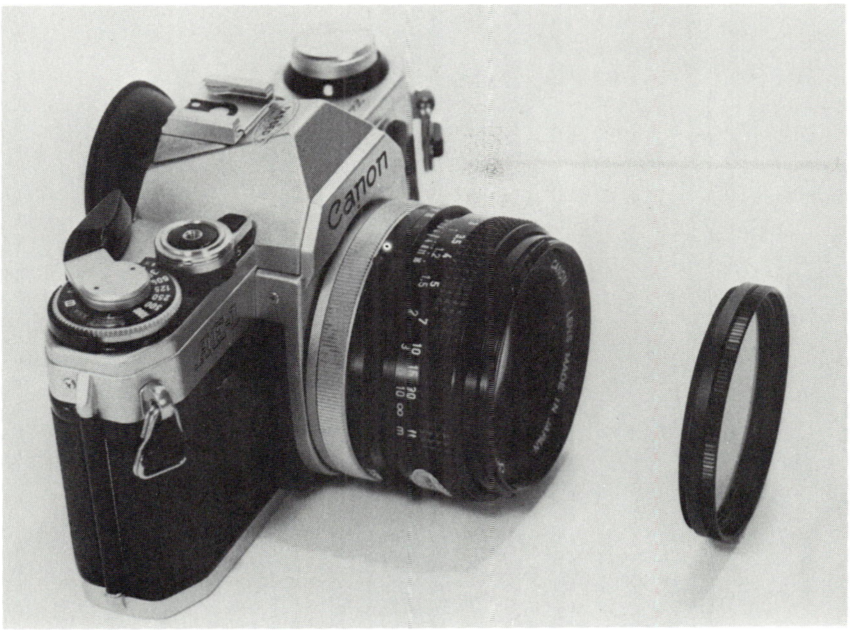

Fig. 19-9. Close-up lens. A magnifying lens that, when attached to the front of the camera lens, allows close focusing and magnification of small objects. These are available in several strengths measured in diopters and may be used singly or in combination.

era than would be possible with the camera lens alone. The strength of the accessory lens is expressed in diopters. The larger the number, the closer one can get to the subject. Close-up lenses can be used in combination to increase magnification. Combining a +1 and a +4 will have the effect of a +5 diopter lens. If you do combine these lenses, place the stronger one closest to the camera lens, then add the weaker one. There will be some loss in sharpness of focus if the lenses are combined.

Although close-up lenses are convenient to use, they have limitations. Because they produce a very shallow depth of field, focusing is critical. Also, distortion may be a problem, particularly with those of higher magnification. It is necessary to remove the close-up lens in order to photograph subjects at a normal distance from the camera, thus these lenses do not have the flexibility of a macro lens.

Extension tubes. Extension tubes (Fig. 19-10) are another accessory that will permit close-up photography with a normal focal length lens. The extension tube is simply a hollow ring which, when inserted between the camera body and lens, increases the focal length of the lens by increasing, the lens-to-film distance, thus increasing magnification. Since this tube has no optics in it, there is less chance of distortion or flare, such as with close-up lenses.

There are some disadvantages to the use of extension tubes. As with the close-up lenses, the extension tube must be removed to take photographs at normal distances. Also, increasing the distance between the lens and film decreases the amount of light transmitted to the film; thus exposure must be increased to compensate for

this. The amount of increase in exposure necessary for various length extension tubes may be determined from a built-in meter in the camera, from tables supplied with the tubes, or from a formula. This formula is derived from the fact that the effective f number is the ratio between the size of the diaphragm opening and the focal length of the lens. For example, a 50 mm lens set at f16 will have an aperture diameter of 3.125 mm (50 ÷ 16 = 3.125). If a 50 mm extension tube is inserted, the effective focal length of the lens is increased to 100 mm. Set at f16 the aperture diameter will still be 3.125 mm, but the effective f stop will be f32 (100 ÷ 3.125 = 32). From these facts the following formula can be used to determine the amount of exposure increase necessary for a given lens—extension tube system:

$$f = FL \div A$$

where

    f = Effective f stop of the lens–extension tube combination
    FL = Effective focal length of the lens-tube combination (focal length of lens plus length of tube)
    A = Diameter of the aperture at which the lens is set

For example, if you are using a 50 mm lens with a 50 mm extension tube and the indicated exposure for a normal lens is 1/60 second at f8, then:

$$f = FL \div A$$
$$f = 50 + 50 \div 6.25$$
$$f = 100 \div 6.25$$
$$f = 14.2 \ (f16)$$

In other words, you must increase exposure by two stops to compensate for the increase in focal length.

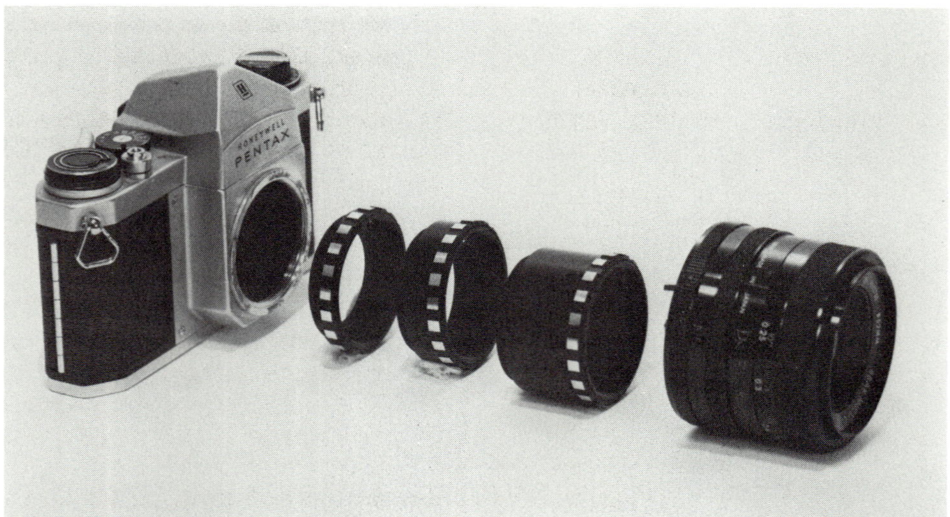

Fig. 19-10. Extension tubes. A hollow tube that, when inserted between the camera body and lens, increases the lens to film distance, thus magnification. These come in several lengths and may be used singly or in combination to vary the lens to film distance.

Extension tubes come in various lengths and may be added together to increase the lens-to-film distance. The greater the extension, the greater the magnification, but remember that as this distance is increased less light is transmitted to the film and exposure must be increased to compensate. When the amount of extension equals the focal length of the lens, a 1:1 reproduction ratio is achieved.

Bellows. A bellows (Fig. 19-11) is another device that can be used to increase the lens-to-film distance for close-up photography. Like extension tubes, it increases the lens-to-film distance; but unlike extension tubes the bellows can vary this distance over a continuous range. The reproduction ratio of extension tubes is usually 1:1. A bellows, however, can give a reproduction ratio of up to 1:4.

Most bellows are manufactured by the camera makers and are designed to fit only their cameras. Others may be adapted to various cameras with a T mount. These mounts, in addition to permitting the bellows to be used on different cameras, allow the use of a variety of lenses, some of which are made especially for ultra close-up work.

As with extension tubes, increasing the effective focal length of the lens will require an increase in exposure. The same formula described for this increase with extension tubes applies to the bellows. Most bellows have a focusing rail with a scale to indicate the amount of extension. From this, the effective focal length of the bellows-lens combination can be determined and used in the formula. Of course, if the camera has a built-in exposure meter, proper exposure can be read from this.

A camera with a bellows attached is somewhat bulky and cumbersome. Also, with full extension a slow shutter speed may be necessary for optimal exposure and depth of field. For these reasons, a tripod is advised to hold the camera steady when using bellows. A good way to start when using a bellows is to set the lens-film extension, then move the camera back and forth until the subject is in focus. If you want more magnification of an object and still want to fill the frame, it will be necessary to increase the lens-to-film distance by moving the lens mount forward on the focusing rail. If the focusing rail prohibits getting close enough to the subject, then the extension can be increased by moving the front mount as far forward as possible, then varying the extension by moving the rear standard backward.

Surprisingly enough, a shorter focal length lens will give greater magnification with the same amount of bellows extension than will one with a longer focal length. Remember that a 1:1 reproduction ratio exists when the amount of bellows extension equals the focal length of the lens. Thus a 100-mm lens with 100-mm extension gives a 1:1 reproduction ratio. Changing the lens to 50-mm with the same extension will give a reproduction ratio of $2 \times$ (100 ÷ 50 = 2).

A bellows system is also useful for copying slides. Many bellows have an attachment that makes this possible. Most of these are mounted on the focusing rail in front of the lens and permit at least 1:1 copying, if not

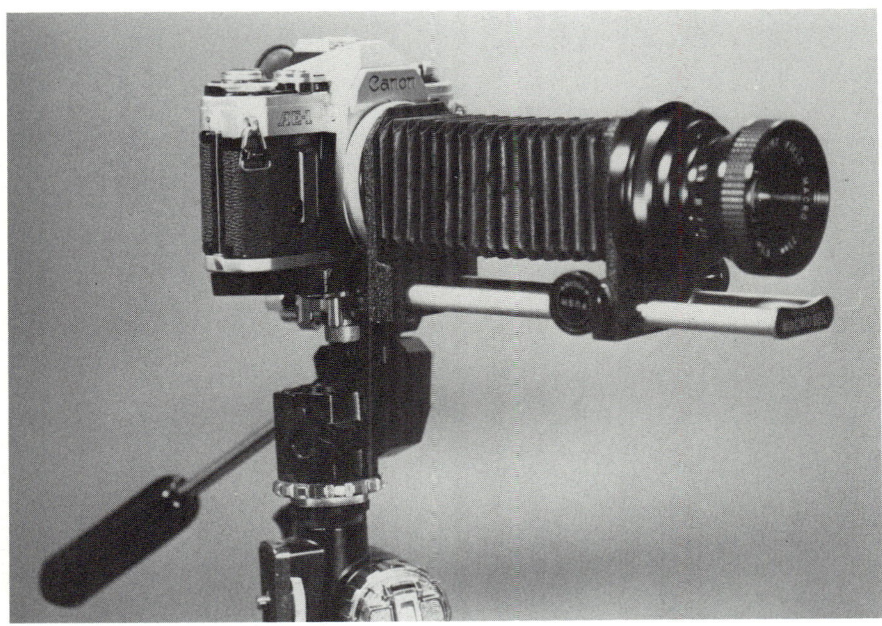

Fig. 19-11. Bellows. A bellows, like extension tubes, increases the lens to film distance, but can do it over a continuously variable range.

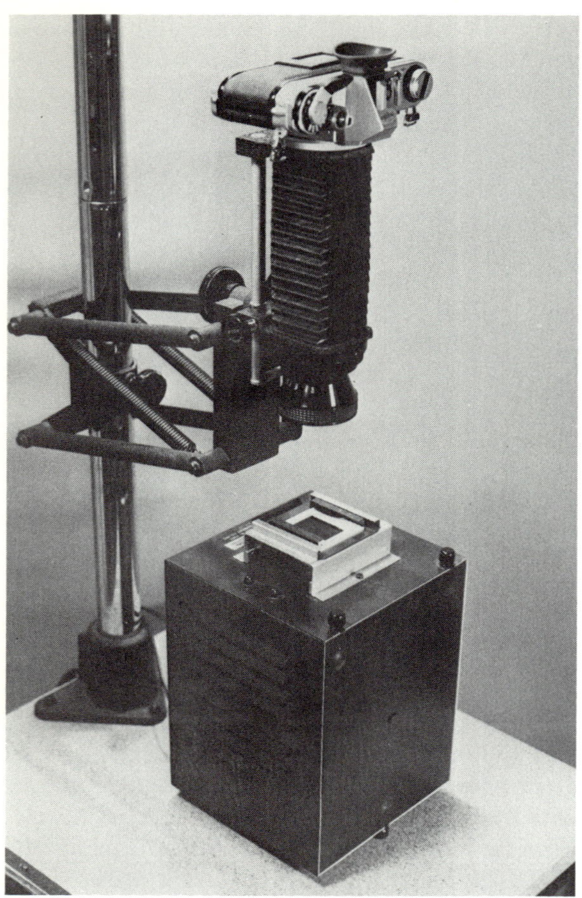

Fig. 19-12. With an appropriate lens and light source, a bellows can be used to copy slides. Since the amount of magnification can be varied with the bellows, this type equipment allows cropping of the original slide.

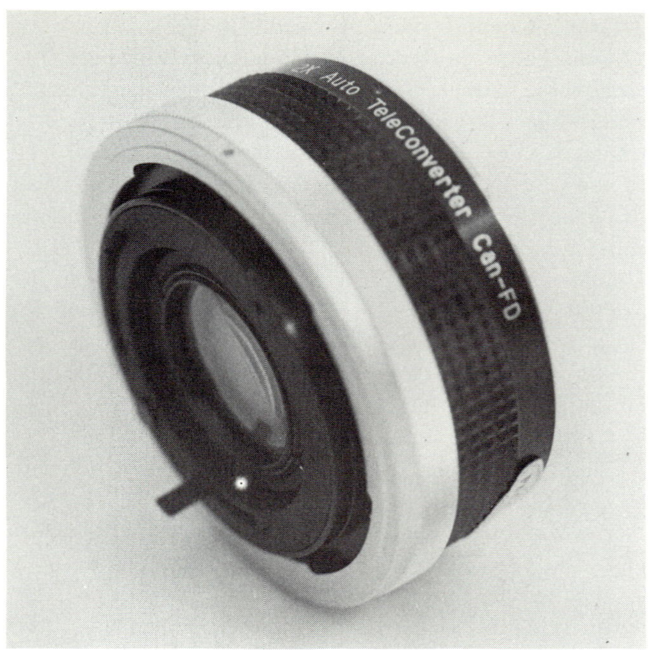

Fig. 19-13. A teleconverter contains a negative or Barlow lens. This is a 2× converter, which doubles the effective focal length of the lens to which it is attached. It also reduces the effective aperture of the lens by two stops.

some degree of magnification or cropping. These attachments are made for a specific bellows and will usually not fit another type. A bellows system may also be used with a copying stand and illuminator for slide copying (Fig. 19-12). For copying slides a flat field lens is recommended, since a normal camera lens may produce blurred edges on the duplicate slide.

Teleconverter. A teleconverter (Fig. 19-13) is another method of increasing the focal length of a lens. This consists of an extension containing a negative lens, which fits between the camera and the lens. These are available in two fixed power or magnification ratios: 2× and 3×. A 2× teleconverter will double the focal length of the lens to which it is attached, while the 3× will triple the focal length. With a teleconverter attached, the prime lens will still focus down to its normal minimal distance.

These facts would seem to make the teleconverter an ideal attachment for close-up photography. A 50-mm lens with a 3× converter becomes a 150-mm lens with the ability to focus as closely as 24 inches. There are, however, some disadvantages that negate much of this apparent advantage. While the teleconverter doubles or triples the effective focal length of the lens without changing the size of the aperture, at the same time it doubles or triples the effective aperture of the lens. Thus a 50-mm f2 lens with a 2× converter has an effective focal length of 100-mm, but its effective aperture is reduced to f4. This not only reduces the amount of light reaching the film, but also results in a dimmer image in the viewfinder, making critical focusing more difficult.

Consider also that most lenses require stopping down to at least f4 for the best definition. Since a teleconverter introduces additional optics into the light path of the image, there may be degradation of the performance of the prime lens, making stopping down even further mandatory to produce optimal definition. This means that the minimal aperture when using a 2× converter should be f8 (f11 for a 3×). Obviously, then, with this combination much slower shutter speed or a faster film must be used.

In general, because the teleconverter sacrifices at least two to three stops in aperture and may seriously degrade the performance of the prime lens, it is not a good choice for clinical photography.

Lighting

Lighting for clinical photography should be such that it will record the subject as accurately as possible. A simple system will accomplish this most of the time, but special circumstances may require special lighting for accuracy.

Most of us are used to viewing objects in sunlight. Good clinical lighting should duplicate this as nearly as possible. Think a minute about how we percieve an object that is illuminated by sunlight. The light source is from above, there is only one set of shadows, all cast in the same direction, and there is discernible detail in both the highlights and shadows.

The characteristics of light about which we are concerned are the quantity, quality, and color. The quantity depends upon the amount of light produced by the source, the transmission efficiency of the light reflector, and the distance of the light source from the subject.

Quality refers to the relative softness or hardness of the light. Specular light is composed of direct, parallel rays and produces crisp, sharp rendering of the subject. This is best for clinical photographs. Diffuse light has a softer quality because the rays have been broken up or scattered. It is flattering for portraits, but not suited for clinical work since it rarely portrays the subject or clinical conditions accurately.

The color temperature of light is measured in degrees Kelvin. This is dependent upon the light souce (Table 19-1). The color temperature is important not only in accurate reproduction of the subject being photographed, but also in the selection of the proper film. Color films are made to be used with a specific light source or color temperature, and these must be matched for accurate color rendition. Daylight color film is balanced, as the name suggests, for daylight or for electronic flash, which has a color temperature of approximately 6000 K. If this film is used with incandescent illumination, the pictures will have a yellow or orange tone.

Two types of color film are available for use with artificial light: type A, which is balanced for use with 3400 K photofloods, and type B, intended for use with 3200 K tungsten lamps. Even the 200 degree difference will make a discernible difference in color rendition if improperly used. If tungsten films are exposed in daylight the photographs will have an overall bluish cast.

Different types of color films can be balanced to the light source with appropriate filters (Table 19-2). If filters are used, remember that an exposure increase will usually be necessary to compensate for the loss of light transmission caused by the filter. Black-and-white film is

Table 19-1. Color temperatures

Light source	Degrees Kelvin
Electronic flash	6000-7000
Blue flashbulb	6000
Average noon sunlight	5500
Clear flashbulb	4000
Photoflood lamp	3400
Tungsten photolamp	3200
100 watt household bulb	2800

Table 19-2. Color correction filters

Film type	Light source	Filter	Exposure increase
Daylight	Daylight	None	None
	Electronic flash	None	None
	Blue flashbulb	None	None
	Photoflood (3400K)	80A	2⅓ stops
	Photolamp (3200K)	80B	2 stops
	Fluorescent	FL-D	1 stop
Type A	Daylight	85A	⅔ stop
	Electronic flash	85A	⅔ stop
	Photoflood (3400K)	None	None
	Photolamp (3200K)	82A	⅓ stop
	Fluorescent	FL-B	1 stop
Type B	Daylight	85B	⅔ stop
	Electronic flash	85B	⅔ stop
	Photoflood (3400K)	81A	⅓ stop
	Photolamp (3200K)	None	None
	Fluorescent	FL-B	1 stop

sensitive to all light sources equally, and usually no filtration is needed unless necessary to emphasize or minimize certain colors.

Three types of lighting are used in clinical photography: flat, contour, and texture. Flat lighting is produced by one light source, usually near and slightly above the axis of the camera. It provides even distribution of light over the entire subject. This type is best for most clinical situations, particularly to accurately depict lesions that might be lost in shadows. It also most nearly duplicates the lighting in which we are used to viewing subjects. In addition, it has the advantage of requiring only one light source.

Contour lighting requires at least two, sometimes more, sources of light. At a minimum a main light source and a fill light are necessary. This type light, as the name suggests, is most useful for recording changes in contour; but if used in other situations may actually distort or eliminate important details, particularly in shadow areas.

Texture lighting is useful to portray certain conditions, such as the scarring of acne, or to emphasize the contours of elevated lesions. This is produced by directing the light source across the surface of the area to be recorded.

Types of lighting

Incandescent or photoflood. This type lighting (Fig. 19-14) allows the photographer to view the effects of light placement before taking the picture. It can be moved or adjusted for optimal lighting of the subject. It is, however, bulky and best used in an area specifically set aside for clinical photography. This type of lighting is difficult to use in the operating room, the patient's room, or even in the average office setting. If this type is used, the film must be balanced to the light source, using either 3200 or 3400 K bulbs and the appropriate film.

Available light. Available light, whether sunlight, incandescent, fluorescent room light, or the operating room light is seldom satisfactory for clinical photography. There are too many variables in both direction and color temperature of the light source to permit accurate and reproducible results. It should be used only in an emergency and with the realization that a less-than-satisfactory photograph may result.

Photoflash. The flashbulb was the first truly portable form of photographic illumination. It is still used in some forms of clinical photography, particularly with the simple systems, such as the Instatech. The newer flashcubes are more convenient than single flashbulbs, but are expensive and inconvenient, and their use should be restricted to those who take only an occasional clinical photograph. These require a film balanced to the proper color temperature.

Electronic flash. By far the most popular and useful light source for clinical photography is the electronic or "strobe" flash. It is relatively inexpensive, portable, and reliable. The duration of the flash is somewhere between 1/200 and 1/10,000 second, thus camera or subject motion is virtually eliminated. It produces a light with a color temperature roughly equivalent to sunlight and its light output is constant. These units derive their power from either an AC source or expendable or rechargable batteries; the cost per flash is significantly less than that of flashbulbs or flashcubes.

Electronic flash units are available in both manual and automatic types (Fig. 19-15). When the manual type is used the exposure is determined from a formula supplied by the manufacturer, and the proper exposure is achieved by setting the appropriate f stop on the camera lens. The automatic type has a built-in sensor that determines the amount of light reflected from the subject, then adjusts the light output of the unit. This type is simpler to use and may result in longer battery life, but may give poorly exposed photographs, since it reads reflectance from the entire subject being photographed. For example, if the most important area to be recorded is in the shadows and if the rest of the field is light, the automatic sensor will read the average reflectance from

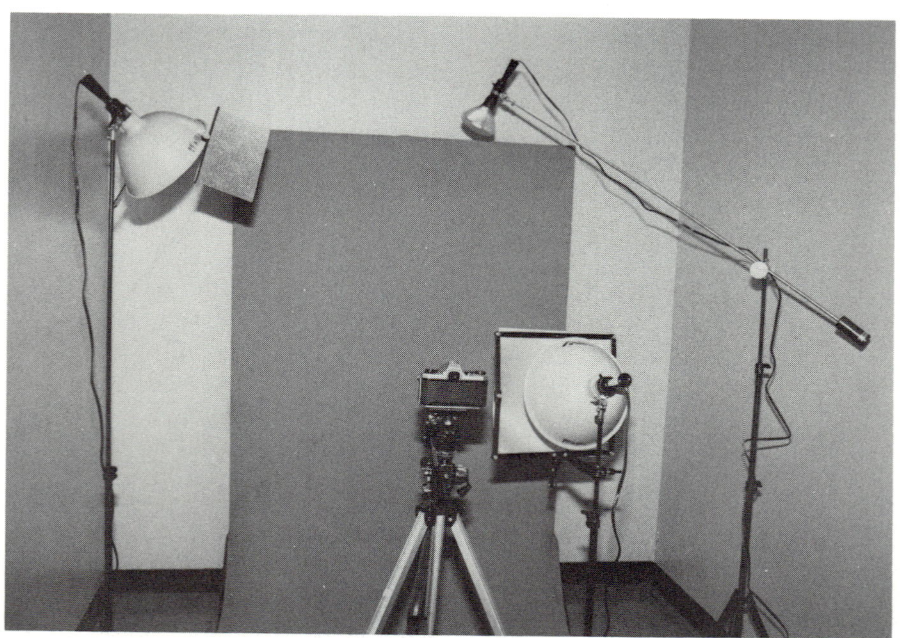

Fig. 19-14. Studio lighting with incandescent lights. This type lighting can produce excellent clinical photographs. Three lights are usually necessary and a special area must be set aside for their use.

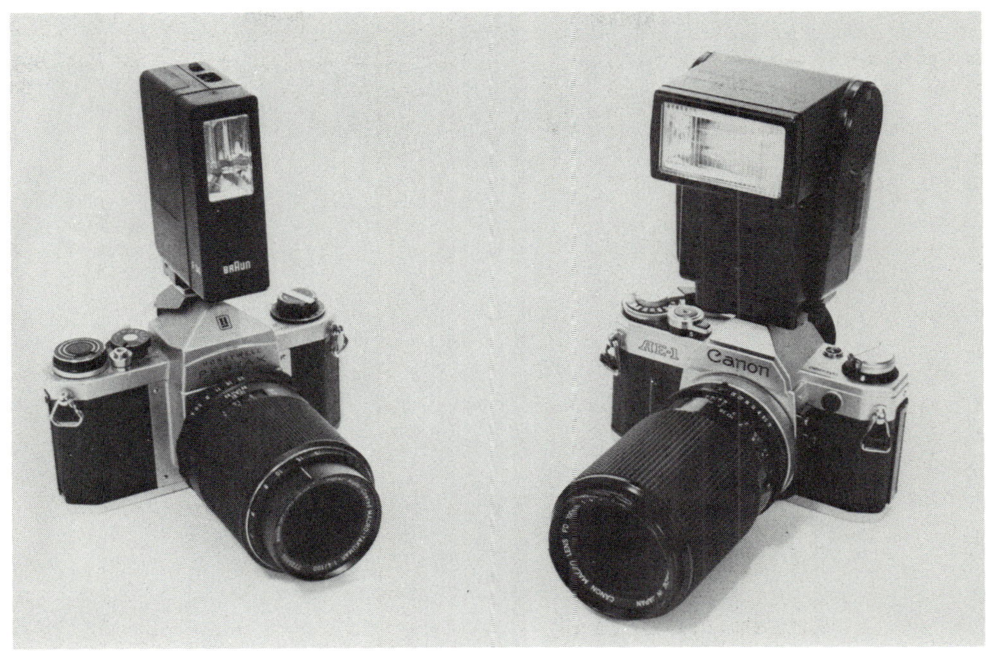

Fig. 19-15. Electronic flash units. The unit on the left is a manual type. Correct exposure settings when using this type are determined by dividing a guide number provided by the manufacturer by the flash-to-subject distance. The one on the right adjusts exposure automatically.

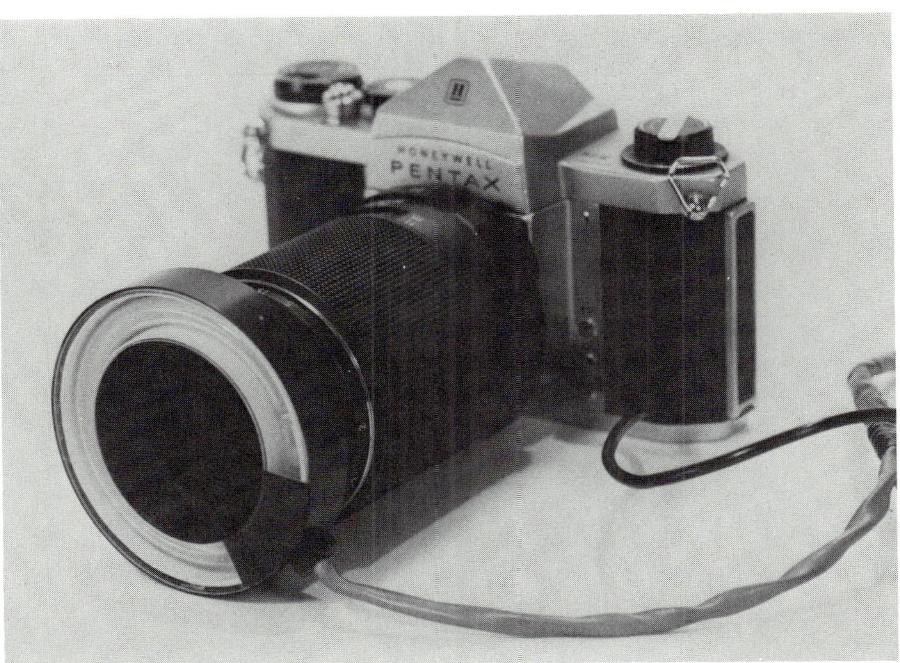

Fig. 19-16. Ring light. A circular electronic flashtube fits around the front of the camera lens. It produces a shadowless light and is particularly valuable for intraoral or cavity photographs.

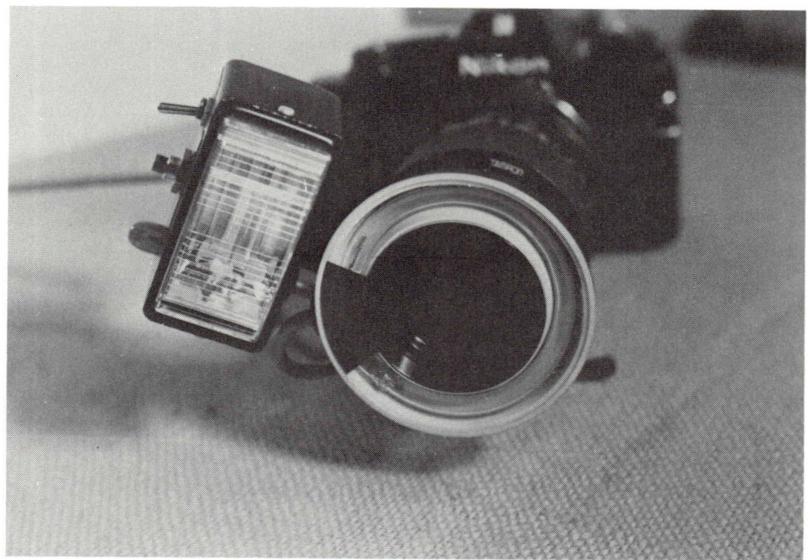

Fig. 19-17. Combination ring and point light. This allows the use of either ring or point light with a single unit. (Courtesy Lester A. Dine, Inc.)

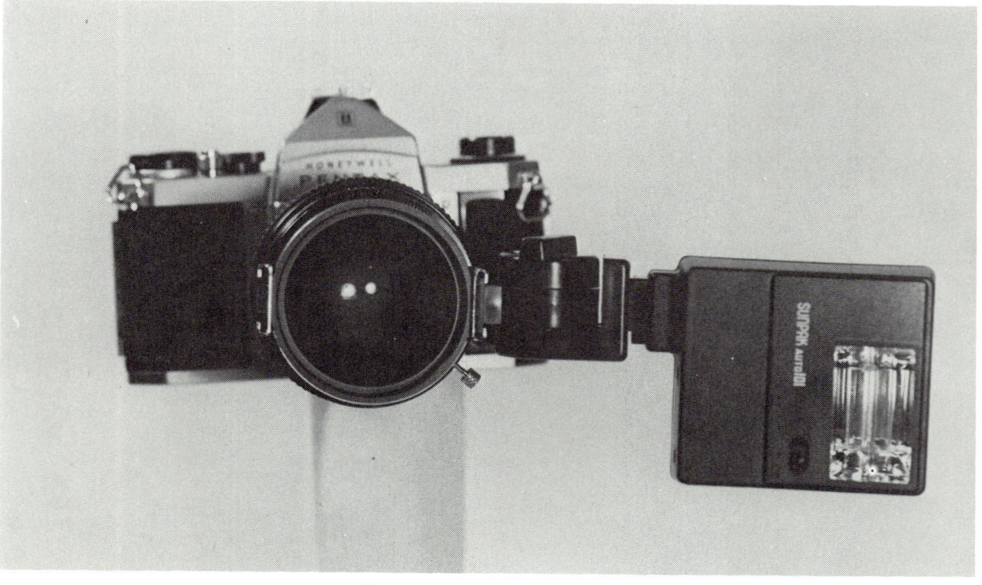

Fig. 19-18. Attachment for close up photographs. One or two small flash units can be attached to this, placing the light source at the end of the lens so that the subject can be completely lighted. This is especially important when taking extreme close-ups since the light from a camera-mounted flash may be masked by the lens when the camera-to-subject distance is short.

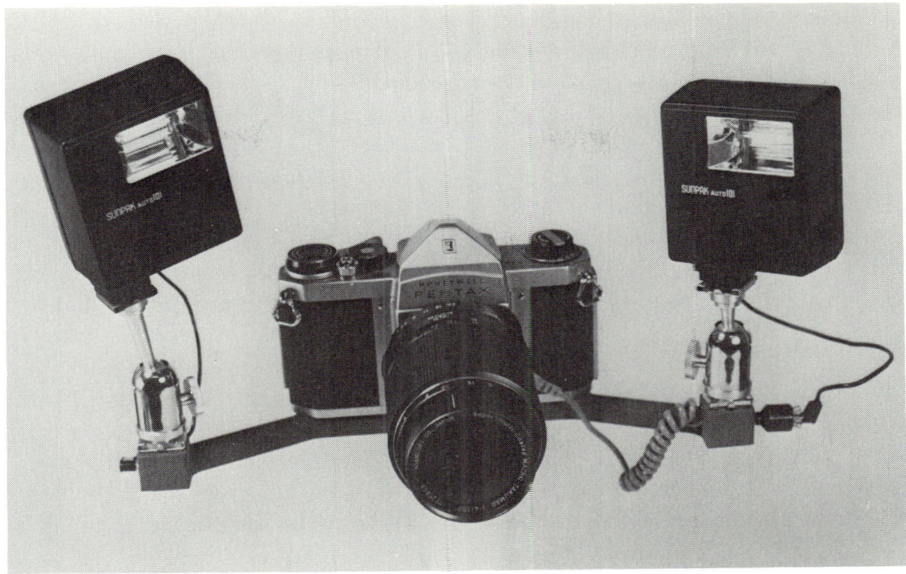

Fig. 19-19. Bracket for mounting two strobe units. This device attaches to the tripod socket of the camera and permits the use of two electronic flash units, one on each side of the camera. This arrangement helps to eliminate shadows and gives even lighting, but the lighting may be too flat to delineate some conditions accurately.

the field and may underexpose that portion within the shadows. For this reason, a manual flash unit is probably best for clinical work. If you do chose to use an automatic system, select one that can be set manually for those conditions in which the automatic function would be unsatisfactory.

A special type of electronic flash is known as the ring light. As the name suggests, the flash tube is circular and mounts around the lens of the camera (Fig. 19-16). This gives even illumination of the entire field and results in virtually shadowless light. This is an advantage when photographing the oral or other body cavities, but its flat lighting may distort raised or depressed lesions, wrinkles, or other contour abnormalities. If a ring light is used and if contour or directional lighting is desired, the unit may be removed from the camera and hand held to one side or the other.

There are other special units. One is a combination ring and point light, which can illuminate cavities but at the same time give enough directional light to provide modeling of raised or depressed lesions (Fig. 19-17). Another is a special mounting bracket that attaches one or two small strobe units to the lens barrel (Fig. 19-18). This, like the combination unit, will both illuminate cavities and give directional light for surface detail. It is particularly useful for extreme close-ups with a macro lens. Another unit has arms on which to mount two small strobes (Fig. 19-19). This gives bidirectional light, some

degree of modeling, and helps eliminate background shadows, but at the same time the lighting may be too flat to accurately portray shadow detail.

Electronic flash is also available as studio units. These are permanently mounted on stands, are somewhat bulky, and are expensive. If these are used, subject-to-flash distance and light placement may be standardized for reproducible results, but their size makes it necessary to set aside a separate area for photography, just as with studio type photoflood illumination.

PHOTOGRAPHING THE PATIENT

The purpose of a clinical photograph is to document—accurately—the status of a patient in a manner that is reproducible. This depends upon the placement of the camera relative to the subject, magnification, lighting, and background. All should be standardized so that subsequent photographs are taken from the same position, the same angle, and with identical lighting. Obviously, all photographs should be taken with a similar type camera and a lens of the same focal length. (See also Appendix C-7.)

The film plane of the camera must be parallel to the plane of the important features to be photographed. The center of the lens axis should be directed to the center of the features to be recorded, and the vertical axis of the subject should be parallel to the vertical axis of the film. For example, when the face is photographed, the center of the lens axis should be along the Frankfort horizontal line. In lateral views the ear should be included and the border on the nasal side should be wider than on the occipital side.

Background

The background should be plain, nonreflective, and of a neutral color, preferably a medium blue. Black and white backgrounds are not good choices. Do not include any distracting features in the background (Fig. 19-20).

Lighting

The lighting for all photographs must also be standardized. The light-to-subject distance should be constant and from the same direction. In general, lighting that is from slightly above and parallel to the lens axis is best. If a shoe-mounted strobe is used, this is assured when the camera is in a horizontal position. If the camera is turned vertically, be sure the light is placed on the nasal side of the patient (Fig. 19-21).

Standards

It is impossible to overemphasize the importance of developing reproducible standards for clinical photographs. This must include comparable camera and lens, subject-to-camera distances, and lighting. One way to do this is to shoot a series of test exposures with your camera-lens-light combination and evaluate the results. Choose the best and then make a table or guide for all subsequent photographs. By doing this and by using a comparable background for all photographs, you can ensure duplicate results each time. An example of such a guide is shown in Table 19-3.

If other than routine frontal and lateral views of the face are taken, establish standards so that all subsequent photographs will be comparable. As an example, for a basal view align the tip of the nose with the eyebrows. By doing this, all photographs will have a similar angle of view. The same technique can be used for reproducible three-quarter views: align the oral commissure with the outer canthus of the eye on the same side (Fig. 19-22).

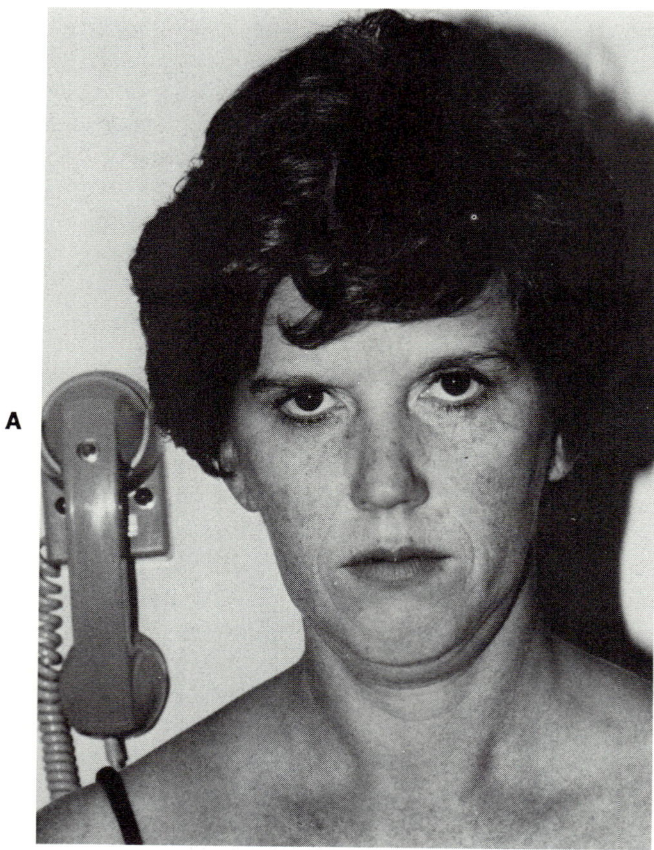

Fig. 19-20. Examples of distracting backgrounds. Compare the distracting backgrounds in **A, B, C,** and **D** with that in **E** in which a plain, neutral background is used.

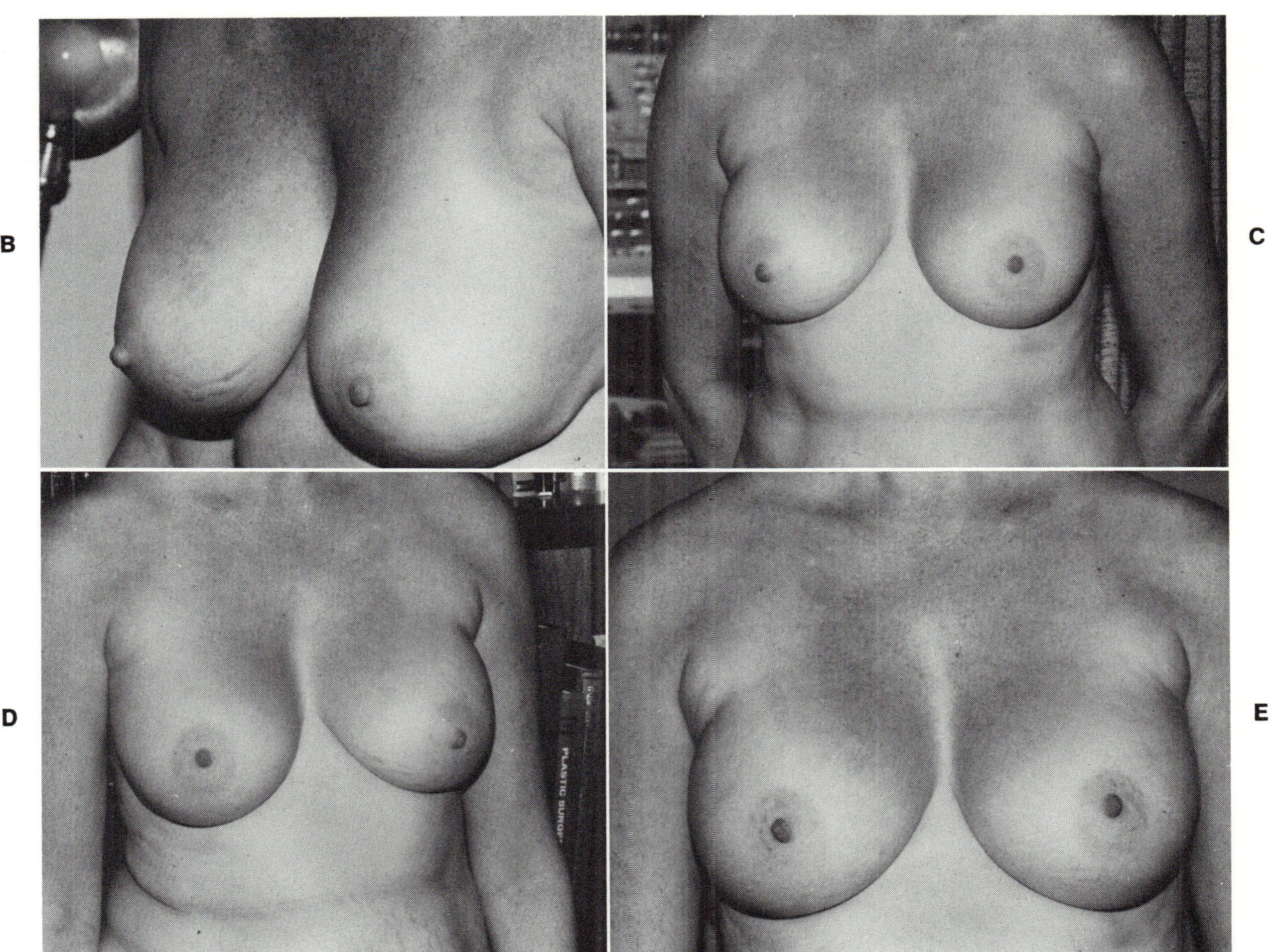

Fig. 19-20, cont'd. For legend see opposite page.

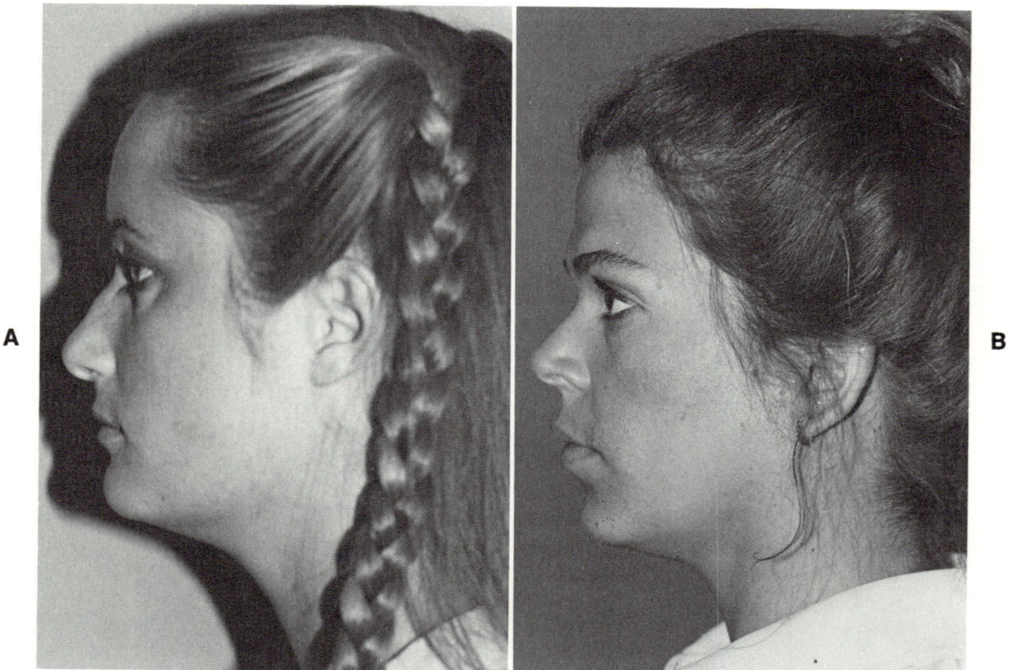

Fig. 19-21. Direction of lighting. **A,** The result of having the light source on the occipital side of the patient. **B,** The light is on the nasal side.

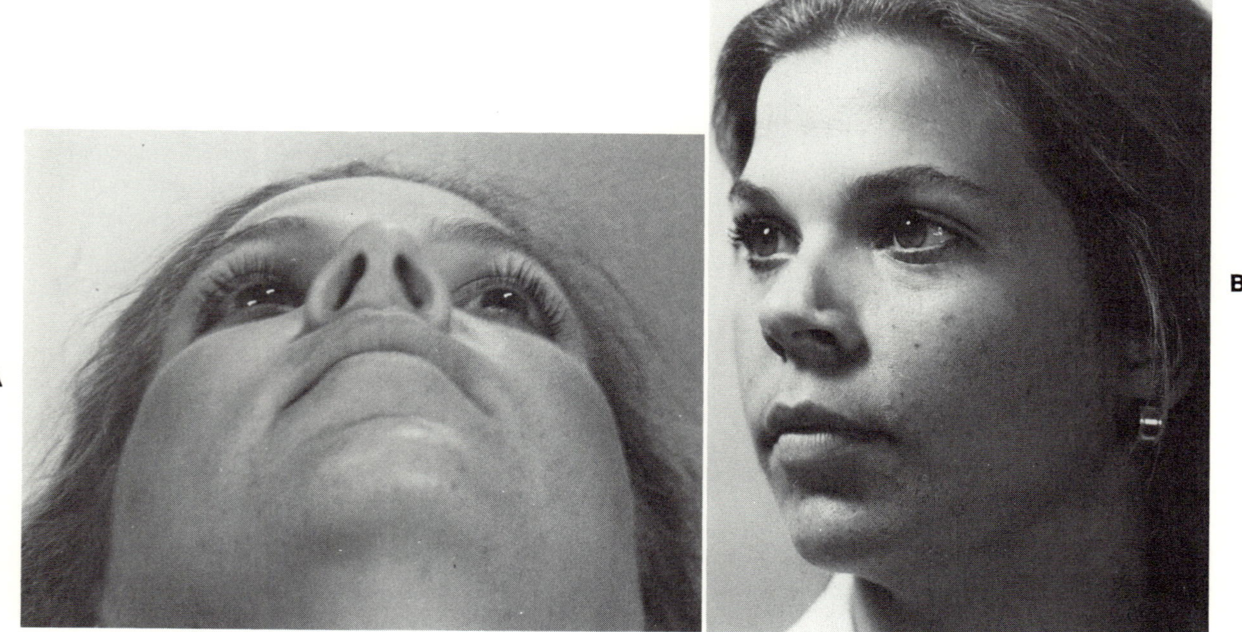

Fig. 19-22. Standards for special views. **A,** For a basal view of the face, align the tip of the nose with the eyebrows. **B,** For a three-quarter facial view, align the outer canthus of the eye with the oral commissure.

Table 19-3. Standardization of clinical photographic views (use with either 50 mm or 100 mm macro lenses)

Area	Ratio
Full body	10 feet (50 mm)
Half body	1:25
Legs	1:25
Breasts	1:15
Arms	1:15
Head or face	1:10
Hand	1:8
Eyes	1:5
Ears	1:4
Nose only	1:3
Mouth or lips	1:2.5
Teeth or intraoral	1:2

OPERATING ROOM PHOTOGRAPHY

Photography in the operating room is essentially the same as any other clinical photography with the exception that the equipment must be portable and that photographs may from time to time be taken by relatively inexperienced personnel. In general, the same equipment that is satisfactory for office photography will be suitable for operating room work. Obviously, multilight incandescent or strobe studio units will not be suitable for the average operating room photography; nor will available light. The best equipment will be a 35 mm single lens reflex, a 100 mm macro lens, and an electronic flash unit.

If preoperative photographs are to be taken in the operating room, pay as much attention to standardized views and to the background as you would in the office. A distracting background can be eliminated by having someone hold a surgical drape behind the patient. If this

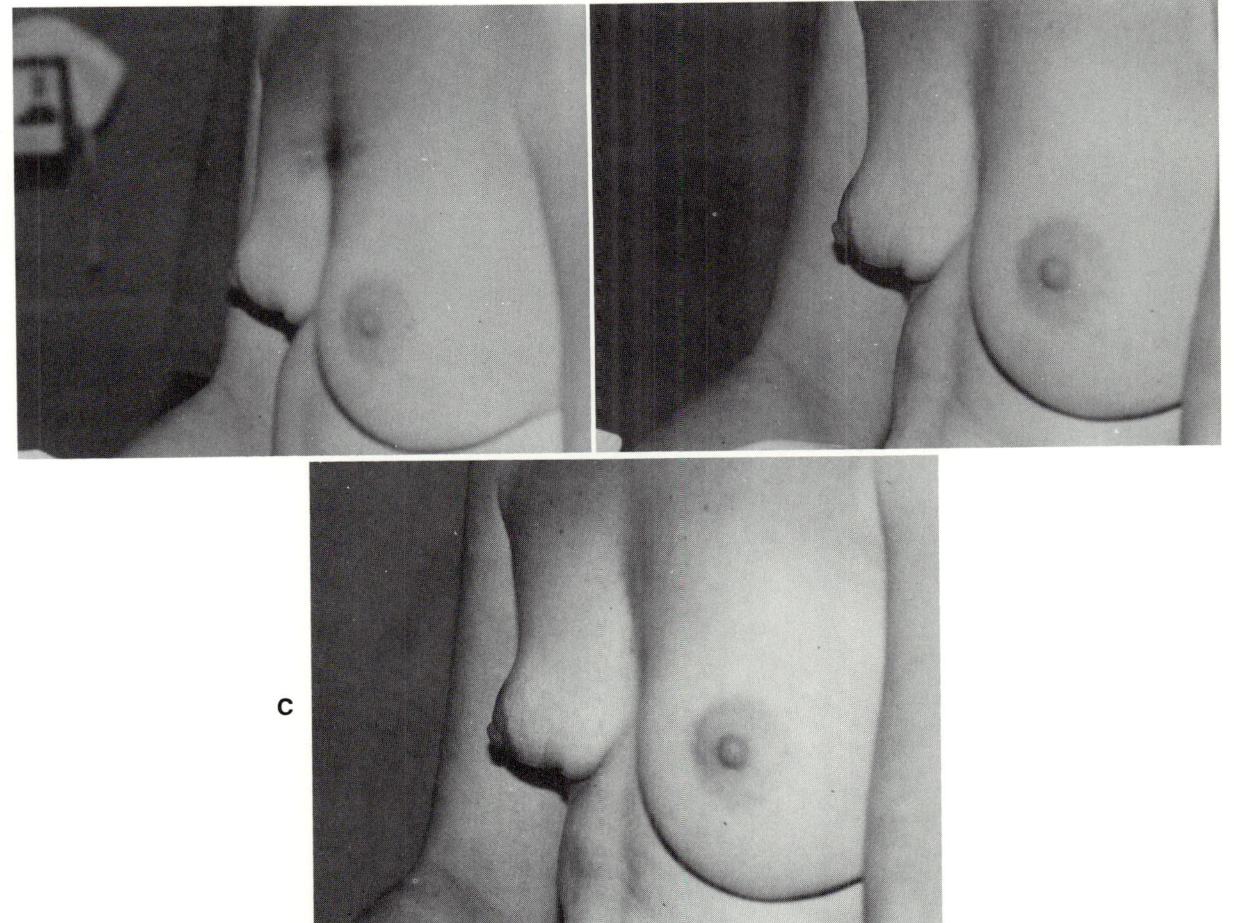

Fig. 19-23. Preoperative photographs in the operating room. **A,** A distracting background. The quality of the photograph can be improved as shown in **B** by either moving the equipment or changing the camera angle. It can also be improved by shooting at the widest possible aperture so that the background is thrown out of focus. **C,** An even better result is obtained by holding a drape behind the patient.

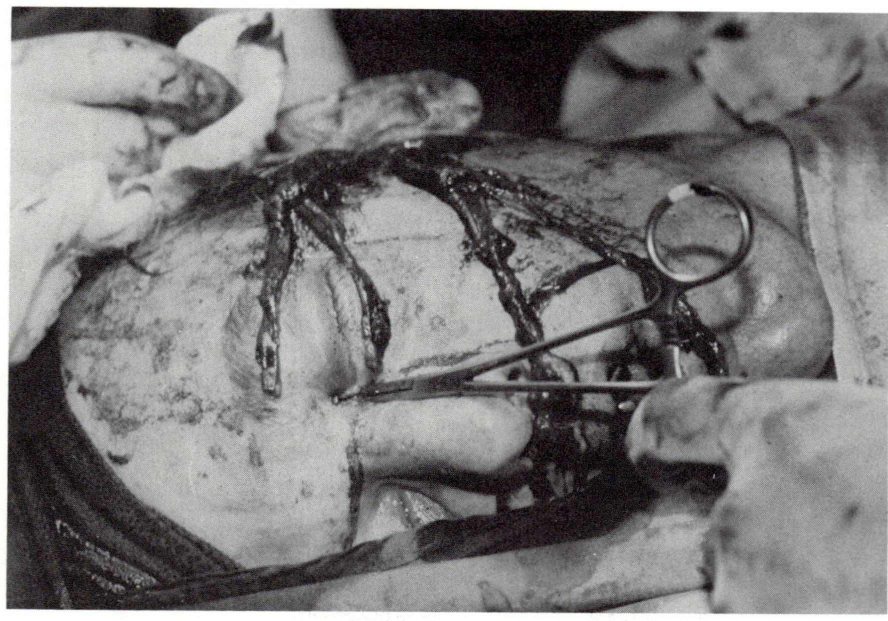

Fig. 19-24. The presence of blood and bloody drapes, instruments, and hands result in a poor intraoperative photograph.

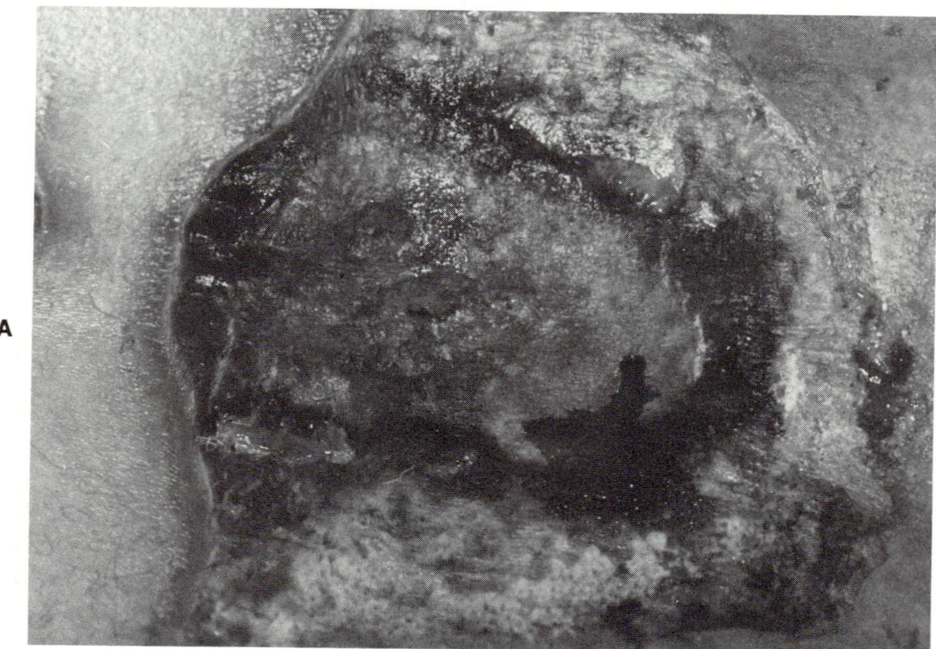

Fig. 19-25. Orientation of intraoperative photographs. **A,** Accurate depiction of the appearance of an electrical burn, but there is no information about its size or location.

is not possible, use as large an aperture as possible on the lens to reduce depth of field and to throw the background out of focus (Fig. 19-23).

Good intraoperative photographs must be done carefully and in good taste. Many of these have details which are, if not offensive, at least distracting. Common faults are the presence of bloody drapes, hands, sponges, or instruments in the field; or the inclusion of an extraneous or distracting background (Fig. 19-24).

A good intraoperative photograph should include enough anatomic landmarks in at least one picture to orient the viewer. Others in the series can be close-ups of the operative site. If no anatomic landmarks or reference points are shown, a ruler should be included to demonstrate the size of a defect or lesion (Fig. 19-25).

When intraoperative photographs are taken, the operative field should be cleansed and clean drapes applied. All extraneous instruments, sponges, and hands should be eliminated from the field of view. A clean drape can be held behind the operative field to eliminate any unnecessary background (Fig. 19-26). If possible, all photographs in an intraoperative sequence should be taken from the same angle and distance, using identical lighting.

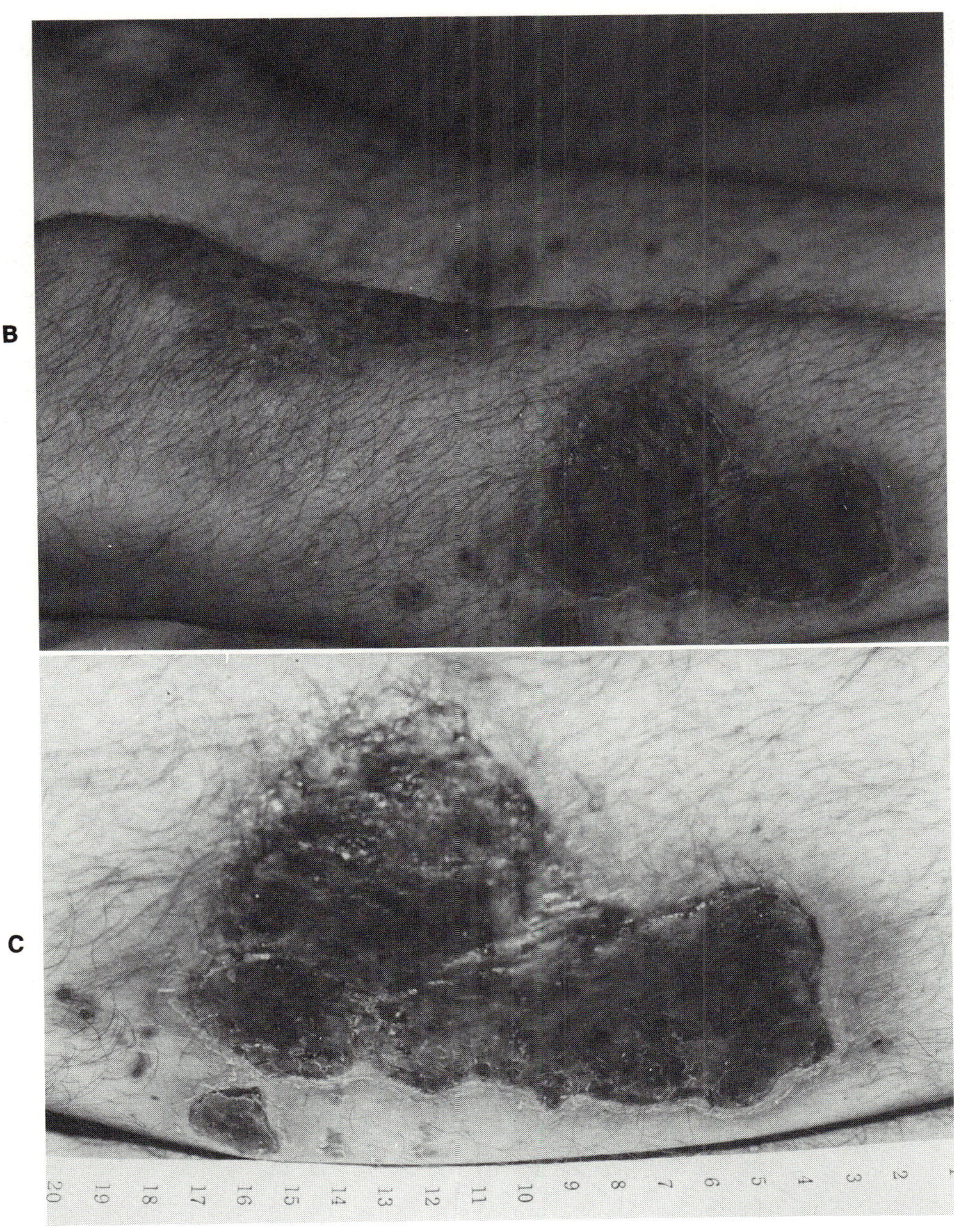

Fig. 19-25, cont'd. B, The location is shown. **C,** A ruler is added to the close-up photograph to indicate the size of the lesion.

Continued.

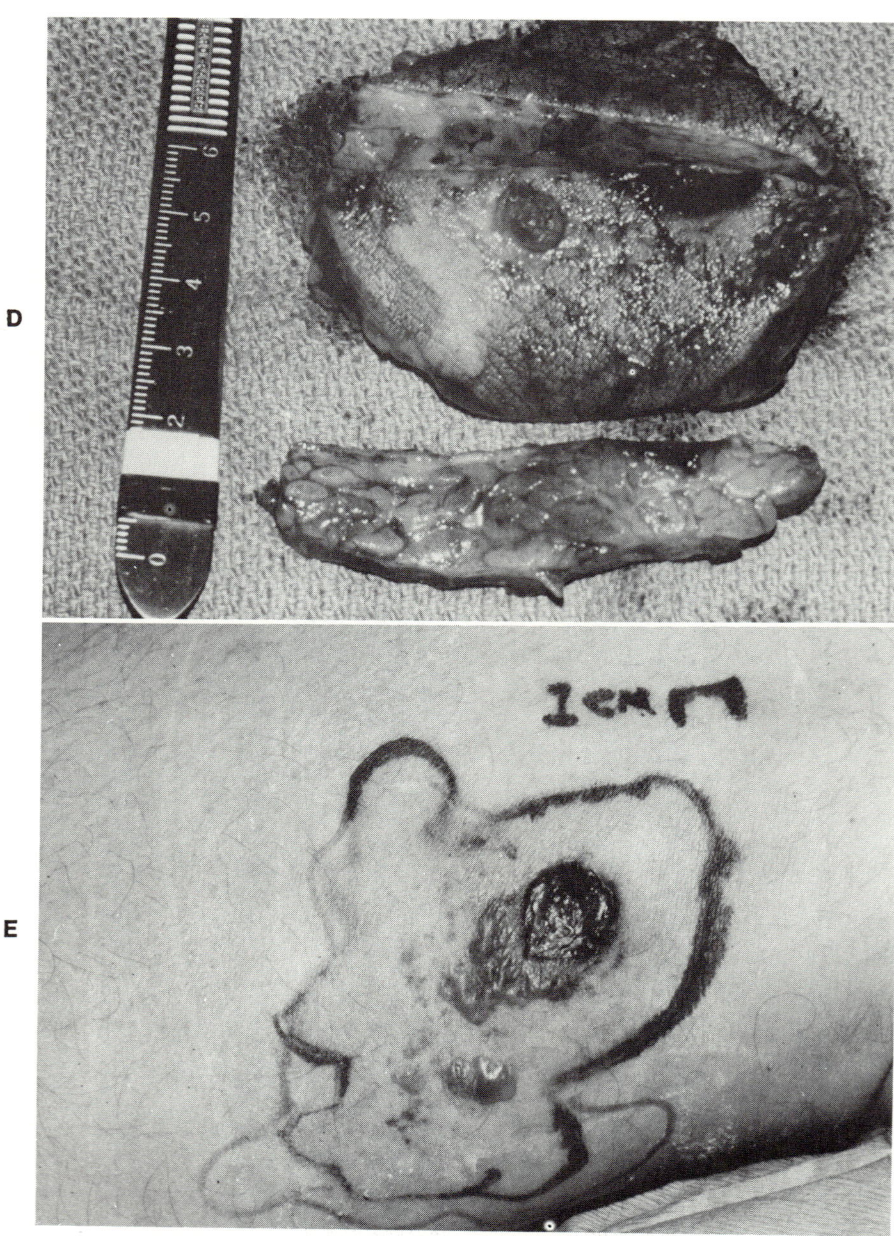

Fig. 19-25, cont'd. D, Similarly, the addition of a familiar surgical instrument to the photograph of the specimin indicates the size of the lesion. If you have no ruler or scale, simply draw an orienting measurement adjacent to the lesion, as in **E.**

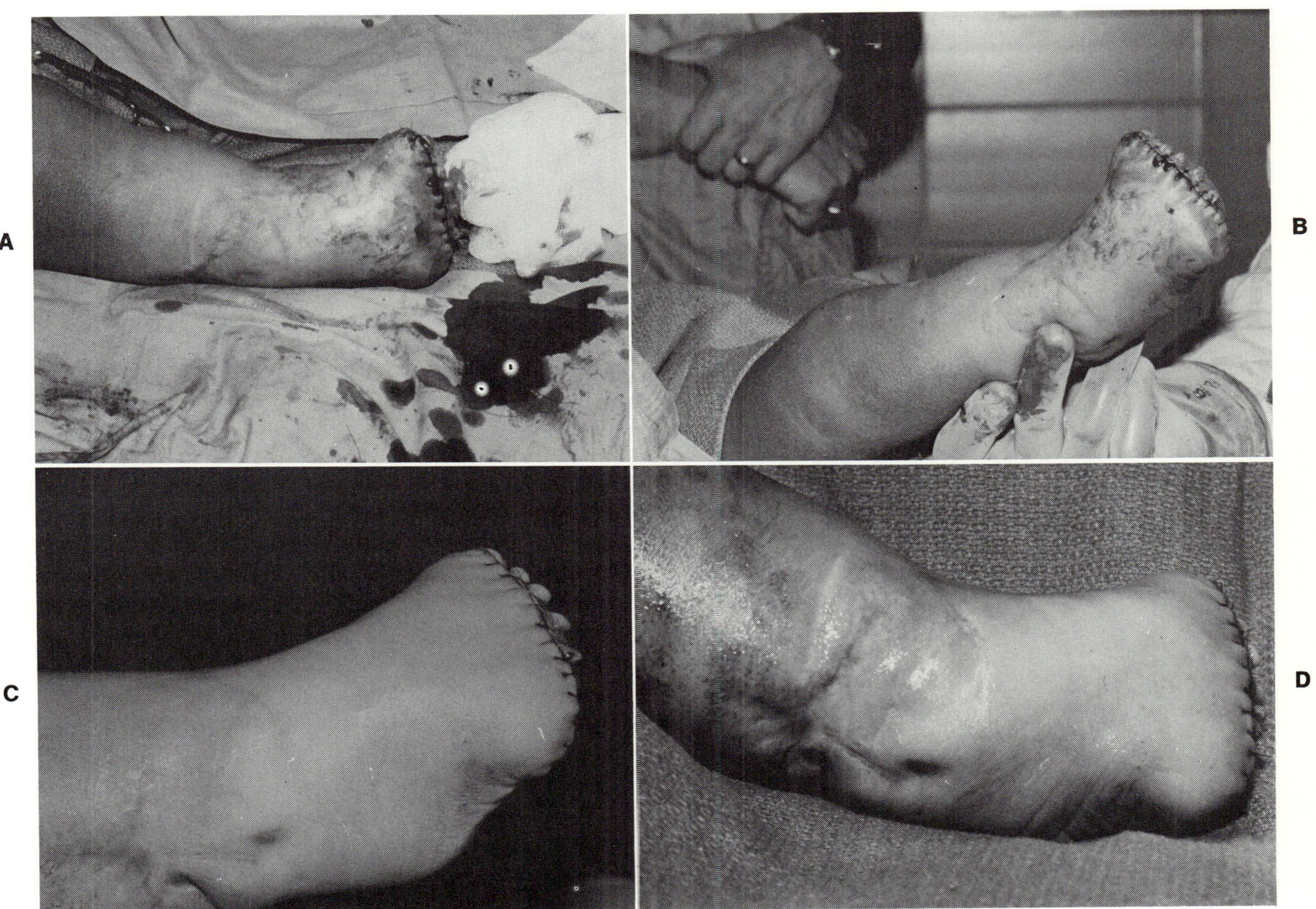

Fig. 19-26. How to improve intraoperative photographs. **A,** A poor intraoperative photograph. Note the presence of blood, dirty drapes, and sponges. **B,** The photograph is little better; there remain, blood, bloody gloves, and a distracting background. **C,** The area has been cleansed and a large aperture has been used to throw the background out of focus. **D,** the area has not only been cleansed, but a drape has been used as a background.

SUMMARY

Good clinical photography depends upon the selection of proper equipment, the selection of an appropriate source of lighting, the use of the proper film, and, most importantly, attention to detail in camera-to-subject placement and establishment of a routine that allows reproducibility of results.

The following are my recommendations for the equipment to be used for clinical photography. These are suggested as guidelines only. Before you buy any equipment, study your needs, determine what equipment is available to fit your budget, then acquire what will best fill your needs. You may want to start with a basic setup, then add additional equipment as the need arises or your budget permits.

Minimal equipment
  35 mm single lens reflex camera
  100 mm macro lens
  Electronic flash
Desirable, but not essential
  50 mm macro lens
  Bellows or extension tubes for extreme close-ups
  Slide copying device
  Copy stand
  Ring light or other special lighting equipment
Luxury
  Special photographic room with studio lighting

CHAPTER 20

Reproduction of photographs and artwork

Robert C. Reeder, M.D.

If a photograph is to be reproduced accurately in print, it must be of excellent quality. A black-and-white photograph is a continuous tone copy with infinite shading from light to dark, but a printer can work only in shades of gray or in densities expressed by the presence or absence of ink on the printed page. The printer uses a process called halftone in which dots of ink represent highlights and shadows. Larger dots of ink reproduce the shadows, medium sized ones the mid-range densities, and smaller ones the highlights. Areas of white have none. Since these dots are very small, the picture may appear as a continuous tone, but when viewed with a magnifying glass the pattern of the dots is apparent.

Two important factors determine if a print will reproduce well: contrast and sharpness of focus.

CONTRAST

The range of difference between the highlights and shadows is known as contrast. Mechanical reproduction has limits beyond which extreme tone ranges cannot be recorded accurately, nor can extremely light or dark tones be reproduced. You should, therefore, look for both highlight and shadow detail in a photograph that is to be mechanically reproduced. An overexposed print will be too light and have loss of detail in the highlights, while one that is underexposed will be too dark with loss of detail in the shadows. Given a choice, a slightly overexposed print is better, since the highlights usually carry the important details.

FOCUS

Medical photography demands that even the smallest detail be recorded sharply. Even the best photograph has but one plane of critical focus. There is often an acceptable range of focus, but still only one plane will be in *critical* focus. This may present no problem when reproduced mechanically unless an extreme enlargement is made, in which case all areas that are slightly out of the plane of critical focus will lose detail.

Sharpness of image depends upon accurate focus, lens aperture, and absence of motion in the camera or subject. The ground glass viewing screen of the single lens reflex camera helps ensure sharp focus. Focusing should be done with the lens at its largest aperture, but exposure made at the smallest aperture consistent with the light source, since smaller lens apertures increase the depth of field.

The area of most importance should be placed in the critical plane of focus. If several features are important, stop the lens down to increase the depth of field. If critical focusing throughout is not possible, those areas toward the background rather than those in the foreground should be out of focus.

Mounting the camera on a tripod will help minimize camera motion. A strobe light, with its very short flash duration, will eliminate motion in both the subject and camera.

FILM

A photograph intended for reproduction should be made on black-and-white film, although acceptable prints can be made from color negatives or transparencies. If you know at the time a photograph is taken that both color transparencies and black-and-white prints will be needed, use color negative film from which both, as well as color prints, can be made.

When making a black-and-white photograph, use a fine-grain panchromatic film, which is sensitive to all colors, rather than orthochromatic, which is sensitive only to blue and green. An exception is if you need to emphasize a faint pink lesion or subdermal blotches. In this case, use either an orthochromatic film or a panchromatic with a number 66 Wratten filter over the lens.

If a color transparency must be converted to a black-and-white print, make a copy negative with Panatomic X film, from which the print can be made. As an alternative, have a color internegative made, then make a black-and-white print on Kodak Panalure paper.

MAKING PRINTS

Be sure that the base color of the paper on which prints for reproduction are made is white. Many papers that are considered black-and-white have a cream or ivory base and thus do not reproduce true blacks and whites. The surface should be smooth—either a glossy surface that has been ferrotyped or a resin-coated paper that air dries to a high gloss. Avoid papers that have a texture or silk finish; they do not reproduce well.

Occasionally you may have a negative which, because of poor exposure or the circumstances under which it was taken, would make a less than satisfactory print for mechanical reproduction. This can often be improved in printing by selecting the appropriate grade of contrast in the enlarging paper, by reducing exposure in some areas by "dodging," or by overexposing other areas. Underexposed negatives can sometimes be intensified, or overexposed ones reduced by chemical methods.

Other techniques to improve print quality involve the use of an opaque medium on the negative to eliminate unwanted background or spotting the negative to remove small pinholes or clear spots. Prints can be retouched to correct other defects, but this must be done with care. Even though retouching has been done carefully and may appear satisfactory to the eye, the camera may view the retouching medium differently and make it obvious when reproduced. This is particularly critical if color prints or transparencies are retouched, in which case the dyes must be compatible with the material being retouched. All of these correction techniques should be done by a professional photographer or photofinisher unless you are skilled in the use of them.

SUBMITTING PHOTOGRAPHS TO A JOURNAL

Before submitting photographs to a journal, refer to the "advice to authors" section. Many journals will specify exactly how photographs are to be submitted. Some will require the prints to be larger than the ultimate reproduced size; others require exact-size prints. Few will accept prints that must be enlarged significantly. Pre- and postoperative photographs should be enlarged or reduced so that the anatomic features are the same size. Positions and lighting should be identical.

Some journals will accept color for publication if it significantly enhances the value of the paper. Color printing is usually done at the expense of the author. Some journals require color prints, while others will accept transparencies. The requirements will be spelled out in the "information for contributors" section of the journal.

No marks should be made on the face of the photograph, except crop marks, and these in the margin only. The name of the author, the figure number, the orientation, and any special instructions should be affixed to the back with a gummed label or pencilled lightly on the back. Pencil marks should not be made with enough pressure to imprint the surface of the picture. If a special layout of photographs is desired, outline this on a separate piece of paper included with the prints.

Photographs should not be mounted, nor should any explanatory material be affixed with paperclips, which might mar the surface. Be sure that the figure number and "top" are lightly pencilled on the back. Protect all illustrations and photographs with a double layer of cardboard to prevent wrinkling or bending in the mail.

ILLUSTRATIONS

Line drawings, graphs, and charts submitted for publication must be of the same high quality as photographs. The originals should be done in black ink on white illustration board and the lettering large enough and of a style that will be legible if the original is reduced in size when reproduced. Some journals require the submission of original artwork, while others ask that high-quality black-and-white glossy prints be submitted.

Crisp prints of black-and-white line drawings or graphs can be made by photographing the original artwork with Kodalith Ortho Film 2556, Contrast Process Ortho 4154, or similar high-contrast films. Continuous tone drawings should be copied with Kodak Professional Copy Film 4125 to retain the highlight gradations.

Problems may occur if a black-and-white print must be made from a colored line original. Because of film sensitivity to certain colors, either the background or some of the information lines may reproduce as gray tones that lack contrast. This type of original artwork should be copied with Kodak Contrast Process Pan 4155 film. If the problem still exists with this film, then copy the artwork through a filter that will cause the specific color to be reproduced as either black or white (Table 20-1).

X-RAY FILMS

X-ray films for publication should be submitted as a high-contrast glossy print with the black areas on the print corresponding to the dark areas of the original film. A good technique for reproducing radiographs is to place

Table 20-1. Filter recommendations for copying colors in black and white

Original color	Filter to render color as white		Filter to render color as black	
	Orthochromatic film	Panchromatic film	Orthochromatic film	Panchromatic film
Red	Not recommended	Red #25	None needed	Green #58 or blue #47
Yellow	Yellow #9	Yellow #9	Blue #47	Blue #47
Green	Green #58	Green #58	Magenta #30	Magenta #30
Cyan	None needed	Green #58 or blue #47	Not recommended	Red #25
Blue	Blue #47	Blue #47	Yellow #9	Green #58
Magenta	Magenta #30	Magenta #30	Green #58	Green #58

NOTE: Consult manufacturer's data sheet for filter factor for film being used to determine the compensatory exposure increase caused by the filters.

the film on a view box, read with an exposure meter the portion of the film that is most dense but still has detail, and expose Plus X film accordingly. The developing time for film exposed by this technique should be reduced approximately 20%.

LEGENDS

Each figure in a published article, whether photograph, drawing, or chart, must have a legend. These should be typed on 8½ × 11 inch paper, double spaced, with one-inch margins. The legend numbers should correspond with the figure number on the artwork and in the text. Legends should be neither affixed to the illustrations nor typed in the manuscript. They should be submitted as a separate document along with the manuscript and illustrations. If any illustrations or tables have been previously published, written permission must be obtained from the original publisher and author and the source indicated in a footnote.

If original drawings are submitted, the labels should be positioned on a tissue overlay, since this material will be edited and set in type.

AUTHORIZED USE OF PHOTOGRAPHS

The specific written consent for publication of photographs must be obtained from all identifiable patients shown in the illustrations. If the patient is a minor, this permission should be obtained from the parents. The eyes should be blocked unless they are the primary reason for the illustration or the blocking will distract from the demonstration of important points. If the eyes are to be blocked, this should be noted on the reverse side of the illustration.

CHAPTER 21

Poster sessions

**Stephen H. Miller, M.D., Martin C. Robson, M.D., and
Richard A. Heimburger, M.D.**

Communication is the interpretation or interchange of thought, opinion, and information. It is the essence of scientific endeavor. Effective scientific communication requires that a message be delivered, that it gain attention from an interested audience, that it be properly interpreted, and that it allow for and encourage discussion between the presenter and the audience.

Audiovisual (slide) presentations and exhibits are the principal methods of disseminating information at most scientific meetings. Unfortunately, with increasing attendance at meetings and the need for multiple scientific sessions, neither satisfactorily fulfills the requirements for effective scientific communication. While slide presentations deliver a message and gain attention, they do little to ensure proper interpretation of that message or meaningful dialogue between the presenter and the audience, especially a large one. Moreover, because of limitations in time and space, the message may not reach all interested parties. Those who miss the presentation must await its publication months later, if ever, in a scientific journal.

During most meetings free-standing scientific exhibits are available to deliver a message, but they are often in locations where they attract little attention. Other disadvantages are that they may be misinterpreted and do not encourage effective discourse between presenter and audience, since the exhibitor is rarely present at the exhibit during the meeting.

Both the formal presentation and the scientific exhibit are effective means of communication and neither should be abandoned. However, a program committee responsible for organizing a large scientific meeting should consider including in its program a third mode for scientific communication, the poster session. We believe that the latter combines some of the best attributes of the free-standing exhibit and the slide presentation.

Poster presentations promote discourse between presenter and audience (Fig. 21-1). The components are made from simple, inexpensive graphic and written materials, which are easily carried to the meeting and mounted on poster boards. Posters of related subject matter are grouped in a specific place and at a specified time selected by the program committee. During each session, moderators chosen for their expertise in the particular subject lead small groups of interested parties to each poster so that the author can present his or her data. The oral presentation is less formal and much shorter, two minutes or less, than the usual slide presentation since the poster should transmit most of the message. Following the formal presentation, the small audience can then discuss the work with the author. Misinterpretation of results and conclusions is less likely since the size of the audience at each poster is small, yet well enough organized by the moderators to allow exchange of information. This mode of presentation allows for and encourages more meaningful dialogue between presenter and audience than does the usual question-and-answer period following a slide presentation to a large audience in an auditorium.

Since the author is present during a specified time to present the work to an organized group, the poster mode has distinct advantage over the usual free-standing scientific exhibit. Also, if a poster presentation is of unusual interest or has not been seen by a significant number of attendants, it can easily be set up again in the same or a new location as an exhibit or repeat poster session. This flexibility is not possible with a slide presentation.

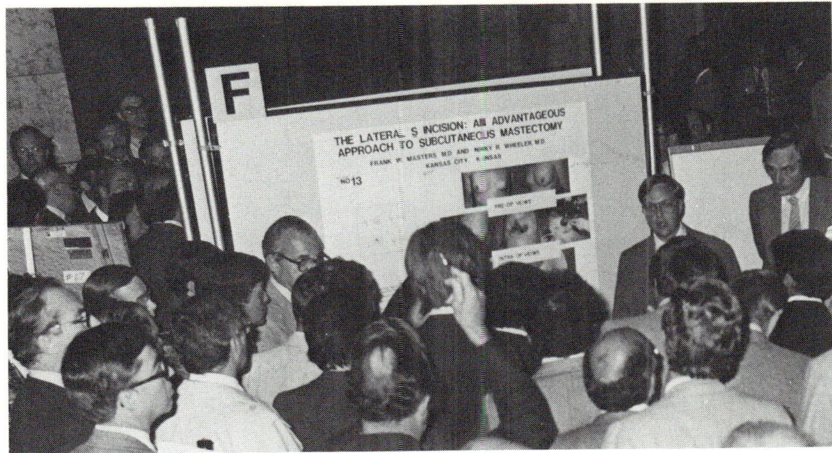

Fig. 21-1. Poster sessions encourage discourse between the audience and the author since a limited number of persons are in attendance and the author is present during the entire time the poster is shown.

PLANNING

1. Enlist the help of a medical illustrator, if possible, to best determine how to effectively present your material.
2. Emphasize visual elements with enlarged color photographs, illustrations, and large color diagrams.
3. Place your material according to importance. The top and center of the poster attract the most attention. The lower left and right attract less and can be left empty. Some blank space will provide visual rest and highlight the main points.

Explanatory text on the poster should be concise and should be readable from 2 feet away. Lettering should be large—3 inches high for titles, 1 inch for major subject headings, and ⅝ inch for the main body of the text, legends, and labels on illustrations. A mechanical lettering device or ³/₁₆ inch IBM Executive typewriter type can be used for the lettering. Because words written in lowercase letters are more easily read than words written in all capital letters, the latter should be used only for emphasis.

PRODUCTION

A poster exhibit can be produced by either a medical illustrator or the author. Poster production requires adequate time and rarely does a good one result when preparations are left for the last minute. Take all ideas for illustrations, photographs ready for mounting, and written copy (title, author's name, text, legends, labels, and credits) to an illustrator at least three to four weeks prior to your departure date. For those who wish to produce their own posters the following steps are suggested:

1. *Draw a plan of the actual size of the exhibit* on Kraft paper and a reduced version on a smaller piece of paper. The latter can be taken to the meeting to assist you in setting up the poster.

2. *Cut out the individual poster components.* Crescent #201 white illustration board and medium weight Crescent color drawing boards, purchased at an art supply store, can be cut with an X-Acto knife, #11 blade, or large paper cutter. Triangles, T squares, and metal straight edges will help make the edges straight and corners square.

3. *Draw the illustrations and diagrams.* Use quality materials obtained from an art supply store. Drafting pens, Chart Pak colortapes, crepe tapes (used to make curved lines), Design Art Markers, Zipatone shading screens and color films, Prismacolor colored pencils, three-ply Strathmore bristol board with high surface finish, and hot-press illustration board are all useful.

4. *Attach the illustrations and photographs to the poster board.* Illustrations can be easily attached with strips of double-faced tape such as Scotch adhesive-transfer tape #465 (1 inch wide) and Tuck carpet bond tape (1½ inches wide).

Photographs should be drymounted. Use Kodak or Seal drymount tissue for black-and-white prints and Fotoflat drymount for color prints. While a drymount press is best, a hand iron will work. Use the tip of the iron to tack the drymount tissue to the back of the print in the center and at two diagonally opposite corners. Trim off the white borders of the print, cutting through both print and drymount tissue. Place the trimmed print on the poster and use the tip of the iron from the center out to the edges in all directions until the print adheres smoothly. Allow the drymounted print to cool under a flat, heavy weight. An alternate method of mounting photographs is to use double-faced tape on the back of the print. Spray adhesives will give acceptable results, but are dangerous when inhaled and are not permanent.

5. *Letter the title.* Use 3 inch vinyl, adhesive-backed letters such as Letrasign Helvetica in either black or white. Rule a baseline in pencil, carefully line up the bottom edges of the letter with the baseline, and press to adhere. White letters stand out against medium and deep colors; black letters stand out against lighter colors.

6. *Attach lettering blocks.* Since it is easy to make mistakes while lettering, lettering is best done on colored paper or cardboard strips that can be attached to the poster after being checked for accuracy. Use double-faced tape or white glue to attach lettering blocks.

   a. *Major headings.* Use pressure-sensitive lettering such as Letraset or Zipatone dry transfer lettering. Helvetica and Futura typefaces in 60 or 72 point sizes are suitable. Rule the baseline in pencil, position the letter on it, and rub the surface with a burnisher to release the letter from the carrier sheet onto the paper or cardboard. Vinyl adhesive letters (1 inch) are also good. Another possibility is to use stencil lettering.

   b. *Text and legends.* Pressure-sensitive lettering in size 24 to 42 point is suitable. It is best to use this in small quantities since the application is time consuming. Sharp typed copy, made with an IBM Executive typewriter can be enlarged photographically to the desired size and the photograph trimmed and drymounted to the poster. A photographic enlargement can be made on graphic arts film and the transparent film positive affixed to the poster with spray adhesive on the reverse side of the film.

7. Poster components should be portable and in sections to make shipping easier. Large components, such as the title strip, can be hinged to fold into a smaller size for carrying.

8. Handout sheets or materials can be used to supplement poster presentations.

PRESENTATION

A check-in room and poster assistance team should be available during the meeting to direct each author to the assigned location and help set up the presentation. Using the previously prepared plan (Fig. 21-2), the poster components should be mounted on the specially prepared bulletin board (Fig. 21-3). The components should be mounted with clear or white push-pins or tacks. Do not use staple guns or nails. All posters should be in place at least 15 minutes before the session begins. They should be removed from the bulletin boards shortly after the session ends so that the next group will have enough time to mount their posters. If a poster proves to be very

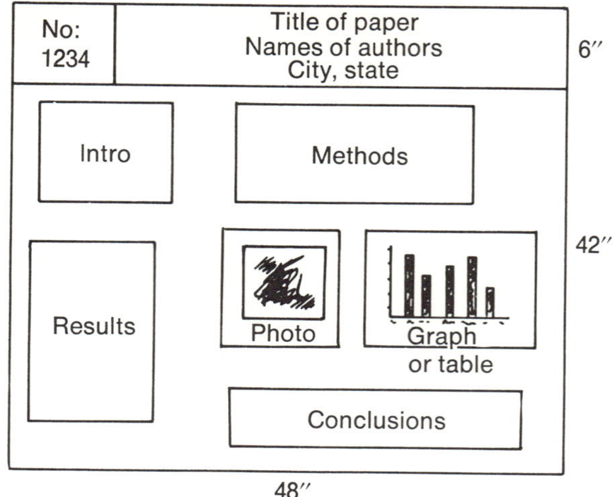

Fig. 21-2. Preliminary plan of a poster. This can be used not only when preparing the components but also as a guide when assembling the exhibit.

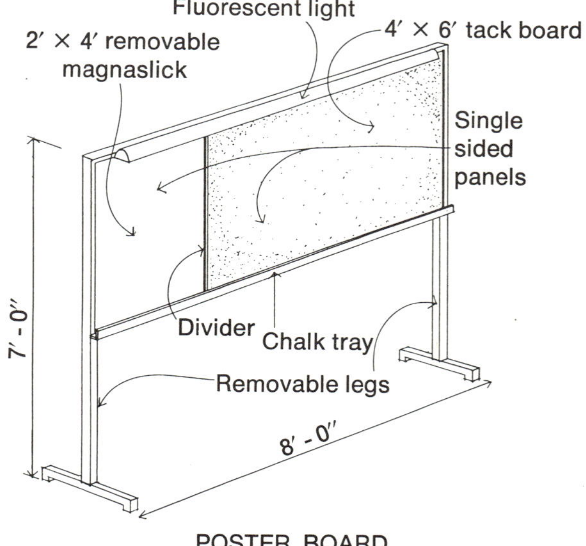

Fig. 21-3. Bulletin board especially prepared for mounting the components of a poster session.

popular, it can be remounted and exhibited at another time.

The room for the poster session should be well lighted and large enough to accommodate the expected audience. The posters should be widely enough separated from each other to allow discussion without interference from the other groups. The moderators should initiate discussion and keep the groups moving along a prescribed course at predetermined time intervals so that all persons may see each poster during the session.

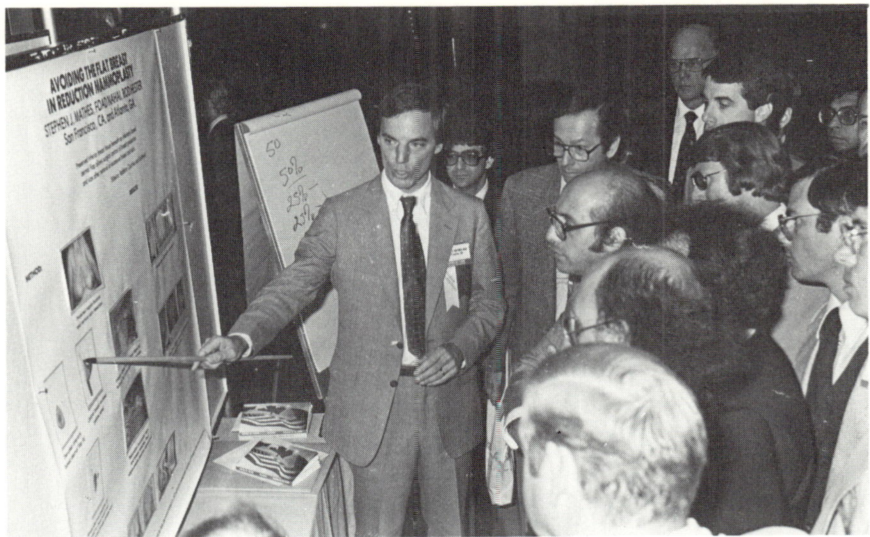

Fig. 21-4. The author should introduce the work with a short presentation to the audience before the question-and-answer period or discussion begins.

As each group arrives at a poster, the author should give a short presentation of two minutes or less to introduce the work and focus the attention of the audience upon the highlights of the poster (Fig. 21-4). After this, the moderator should encourage discussion and interchange of ideas between the author and the audience.

SUMMARY

Poster sessions are an important mode of scientific communication. The ability of posters to deliver a message, gain attention for that message, and encourage small group dialogue between presenter and audience is the advantage of this type of communication.

CHAPTER 22

Scientific exhibits

Richard Mladick, M.D.

For the past thirty years, scientific medical exhibits have played an important role in continuing medical education. During this time, exhibits have graduated from out-of-the-way side rooms and hallways to prominent display in the large convention halls of national meetings. The quality of exhibits has also been improved by the profession's creativity and the technical advances of the exhibit industry. Unfortunately, the inflationary costs of fabricating new exhibits and strong labor controls over convention centers are making it increasingly expensive and difficult for the casual exhibitor. Therefore, before you make a commitment to exhibit, it is extremely important to become familiar with the exhibit concept and principles of the design and construction of a scientific medical exhibit.

THE EXHIBIT CONCEPT

The scientific medical exhibit is a portable, multimedia display that is adaptable and convenient for communication to both large and small groups. The exhibit is still considered by many to be one of the best and most enjoyable forms of medical education, and its popularity has continued over the years. An exhibit offers unlimited viewing time for the observer—a definite advantage over other types of audiovisual presentations. The self-explanatory feature of exhibits means the author need not always be in attendance.

This advantage does not make exhibiting easy, for there can be hard work, long hours, demanding questioning, insistent viewers, audiovisual breakdowns, and assembling and disassembling difficulties. The total commitment to an exhibit begins with the idea, follows with the construction, and culminates with the successful showing at the meeting. This will mean time, money, and other sacrifices, but the rewards will be numerous. The exhibitor will learn more from the exhibit than any other person, as there is more personal interchange than in any other type of medical education. There is also the fun and satisfaction of creating your own work of art and successfully communicating your message; considerable respect and prestige are gained from presenting a top-notch exhibit.

PLANNING AN EXHIBIT

As a preliminary step in planning a medical exhibit, write to the scientific association where the exhibit will be shown. It is advisable to determine the size of the exhibit space allowed, whether there will be adequate lighting, whether chairs and tables will be provided, and what the meeting's requirements are in regard to the exhibitor's attendance. Most associations require a sketch or photo of the exhibit or an abstract regarding its content.

A scientific exhibit should be designed for quick and easy communication. It should be concise and without excessive details, statistics, or examples, and should be designed around a central idea or theme. If possible, it should have a definite conclusion, summary, or statement as to future application. The average viewer will spend only four minutes in front of the typical medical exhibit and many viewers will spend much less initially, merely glancing at the exhibits the first time around looking for that central idea or theme that will bring them back for later study. An exhibit that is loaded with minute details and myriad diagrams and transparencies but lacks a central theme may discourage these viewers. A simplistic, clear, and attractive exhibit will generate more interest than a complicated and crowded one.

If the services of an experienced medical illustration department are available, it is advisable to use their expertise in designing and constructing the exhibit. A medical illustrator is conversant with medical terminology, usually has exhibit experience, and has the artistic and design knowledge to organize the material as an effective teaching unit.

While there is no one right way or typical format for a medical exhibit, a proved way is to use a medical manuscript format; that is, introduction, material and methods, case examples, statistical analysis, discussion, and summary or conclusion. Since it is customary to read from left to right, the introduction should be located to the left, case examples and statistics and possibly some discussion in the center, and the right panel used for final statistical analysis, summary, and possible future application of the work. Any layout should be designed to keep the traffic flow moving in one direction so that traffic jams are not created in front of the exhibit.

A concise, easy-to-read diagram, chart, or graph that summarizes the material will help the viewer analyze the work much faster than rows of statistics or tables of numbers. Eliminate all unnecessary words to conserve space, retain the viewer's interest, and minimize printing and lettering costs. It is neither necessary nor desirable to try to display a great deal of the experience, cases, or work on a particular topic. Rather it is important to select some typical examples. If a thousand cases have been done successfully, the exibit need show only a few outstanding examples with reference in the statistical analysis to the number of cases done.

Color prints or transparencies are preferable to black-and-white when possible. Very large color prints can be quite costly; 8 × 10 inch prints are effective and still fit easily into the budget. It is best to use color print film from the beginning, rather than use a negative printing method to go from color transparencies to color prints. To change color transparencies into prints is costly and the print quality will suffer.

X-ray films may be used as transparencies themselves with back lighting or they may be photographed and used as black-and-white prints. X-ray films must be of good quality, must be easily readable from a distance, and should have labels to identify important details to increase the interest and clarity of an exhibit.

Three-dimensional models are excellent (Fig. 22-1). They should be made lightweight if possible and not be overly fragile. In some cases, even live models may be a useful addition to an exhibit.

Supplementary brochures at the exhibit site are also helpful to present a more complete and detailed exposition of the work and may include many more examples.

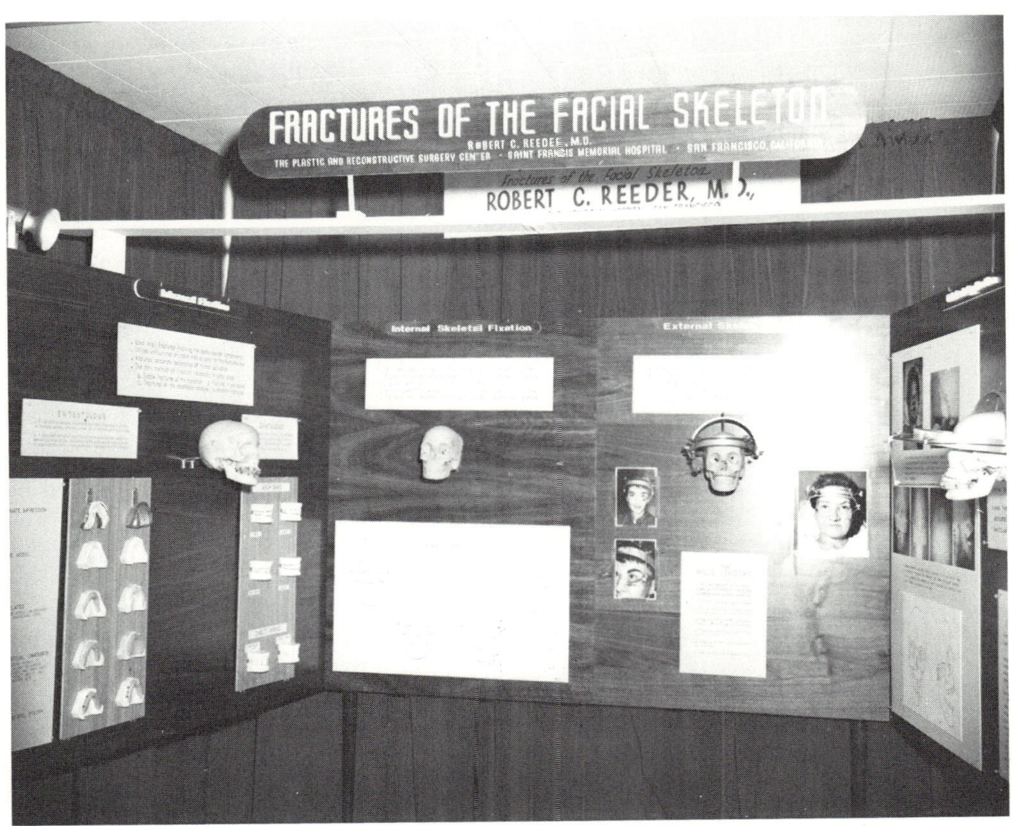

Fig. 22-1. An example of the use of three-dimensional models on a scientific exhibit.

Lighting is frequently the number one problem with an otherwise excellent exhibit. While most exhibit halls have massive overhead fluorescent lighting, this type of lighting can be poor for an exhibit. Shadows, dark spots, and reflections may all seriously jeopardize the quality of the exhibit. It is advisable to bring your own floodlights or overhanging lights or to build them into the exhibit unless you are personally familiar with the exhibit hall and can be assured of proper overhead lighting. Front illumination may cause glare on color prints or graphs. This can be avoided by changing the location or type of lights.

Another way to avoid front glare is to design the exhibit for back-illuminated transparencies. This will increase the cost and technical difficulties of construction and will also increase the chances for electrical breakdowns, burned out or broken lights, or damage to the transparencies, but can make a truly excellent and attractive exhibit. Be prepared to add $500 to $1000 for building in the back-illuminated transparencies.

TYPES OF EXHIBITS

A rough sketch of the proposed exhibit or a working model is a most helpful step before beginning the actual construction. Complete the prototype exhibit in detail with all writing, photographs, and visual parts sketched in place. At this time, you can determine whether your exhibit should have an audiovisual component, what type of construction will best provide you with a sturdy, lightweight exhibit, and an estimate on the cost. The discussion of the types of exhibits in the following section should provide useful information regarding these aspects.

Visual exhibits

Poster exhibits. A poster exhibit is the simplest type. It may be a simple collection of black-and-white sketches, prints, diagrams, graphs, or photographs pasted on plain white artboard. These large posters can be packed easily in a suitcase or light package. At the meeting, the exhibit boards are usually placed on a table or rented backpanel. This type of exhibit requires the attendance of the author or someone who can narrate the purpose of the exhibit and answer questions. If this is the type of exhibit chosen, someone should be prepared to spend considerable time in attendance during the meeting.

This type of exhibit will cost between $500 and $1000. Very large color prints alone, however, may cost up to $200; so even this type of exhibit can be expensive. Diagrams, photos, and all lettering should be readable at 4 feet. Excellent rub-on or adhesive letters can be purchased in many sizes, along with the artboards, at an art supply shop. There is a recent trend for poster sessions to be scheduled as a separate session of the meeting and in a location different from the other scientific and commercial exhibits.

Folding panel exhibits. The folding panel exhibit is more elaborate and durable than rental background boards or table-top poster exhibits. This type of exhibit is usually designed to fit within the standard 8 × 10 foot exhibit space. It usually has three to five background panels approximately 2 feet wide and from 6 to 8 feet tall (Fig. 22-2). The display area usually starts approximately 3 feet from the floor. These exhibits may have a built-in shelf or counter onto which may be placed models or brochures. Folding exhibits may also be half the usual height, in which case they are designed to rest on a table. This type of exhibit may be constructed with each 8-foot panel made to fold in half into a 2 × 4 foot size. A shipping crate would, therefore, have to accept at least four of the 2 × 4 foot panels plus the supporting struts, lighting, and electrical equipment. Nevertheless, a properly designed shipping case can still be quite compact and of manageable size for two people.

The folding panel exhibit is one of the most popular types for the exhibitor who has plans for many meetings. It may be shipped in its own crate but this may cost from $50 to $150, depending on the means of transportation; there can be additional labor fees for assembling and disassembling. This exhibit will move the budget from the $1000 range to the $3000 to $4000 range.

The folding panel exhibit should be sturdy but lightweight. These two aspects are not contradictory if plastic, fiberglass, or tubular aluminum is used in construction. Wooden frames and plywood structures are more or less obsolete and usually are too heavy and cumbersome for shipping and handling. It is helpful if the shipping size of the crated exhibit can be fitted into the back of a standard station wagon. However, if there is unlimited budget and plenty of help with lifting, moving, assembling, and disassembling, the size of the exhibit need not be of concern.

Some associations and meetings may allow two 8 × 10 foot spaces for oversized exhibits, but this is not a general policy and is usually not the rule if there are many applications for a limited number of exhibit spaces.

As an alternative to constructing your own folding panel exhibit, consider one of the currently available prefabricated exhibits (Fig. 22-3). There has been a big market for these prefabricated exhibits in commercial fields, and they have been developed with a high degree of success. Lightweight folding panels that fit nicely into custom designed cases are used. They are of high quality in their finished details and there is an excellent selection of attractive colors for background panels. A nice feature of the prefabricated exhibits is the Velcro surface

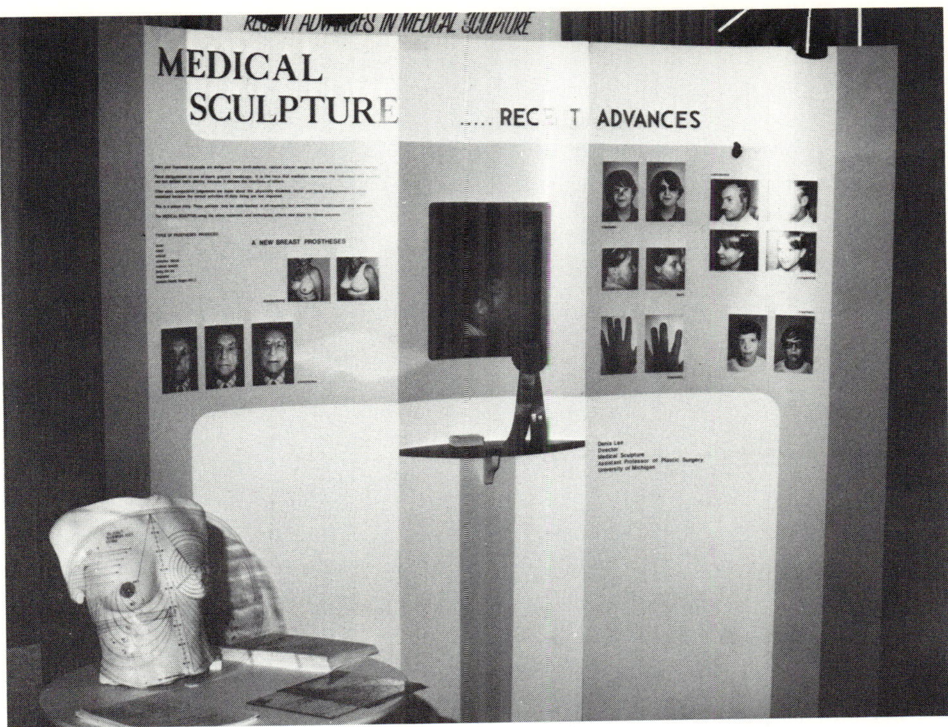

Fig. 22-2. A custom-made folding panel exhibit. This will pack into a 4 × 8 foot shipping case when disassembled.

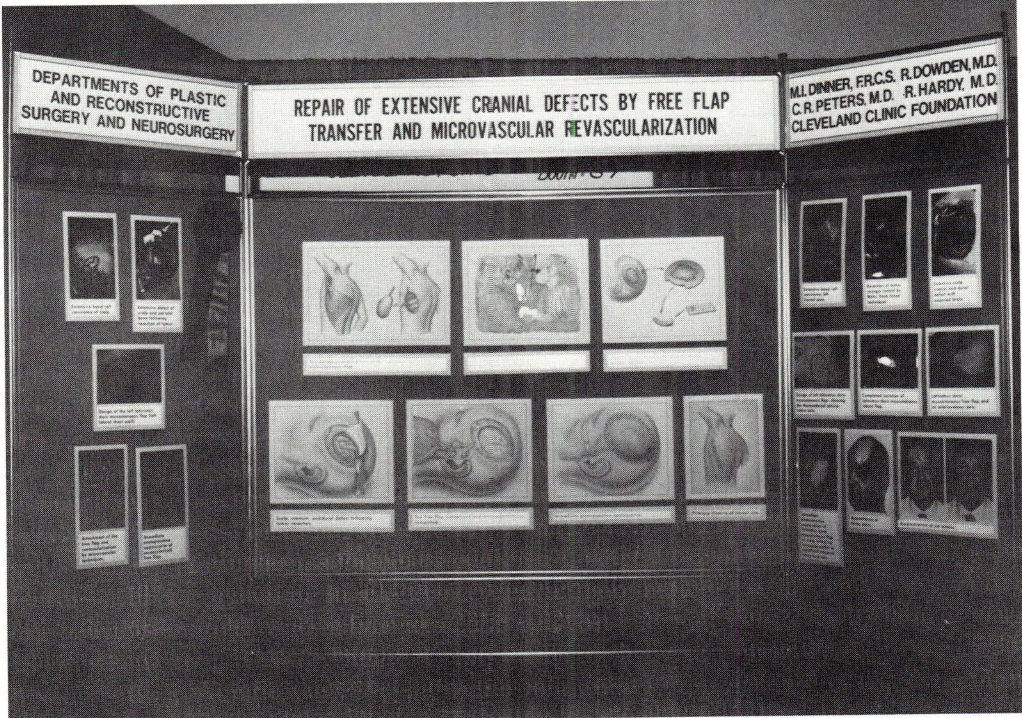

Fig. 22-3. An exhibit constructed on a commercially available modular exhibit frame. This type exhibit is lightweight, easily transported in its own case, and easily assembled. The display panels are attached with Velcro tabs or push pins.

covering the panels. By applying small Velcro tags to the backs of graphs, photos, and so forth, the exhibitor can easily attach and rearrange them. These exhibits are quite simple to assemble and take down and have light, custom-designed, sturdy shipping cases. They can save the exhibitor a great deal of time and effort which can be spent on other elements of the exhibit.

Audiovisual exhibits

There are a number of different ways to add the audiovisual element to your exhibit: from the simple remote slide projectors with synchronized slide-audio-cassettes to the continuous super 8 or 16 mm reel type film or even the more modern videotape exhibits. All of these modalities will add anywhere from $500 to $5000 to the cost of the exhibit. The audio part of the exhibit may be brought out through a central speaker, or preferably through the use of headphones or telephones so that adjacent exhibitors are not disturbed. The obvious advantages of this type of exhibit is that you are getting your message across more effectively to anyone who stops to listen, whether you are there or not. Even with a totally automated audiovisual exhibit, many meetings still require the author's presence at the exhibit site, and you must be prepared to make this commitment. Of course, the impact of the audio plus the visual component has been proved to be more significant than only the visual element.

The most popular and basic audiovisual modality is the synchronized audiocassette with rear screen slide projector. This type of exhibit will need a little more depth in the back of the exhibit space to allow room for the projector. With this type of exhibit, it is advisable to add an off/on button so that when no observer is present, the projector will not be playing and wearing down the tape, slides, bulbs, and so forth. There may be an occasional equipment problem with this type of exhibit so it is advisable to bring along extra bulbs for the projector and even extra audiocassettes. It is also necessary to have regular times throughout the day to check on the exhibit if someone is not in attendance. The audio part of the exhibit should be synchronized with the slide show and should be concise, clear, and last no more than 5 minutes. Rarely will an observer pay attention to a slide show for longer than this.

With continuous-reel super 8 or 16 mm movie or videotape equipment, it is possible to present a longer and more interesting program that can hold the audience's attention for up to 10 minutes. Videotapes will wear out after many uses and are not as durable as 16 mm movie film. To be safe, have an extra copy of the film or videotape in case the tape should break, become stuck, or damaged.

TRANSPORTATION AND MEETING ARRANGEMENTS

It is important that transportation and plans for assembling and disassembling be made well in advance of the meeting. Check with the airline, rail, or bus company about the size of the exhibit. Confirm with the exhibits coordinator or the decorator of the meeting the regulations for assembling and disassembling.

The standard space at most meetings is 8×10 feet. If this crowds the exhibit, ask for additional space, end space, or some other type of arrangement that might give a little extra room. (A telephone call to the exhibit coordinator may help get that extra space.) While it is cumbersome to travel with a projector or other audiovisual equipment and is somewhat risky to ship it, it is often more of a gamble to rent audiovisual equipment. To be on the safe side, it is best to bring your own projector.

The cost of transportation will vary a great deal between air freight, parcel service, bus, moving vans, or car. The quickest move is by air freight but this is also the most expensive. Bus companies are readily available but they do not have pick-up or delivery service.

No matter what type of transportation arrangements are made, the exhibit must be clearly labeled with waterproof labels. It should be securely packaged and insulated against the usual trauma of rough handling. If the exhibit arrives damaged at the meeting, you will most likely not have the material or time available to fix it. Self-contained shipping cases are the ideal form of packing.

For exhibiting in foreign countries, it is best to work through a customs broker, usually preselected by the professional association holding the meeting. The broker will save you time and money and expedite getting your exhibit through customs—an otherwise, slow, painful, and costly process in many countries.

Exhibiting can be a most enjoyable experience as long as you have made your plans well in advance and are prepared to put in considerable time and effort at the meeting.

ACKNOWLEDGMENT

Thanks is given to Mr. Larry Gaskins, former Director of Medical Illustrations Department at the Hampton Veterans Hospital, for the help he gave in preparation of this paper.

CHAPTER 23

Sound-slide presentations

Martin C. Robson, M.D., Robert W. Parsons, M.D., and Joel W. Cole

Medical communication can be effectively enhanced by providing information both aurally and visually using an integrated series of narrated slides. Such a sound-slide program uses the medium of projected transparencies. A slide projector, screen, and cassette tape player are the only equipment required, and these are readily available. Sound-slide programs are easy to create and use, inexpensive, and are effective for both individual self-teaching and presentation to larger groups.

APPROPRIATE SUBJECT MATTER

The first step in planning the sound-slide program is to be sure that the topic is appropriate for this mode of communication. Not all subject matter is suitable for a sound-slide presentation. Dynamic subjects such as the intricacies of a specific surgical procedure are often better presented in the more dynamic media of films or videotapes. Sound-slide programs provide an ideal communication aid for more static material, such as the anatomy of the various myocutaneous flap territories, surgical pathology, and presentations of the overall approach to clinical problems. Often the information in such material must be committed to memory and the sound-slide program can be adjusted to the student's individual speed. Another advantage of this format is that a program can be updated or modified for different uses by adding or subtracting slides as needed.

PLANNING THE PRODUCTION OF A SOUND-SLIDE PROGRAM

After the decision is made that the subject is suitable for this medium, the presentation must be planned carefully. The sound-slide program should be specifically designed for the intended audience and teaching objectives. For example, a self-teaching program for medical student on the management of leg ulcers might be designed quite differently from a program on the same subject for continuing medical education of practicing surgeons. This is true even though the illustrations might be the same for both. The content of the sound-slide program must be relevant to the needs of the intended audience and organized for understanding and retention.

The next step is to prepare an outline of the proposed content of the program, keeping the audience and objectives in mind. This should be sufficiently detailed to include all of the significant points to be emphasized. The outline will serve as a guide for selecting clinical slides to illustrate the major points. The need for drawings, tables, graphs, and slides containing text can be determined.

A title slide with the author's identification should begin the program. The slides should be selected and prepared with careful attention to the technical points discussed in the next section of the chapter. Finally, the slides are put in sequence following the outline.

The script for a sound-slide program should be prepared as a lecture, not as a manuscript. Although some speakers are more natural when talking from an outline, it is best to prepare a carefully written script. This assures that all of the points the author wishes to make are included and that they receive the intended emphasis. Also, using a script requires that the slides follow the author's ideas and prevents a presentation in which the ideas are merely comments on the slides. Sentences should be precise, direct, and brief. Long compound sentences are difficult for an audience to understand. One should not use three sentences where one will suffice. At this point it is helpful to record the script on a tape recorder or dictating machine and listen to it without the slides, to judge the overall effectiveness of the words.

TECHNICAL REQUIREMENTS
Audio

Whenever possible, a taping studio should be used. This removes all background noises and provides the added benefit of professional guidance. For the best sound-slide program, a professional narrator should be used. This requires the author to go over the script carefully with the narrator to help with the correct pronunciation of medical terms and to emphasize specific points or concepts. The narration can be recorded directly onto a cassette, but it is better to use ¼ inch reel-to-reel tape at 7½ inches per second. Once the master recording of the audio portion has been accomplished on quality tape, it can easily be transferred to a cassette.

Slides

Whenever possible only original slides should be included in the master copy of the sound-slide program. This is especially true of clinical illustrations. If copies must be made, a low-contrast copy film such as Eastman Kodak 5071 should be used. This helps to prevent the sharp increases in contrast and corresponding decreases in quality seen with multiple copying of slides. The slides must be of good quality as far as exposure and clarity are concerned. It is very important to avoid distracting backgrounds or an untidy surgical field.

In the preparation of slides containing text, illustrations, or graphs and tables it is helpful to work with an expert. The width of the material should not be more than 1.3 times the height. The layout of the slides should be kept simple, with plenty of open space. For text, the space between lines should be at least the height of a capital letter. Ideally, title slides should be five words or less. In a sound-slide program, the title need not fully describe the content of the program. Slides containing the text should have uniform printing, and color should be used for emphasis only. White lettering on a blue background is attractive and easy to read. Data can be grasped more quickly when presented in graph form. If tables are used they must be kept simple and uncrowded.

The amount of information on each printed slide must be limited. When multiple points are to be emphasized, it is better to use several slides with a progressive revelation of information. A good rule of thumb to follow when preparing the slides is to use no more than seven lines of text per slide, with three to five words per line. Plan that each slide is on the screen no longer than twenty seconds and no less than five seconds. A printed slide with the author's conclusions should follow the main body of the program. Finally, a slide with the pertinent references will often be appreciated by the audience.

COMPLETING THE SOUND-SLIDE PROGRAM

If the planning steps for production of a sound-slide program have been followed and the technical considerations adhered to, completion of the program should be simple. The presentation should be rehearsed with the narrator, script, and slides. If possible, the rehearsal should take place before representatives of the intended audience. Once the author is pleased with the effect, the final taping can take place.

After completion of the audiovisual program the author may wish to prepare six to ten questions covering the key points to be gained from the program. This permits self-assessment of the information learned by the viewer. This step is especially important if the sound-slide program is to be used for continuing medical education credit.

The finalized set of slides with the accompanying cassette is easy to store for use as needed. The viewer needs only a projector, screen, and a cassette player, or a convenient combination projector such as the Caramate. Thus the sound-slide program provides an inexpensive, easily prepared means for medical communication when used for properly selected subjects.

CHAPTER 24

Videotapes

Programming for medical students

Norman E. Hugo, M.D.

A videotape for educational purposes should be just that—educational. Simply taping a lecture or an operation and presenting it as a spontaneous happening invariably results in an inferior performance by those involved and a slow-paced presentation. When designing a presentation the authors should consider how best to portray their message. Conceptual material that is best exposed by motion is the ideal subject matter for videotape (or film). But it should clearly be *in motion*. Otherwise, the material is better presented as a manuscript, sound-slide program or audiotape. Highly detailed material is more efficiently presented by manuscript.

EDUCATIONAL CONSIDERATIONS

The second consideration after deciding that videotape is the proper and most effective means for transmitting your educational message is to write down the *instructional objectives*. Two excellent monographs on this subject have been prepared by Gronlund and Mager. (see Bibliography). Determining the instructional objectives is clearly the most important aspect of the entire undertaking because they help the creator to clarify the message and shift emphasis from the teaching activity to the learning outcome; that is, the focus is shifted from the teacher to the student. Preparation will force the teacher to concentrate on the learning process rather than the teaching process. Thus the teacher will determine what *behavior* the student will demonstrate to illustrate that he or she understands the material presented. Once this is established, the result can be easily tested and the validity of the instructional program established.

For example, when suturing techniques are taught to the surgical student, behavioral objectives could be to:

1. Gain appreciation of suturing techniques
2. Discuss suturing techniques
3. Demonstrate the correct suturing on the abdominal wound of a pig

Each one of these objectives evokes a behavior but the third one is the most specific, requires application of the techniques, and is the easiest to test. After the main objective is determined, it is broken down into more specific objectives. For example, these could include (1) demonstrating the proper grip of a needle holder, (2) demonstrating the correct angle of introduction of the needle into tissue, (3) demonstrating the retrieval of a broken needle, and (4) demonstrating the length at which different sutures are cut. Proper compilation of these objectives will dictate the content of the videotape and will force the teacher to present the information in a way that will compel the student to learn the material and be able to demonstrate the required skills.

Clearly, the selection of the proper "motion" subject for videotape and the compilation of instructional (behavioral) objectives are the keystones for producing a videotape.

After the objectives are clearly formulated a story board is created. This requires production of many illustrations to portray all of the objectives that have been delineated. The illustrations are then applied to a large surface so that they can be viewed in sequence. The main purpose of the story board is to organize the objectives in logical sequence and thus prepare a script. Its use will allow the teacher to evaluate the proper flow of the presentation. To return to the previous example: The story board could consist of several types of sutures and needles, several needle holders, forceps, a porcine abdominal wound with the several abdominal layers, an area of devitalized tissue, a hematoma, a broken needle imbedded in the tissue, and a well-closed incision with sutures tied at the proper tension. The teacher can then arrange these conceptual illustrations into the sequence that will emphasize the selected objectives.

TECHNICAL CONSIDERATIONS

The technical crew should be consulted on the story board so that they can offer suggestions. For example, they might suggest a different sequence because of required camera angles or lighting. The importance of consulting the video technical crew at this point cannot be overemphasized. Other technical considerations include using blue or green drapes and gowns and using nonreflective instruments. The use of a cautery during actual filming causes the image to disintegrate and should be minimized. Clean drapes and an operative field unobscured by blood are, of course, mandatory.

The script is written after the story board has been approved. The script is created around the story board and is not unlike that of a play with the insertion of specific visual points to be made. For example:

NARRATOR: . . . and the curved needle is introduced into the tissue at an angle so that more of the deeper layer is included to create eversion of the upper layers. (VIDEO: Surgeon to illustrate insertion of needle.)

The script is reworked until all extraneous material is removed and then is reviewed to ensure that it clearly includes all instructional objectives.

If the narration is done even in part on camera, re-editing after completion of the tape requires very expensive and time-consuming use of a computer in order to achieve lip-audio synchronization. Therefore, it is preferable to either add the narration as a voice-over or to edit the tape on site so that it is in final form. The advantage of videotape over film is its ability to be reviewed immediately and edited and corrected without delay. Proper lighting, narration, and visualization are thus ensured. This, perhaps, is the major advantage of videotape over motion picture film.

COST

As recently as a few years ago good quality reproductions were possible only by recording on a 2 inch master tape. That no longer is true and excellent quality master tapes can be obtained with ¾ inch tape. All tapes have two audio channels, A and B, so that two separate narrations can be entered onto a single tape. This has application if a tape is to be bilingual or if a tape has been recorded live and a second narration is desired as an over-voice. Once the master tape has been completed, duplicates can be made at any of several centers, including the National Audio-visual Center in Atlanta, Bell and Howell in Chicago, and 3M Co. in Minneapolis.

A two-camera setup allows for greater versatility and a clarity of expression not obtainable with a single camera. As with all optical systems, the final results are in large part dependent upon the quality of the lenses and cameras utilized. Small, relatively inexpensive ($2000 to $7500) color cameras are satisfactory for home use but do not give professional quality or the definition required for an educational film. The best type of camera to use is of broadcast quality. Many medical centers and Veterans Administration hospitals have such equipment in their audiovisual sections, and it is wise to consult them. A maximal rate of approximately $2000 per day is charged to those outside the university. Another source is the local UHF channel, which can be hired to provide camera and crews at a cost approximating $3000 to $5000 per day. If none of these is available, private concerns are available at a cost ranging from $2000 to $5000. In-house production is the most flexible and least expensive.

The creation of an educational videotape rests squarely on the establishment of explicit instructional objectives, which will determine its content. The actual filming occurs only after the story board and then the script have been completed. At this point filming should be a relatively straightforward exercise.

Programming for continuing medical education

Charles R. Van Winkle

DEMAND FOR PROGRAMMING

The health and welfare of the American People continues to be the most controversial domestic issue facing our society. No other issue precipitated more governmental hearings and legislation, generated more news, or had a greater influence on our daily lives in the 1970s, and that influence will continue in the 1980s. The impact of all of this attention on organized medicine, in particular, has been profound as requirements for physicians to keep up to date with the practice of medicine are increasing at an exponential rate. Essentially, these pressures on physicians to keep current have been generated by a greater public awareness of health care matters, mounting numbers of malpractice actions, and the establishment of a Physician Recognition Award (PRA). The physician's continuing quest for up-to-date information coupled with the rapidly expanding electronic communication technology signals important opportunities for medical video programming.

Physician Recognition Award

The Physician Recognition Award, established by action of the AMA House of Delegates in December 1969, is the nationwide standard for continuing medical education (CME). The award is given on the receipt of 150 credit hours of approved CME activities within a three-year period. The physician has a great deal of flexibility if he or she meets the 150-hour requirement. Not only has the PRA become common currency for CME credit for many organizations, it has assumed legal and quasilegal status in many situations that affect the physician's access to reregistration of licensure, membership in the state medical society, availability of malpractice insurance, hospital privileges, and admission to medical specialty societies.

As pointed out by the *American Medical Association News,* physicians spend from $1.4 to $1.9 billion annually on continuing medical education. More than 300,000 physicians from every specialty enrolled in at least one CME course during the 1977 academic year, and well over 140,000 physicians have now qualified for the PRA award. In 1977 the number of courses was up 20% over the year before as the requirements and availability of continuing medical education continued to increase at a startling pace. Because of the steady increase in the number of physicians trained each year, soon over 400,000 will be practicing medicine. If each physician takes fifty hours of postgraduate education per year, which is the most common goal, approximately 20 million manhours are lost from practice. This cost in lost time is over and above the cost of providing these education programs, which can be high particularly if training involves travel expenses.

According to Dr. Jackson W. Riddle, director of the AMA Division of Educational Policy and Development, "Continuing medical education credits have assumed more significance than anyone ever anticipated. Physicians struggling to get Category I credits are reminiscent of the crusaders out after the Holy Grail."*

Acceptance of electronic journalism

Electronic journalism is developing rapidly as a major supplement to the traditional teaching techniques of lectures and print. In particular, video players, which can be connected easily to any standard television set, are a technologic advance whose time most certainly has come. General acceptance of the video medium is increasing rapidly. The total number of videocassette recorders (VCRs) in use by the end of 1982 will reach 3.6 million. Research indicates that by mid-1980 approximately 50,000 physicians owned videocassette recorders. Based on the most current market data it is estimated that the number of physicians owning VCRs by the end of 1981 may reach 90,000. Many medical associations and teaching institutions are establishing video "networks" for disseminating CME material both at the physician's homes and at hospitals.

DEVELOPMENT OF A VIDEO PROGRAM

While electronic journalism is rapidly becoming accepted because of its dramatic capabilities and conve-

---

*Riddle, J. W.: American Medical Association News, July 14, 1978.

nience, it is not without problems, the first of which is related to the quality of programming. In general, the degree of viewer sophistication has been established by network television broadcast standards, and, unfortunately, some medical video programming currently available is commonly described as on a par with home movies. As the use of video grows in the medical field, more quality programming sources will develop. However, until a broad spectrum of video programming becomes available from specialty associations and medical schools, physicians may want to produce their own programs.

Equipment

The basic components required for producing a program on videotape are a video camera, videocassette recorder with high-speed picture search and freeze-frame capabilities, and a standard color television set. These components can be easily interconnected to provide taping, instant replay, and editing functions. The cost of these three basic components is about $2,500, depending, of course, on the features of the individual equipment. Before beginning serious shopping, a prospective buyer should obtain the relative advantages and values of the equipment from video hardware magazines and consumer guides.

Before purchasing any equipment, consider where the program will be produced and also which format should be used for the tape programs. Most large hospitals have ¾ inch player equipment; however, most physicians are now purchasing ½ inch VHS and Betamax VCRs and equipment for home use.

Price should not be the overriding consideration when deciding to buy video equipment. Where practical, it is most advisable to buy equipment from an authorized franchise dealer offering on-site or convenient servicing. Having equipment repaired, even if it is under waranty, can take months if a discount dealer has to return a unit to the manufacturer or a regional repair plant.

Any investment that will exceed $3000 should be considered carefully and with the help of a professional. The video industry is in a highly dynamic stage, and rapidly developing technology creates the very real possibility of equipment obsolescence. Industry sources forecast there is little chance that standardization or increased compatibility of equipment is likely for years, if ever. Instead it is more likely the major formats—VHS, Betamax, and the video disk—will coexist, with programming and equipment available in each format. Therefore, any substantial purchase of even basic equipment must be weighed against the risk that it may not be state-of-the-art or even compatible with state-of-the-art technology in the very near future. Consequently, before purchasing equipment, a person would be prudent to consult an objective resource—video journals, video production consultants, etc., as opposed to a retail salesperson—about the compatibility of the equipment under consideration and whether or not it will be compatible with developments on the horizon.

Focus on planning

Regardless of the format in which a program will be presented, the fundamentals for planning an effective video program remain the same.

Outline to story boards. The first important stage in developing a video seminar involves outlining program objectives. Major points to be covered, proper degree of emphasis for the presentation, and level of audience sophistication should be determined.

By outlining the specific objectives of the proposed program, one can prepare a schematic for delivering information efficiently. Establishing a priority order for the major and minor points of information helps to keep a program concise and consistent with the goals of both the presenter and the audience. It is also critical to consider how much of the presentation the audience will remember and to what degree they will be able to apply the information after viewing the video seminar.

After a decision is made about intended audience and the information to be included, the presenter for the video presentation should be selected. When choosing participants consider individuals who, of course, have the proper credentials, but—just as important—can relax while speaking to a camera and following a cue card or teleprompter. It is surprising how many experts are anxious to appear on "television" and how quickly many become at home with the video medium. However, attention to some basic guidelines will help both novice and veteran performers make an effective presentation.

Preparation of a script. There is a great temptation for speakers who are familiar with a subject to "wing it." Preparing a script, or at least an outline, will help organize the material and keep it on track in terms of emphasis, order, and time.

The script or outline can be transferred to cue cards or a teleprompter to help guide the presentation. In addition, the script will guide the development of story boards, which are simple handdrawn illustrations indicating major scene changes, position changes of participants, insertion of graphics, etc., as seen from the "eye of the camera." A script plus a story board developed with the project director will help with camera positioning and lighting for each major scene.

If there is more than one participant or presenter, they should exchange scripts in order to avoid redundance or unintended controversy.

Using graphics. The thoughtful interspersion of graphics (clinical photos, patient examinations, laboratory reports, X-ray films, etc.) can make a dramatic contribution toward a successful video presentation. However, a word of caution about using slides from "live lectures," particularly those with massive amounts of type or numerals. Assume that each member of the audience is in the back row and provide simple, well-spaced, easy-to-read graphics. It is also important to leave visual material on the screen as long as it pertains to the voice-over presentation. (Chances are the slow readers are the ones who will need the information the most anyway.)

For panel discussions on-camera graphics can relieve the tedium of "talking balloons," providing material that takes the audience closer to the clinical situation.

Use of restraint. A final word about scripting and graphics: Understatement can draw the audience in; overstatement can drive the audience out. Remember that the standard for the average viewer is network television, which is very difficult competition in terms of special effects.

Limiting the "fidget factor." The most common video program formats are the single presenter and panel discussions. Both of these formats can be made more dramatic with the use of an off-camera voice-over to amplify or summarize points. The use of an off-camera voice-over also permits a rationale for moving the audience to more interesting situations, adding variety and depth to a program.

Another means of enriching a program is the use of a photodocumentary format in which the presenter is the voice-over and appears on camera only at the beginning or close of a program—or not at all. The voice-over in this case serves as a means of transport from one scene to another, offering appropriate comments.

An interesting variation of the photodocumentary format is to use a patient as the primary voice-over to present the program from a different perspective interspersed with dialogue with the attending physician.

It is most important to plan a program according to the length of time it takes to present the material and *not* with a fixed program length in mind. Certain natural subject break points in most programs will provide the opportunity to divide the tape into segments.

Ideally, no program should exceed 30 minutes without some form of break. As a rule of thumb the optimal effective attention span of audiences for nonprofessional programming is 20 to 30 minutes.

Any exceptionally important information should *not* be presented at the beginning or very end of a presentation to avoid having it overlooked because of the "settle-in" and "fidget" factors. If possible, a videocassette program should have a break for a live question-and-answer session as a functional measure at least after 40 minutes of programming. Obviously, some subjects do not lend themselves to such segmented programming, but planning some audience respite from heavy programming will increase the program's effectiveness.

Production

If production is not being done in the facilities of a hospital or teaching institution, it is necessary to get budget estimates from a supplier. Until good working relationships and cost ranges have been developed, it is most desirable to get several bids on the production.

Budget is usually the main factor in determining whether the program is produced in the production facilities of a hospital or teaching institution or at a commercial production company. Before making a judgment, however, it is advisable to view representative examples of work from each facility and discuss both the production and cost. The following rule-of-thumb can be used as a guideline for budgeting commercially produced programs, although these percentages may change, based on the actual budget base:

Scripting/graphics	25%
Shooting	50%
Editing	25%

If the budget is not particularly tight it is helpful to remember that resistance to prerecorded, nonprofessional video programs is related to the degree of viewer sophistication. As indicated earlier, most audience standards have been established by network television. Therefore, the goal of a production is to get as close to that performance level as budget, talent, and resources permit in order to gain and sustain audience interest. Obviously, experience and equipment play extremely important roles in achieving this goal.

Standard release forms

Once each segment of the program is completed, each participant should be asked to sign a standard release form subject to viewing the rough cut of the program. The standard release form should include the following basic elements:

Participant release

Date of production: ______

Sponsoring organization: ______________________

Producer: ______________________

Participant: ______________________

Purpose of program: ______________________

Intended audience: ______________________

It is understood that this program is being produced for ______________ and being distributed to ______________. Neither my presentation nor any segment thereof may be used without express consent.

Signature: ______________________ Date: ______

Signature of producer: ______________________ Date: ______

Editing

Noncommercial editing in its most rudimentary form involves merely erasing or taping over the actual working tape. If the tape is being edited commercially for the replication of a number of copies of the program, it can be converted to a master tape and should be kept in a temperature-controlled, secured area for possible future use. Depending on the length and format of the tape, professional editing for a tape 30 to 45 minutes long could cost several hundred dollars. Copies of the duplicated program tapes would cost about $45.00 each depending on the format of the tape, length, and quantities ordered.

Editing a one-half hour show commercially should take from 1½ to 2 hours—which is one of the many advantages of working with tape versus film. A rule-of-thumb for tape editing is usually 2 to 1:two hours to edit each hour of program.

Before reaching the final editing stages, it is important to determine who will have the right of final approval in terms of content, the participant or the organization under whose auspices the program is being presented. Determining this prior to final editing will help reduce misunderstanding.

WAVE OF THE FUTURE: SATELLITE PROGRAMS AND MASS COMPUTER RETRIEVAL

During the next decade, it is estimated that over 70% of American homes now using television will also be equipped with some type of video recording and/or playback unit. In conjunction with this trend other advances in communication devices are under development, such as request and demand video programming using mass-computer retrieval. This technology combines all the advantages of videocassette programming with the simplicity of delivery comparable to the current over-the-air systems.

Request TV

The viewer would receive a catalog with a list of available programs. Code numbers would replace time schedules for each program description. By pressing a predetermined sequence of control buttons the viewer would have access to a particular program at any time of the day or night because the programming runs continuously.

Demand TV

By mid-1990 it is projected that viewers will be able to phone a regional video library guide to request a specific program. The program would be transmitted immediately into the viewer's home via cable. If the person wished to inventory the program for later viewing it could be automatically recorded by a videotape unit. It has also been estimated that by the mid-1990s there will be over 60 million subscribers connected by cable—all potential customers for this new technology. With this burgeoning appetite for specific programming, it is not inconceivable that a modest but well-planned program originally intended for a relatively small audience could find its way into a mass retrieval program bank to be shown before sizable and geographically diverse audiences.

CONCLUSION

It seems extremely appropriate for the health care community with present communication capabilities to re-evaluate their use of audiovisual media. Computer and video technologies have vaulted medical communication capabilities into a new generation—the era of electronic journalism, an era futurists now describe as medical schools without walls. This new era will profoundly increase the options of those with the tasks of informing and keeping informed.

Planning a meeting

CHAPTER 25

Setting up a scientific program

Joel Mattison, M.D.

A scientific program may be compared to a sit-down dinner to which guests come and are obliged to eat whatever is set before them; or it may be like a cafeteria meal at which no one is expected to eat everything offered, but, instead, picks and chooses according to personal needs and desires. The single-offering event, whether a dinner or a scientific program, is the more difficult to plan since the program chairman or chef must decide what the fare for everyone is to be. This involves making arbitrary decisions regarding what others should like and even what is good for them. In multiple or simultaneous sessions, however, the responsibility falls, at least in part, on the attendee rather than on the program chairman. As all branches of science grow more complex and tedious, simultaneous sessions become increasingly necessary.

To carry the analogy further: (1) Everyone presumably needs a balanced diet. (2) Not everyone likes the same things and in the same quantity. (3) Some are faddists; others are on diets. (4) The offering must not only be balanced, but also it must be palatable and must even look attractive. The setting, background sounds, temperature, coloration, lighting, and hardware all affect one's appetite and digestion (or absorption of information). In the eighteenth century, when dining was grand and occupied much of an afternoon and evening, it was important to change the scene and to serve the coffee in another setting. (5) At the risk of carrying the analogy too far, there is a certain order of presentation for a meal and for a program. If this order is observed, hunger is satisfied and digestions are unruffled.

Good programs, like good meals or other events, never "just happen." They represent good planning and hard work by persons who are well aware of the frailties and limitations of human behavior. Nothing can be left to chance. A poor program cannot become a good one by chance, but a good one can become intolerably poor if left to chance. It is an undeniable fact that chance cannot help but can occasionally hurt.

Most of us assume that some magic may happen with a gathering of persons, whether at a meeting or party. This ill-defined "something" that is hoped for involves feedback, expectation (self-fulfilling prophecy), and good public relations. Do not leave this to chance. A program must fall upon fertile soil, which means falling upon minds expecting something worthwhile to happen.

THE PROGRAM CHAIRMAN

A program chairman in most organizations will not be a first-timer, but will usually have previously served on the program committee. This, of course, does not apply to a symposium that has been set up as a one-time affair. There are several principles that a successful program planner should follow:

1. No matter what your experience, talk with whomever had the responsibility last. If your organization has a job description, read it carefully; it will make your job easier.

2. Get your instructions from the executive committee, president, or sponsor of the meeting. Have a definite idea of what you are to get across or what your theme will be. Even in an annual national meeting, it is helpful to have some idea or theme (a subject for emphasis, a historical thrust, an examination of a new frontier, or a common problem for exploration).

3. Get a firm date for the meeting from which you can plan your schedule. Be as certain as you can that there are no conflicts that your potential registrants will have to choose between.

4. Plan to use your program committee and get it together early. Go to this meeting with a plan, but be prepared to lay everything aside for something better. Have an agenda and keep a record or you will forget or overlook important details.

5. Plan to balance the program as much as possible. Sample all varieties of experience, represent all fields of your discipline; try to have a balance of personalities as well. This may mean letters to solicit papers from certain individuals whom you feel have something unique to offer.

6. Get last year's program and, if possible, those for the past three years.

7. Be familiar with other programs offered to your potential registrants in order to meet the needs of your registrants uniquely.

8. Visit the meeting site early. Know what facilities are available.

    a. Evaluate the rooms and chose those suitable for your needs.

    b. Evaluate the audiovisual equipment and the personnel who operate it.

    c. Know what recreational potential there is.

    d. Evaluate the break facilities: how much, how good, and if served on time. (It is important to negotiate price for refreshments prior to the meeting since coffee and soft drink breaks may run to $2.50 per person.)

    e. Evaluate the eating facilities: dissatisfaction in the dining room usually spreads elsewhere.

9. Set a schedule and stick with it. Work backward from your meeting date, preferably a year away.

Meeting date	12 months
Call for abstracts	9 months
Abstracts deadline	6 months
Circulate abstracts to program committe immediately	
Notification of acceptance or rejection	5 months
Publish and circulate by mail:	
Abstracts booklet	2 months
Detailed program	2 months

10. Check with program chairmen of other organizations for any papers or topics that they might not have used but that might be suitable for your needs.

11. Plan a questionnaire to be circulated at the conclusion of the meeting to evaluate the effectiveness of the program. This should include:

    Presentation attended
       Speakers
       Panels
       Movies
    Breadth of coverage
    Depth of coverage
    Shortcomings
    Suggestions for future programs
    Comments about the site

This may well be your most significant contribution and will make the job easier for those who follow you.

12. Be aware of continuing education requirements.

Someone on your committee should investigate this early in your planning so that an announcement may be made at the meeting regarding the amount of credit due and how it is to be reported.

There are several items that the program chairman normally need not be concerned with, but should be certain that someone in the organization is responsible for:

    Local arrangements
    Registration
    Transportation
    Recreation
    Sports
    Entertainment
    Meal planning
    Banquet, if any
    Audiovisual equipment (including slide check-in)
    Certificates, if any

Identify the person responsible for each area and make a mental note as to whether or not you need to recheck. If one particular area is unassigned, delegate it, if possible, to someone in the organization or to someone on your committee.

Most hotels or resort facilities have an office that handles conventions or commercial sales. Here you will find a gold mine of professional assistance, including printed brochures, reservation forms, instructions on how to get to the hotel, and so on. Identify one person in that office, establish contact, and check back with this same person as frequently as necessary. Avail yourself of this professional help and experience.

The program chairman will already have enough to do and should see to it that the above mentioned list of responsibilities is delegated to dependable persons. If the chairman is overworked, he or she will do a poor job, overlooking things that someone else might see readily. In addition, someone else who is willing and capable may be deprived of an opportunity to serve the organization and to share in the enthusiasm.

ABSTRACTS

In many organizations abstracts are called for on the same schedule every year. If this is not the case, the program chairman should set up a schedule or timetable. A deadline should be set and announced at least two times: (1) Initially it is announced in either a newsletter or some other correspondence. The purpose is to provide a tickler that will start members thinking about something that they may have on a rear burner. Announcing the deadline at the annual meeting is also helpful but, of necessity, is missed by many of the members. (2) There should be an official letter announcing the call for abstracts and deadline, enclosing an abstract form and an explanatory letter (Fig. 25-1).

The chairman should require that abstracts be sub-

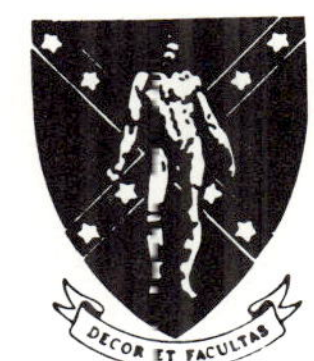

SOUTHEASTERN SOCIETY OF PLASTIC AND RECONSTRUCTIVE SURGEONS

PRESIDENT
  William E. Huger, Jr., M.D.
  Atlanta, Georgia
PRESIDENT-ELECT
  Eugene Worthen, M.D.
  Monroe, Louisiana
VICE-PRESIDENT
  Joel Mattison, M.D.
  Tampa, Florida
SECRETARY
  John R. Reynolds, M.D.
  Chattanooga, Tennessee
ASSISTANT SECRETARY
  Leon Block, M.D.
  Falls Church, Virginia
TREASURER
  Robert C. Reeder, M.D.
  Memphis, Tennessee

HISTORIAN
  James M. Carraway, M.D.
  Norfolk, Virginia
TRUSTEES
  John R. Royer, M.D.
  Winter Park, Florida
  William J. Pitts, M.D.
  Birmingham, Alabama
  Andrew W. Walker, M.D.
  Charlotte, North Carolina
  Thomas J. Zaydon, M.D.
  Miami, Florida
  James H. Fleming, Jr., M.D.
  Nashville, Tennessee
  Phil D. Craft, M.D.
  Chattanooga, Tennessee

October 27, 1979

To All Southeasterners:

Your Program Committee needs your 75 word typed (camera ready) abstracts of papers proposed for submission to the Program Committee by Thanksgiving of 1979. Please mail them to me as Chairman of the Scientific Program Committee (4700 North Habana Avenue, Tampa, Florida 33614.) For papers selected, these abstracts will be printed without editing "as is" into the booklet of abstracts to be distributed at the registration desk at the Greenbrier (May 25 to 29, 1980).

Your Program Committee has grappled with a problem and proposes a solution which it has taken via the Executive Committee: Each person submitting an abstract should understand that no papers should be submitted for consideration that have been <u>presented in the same form</u> within the past year prior to the date of the annual meeting. This is not intended to discourage presentation of a significant advancement or new material on a previous subject, nor a more intense exploration of the subject.

The submitted abstracts will be mailed out just after Thanksgiving to the members of the Program Committee who will vote on including them in the program. It is anticipated that authors will receive some kind of information from the Program Committee shortly after the first of the year.

Program directors and residents should please note that papers for the resident's competition should be submitted directly to Dr. Charles White, 220 South Claybrook, Memphis, Tennessee 38104. As in the past, six papers will be selected for the resident's competition; these will be selected by Dr. White's committee and handed to the Program Committee for automatic inclusion into the program. Any papers not accepted for the resident's competition may be resubmitted to the Program Committee for consideration in the program apart from the competition.

Again, this year there will be an adequate amount of time for problem case discussion. These should be submitted to Dr. Cauley Hayes, 1010

Continued.

Fig. 25-1.

Southeasterners   -2-   October 27, 1979

East Third Street, Chattanooga, Tennessee 37403. There will be time
set aside for Southeastern Society Pearls (otherwise known as SES
Perls. This segment of the program will be under the direction of
Dr. John McCraw, 400 West Brambleton Avenue, Norfolk, Virginia 23510.
This will include categories previously entitled "A Case I Am Proud
Of," "How I Do It", "Something That I Tried That Didn't Work", or
"Something That Has Worked Well For Me." This is intended to be a
high powered session of Pearls, brief in length, which although
important and extremely significant may not have inspired the author
to present them as a paper. Please contact John directly.

Any items to be selected for inclusion under the category of Socio-
Economics should be submitted directly to Dr. Michael Bryant, 6577
Superior Avenue, Sarasota, Florida 33579.

As in the past, movies will probably begin each morning's
session except on the first day. Anyone wishing to submit
a movie of his own or wishing to suggest a movie for inclusion
in the program may do so by using the abstract blank attached
which will apply to movies as well as papers.

Thank you.

                              Sincerely yours,

                              Joel Mattison, M. D.

JM/bhm

Fig. 25-1, cont'd.

mitted on a standard form to avoid receiving an incredible miscellany consisting of everything from pencilled scraps of paper to full presentations complete with illustrations. The information needed is:

Title of paper to be presented
Names of authors, with presenter listed first
Addresses of authors
Institutional affiliation, if any
Abstract, with word limit specified. It is convenient to provide a rectangle within which the abstract may be typewritten. The entire form may be printed in nonreproducing blue ink so that the abstracts can be cut and pasted in a printed abstract booklet, placing the onus for neatness and accuracy on the presenter and saving time and money for the program chairman.

Helpful information to have from authors includes the following:

Type of audiovisual equipment required:
35 mm single projection
35 mm dual projection
16 mm silent
16 mm sound
Length of time requested
Information about the sampling upon which the paper is based
Suggested discussants

A covering letter should include at least the following information:

Date of meeting
Place of meeting
Restrictions as to whether the paper may have been previously presented or published
Abstract deadline
How papers will be chosen
When notification may be expected

CORRESPONDENCE

By now it is obvious that you will need several form letters unless you have unlimited secretarial help. Not only do form letters save time, but they assure that each participant receives adequate and uniform information.

You need a letter to your selection committee. This will accompany the abstracts and should include the following minimal information:

A uniform grading system (the simplest is 0-10)
A list of the abstracts with a blank for the grade for each
A request that all of the abstracts be read and graded at a single sitting, if possible, to assure uniform judgment
A deadline for returning the grading sheet

Program selections are made as frequently on the basis of the submitting author's abilities as upon the material itself. This is probably inevitable and not altogether undesirable. It is probably well, therefore, to leave the author's name attached rather than to have the abstracts evaluated blindly.

You will, of course, need a form letter of acceptance (and one for rejection). The acceptance letter should include:

Abstract title and author
Date and approximate time
Time allowed for presentation
Suggestions for speakers (see box on p. 196)

The rejection letter should be brief; attempts to soften the discomfort are probably not helpful. Be on the lookout for papers that might be used in other ways, such as problem case presentations.

A form letter will also help to recruit those persons whom the authors have suggested to discuss their papers. It should be made clear that these persons should be prepared to discuss, but should be willing to either be brief or silent in the event that spontaneous discussion is generated. Spontaneous discussion is more natural and is usually more successful and more appreciated. Again, however, designating persons to initiate discussion is essential and the effort will pay off.

ASSEMBLING THE PROGRAM

Once you have selected the abstracts, by whatever means, you now have to decide how to put the program together. Up to this point you have merely been gathering data. You have to decide how to group the papers for purposes of organizing the information, for discussion, and for sustaining interest.

One question that always arises is what to do with the first spot each morning, the last spot each afternoon, and the entire last day. The best advice is to ignore, insofar as possible, what time and what day it is. Otherwise, if you place what seems to be your weakest material in the most desirable spots, you will encourage poor attendance at these times even more. Your audience should be assured that the schedule is consistent and will be followed. This will encourage them to be on time and stay until the end. Try to cultivate this trust. Be aware of transportation schedules, however, and do not expect people to stay after the last plane of the day has left for an area accessible only by that route.

The program should be distributed to prospective registrants as far in advance as possible. Although some members will attend without regard to the program quality, others will be encouraged to attend after perusing an excellent and exciting program.

A letter to the membership or an article in the newsletter will also help to develop interest and enthusiasm. There should be something from the program chairman in every newsletter, if possible. Repetition is the soul of advertising, and if you do not think of yourself as somewhat of a salesman, you may be overlooking part of your job.

1. Please be certain that your paper falls within the time limits indicated. We will use the ingenious Worthen timer: A green light indicates that there is plenty of time left. When one minute of speaker's time is left, a yellow light comes on and the green light goes out. When the speaker's time is completely used up, a red light comes on, the yellow light remains lit, and a buzzer sounds. Each speaker should be prepared to conclude his or her remarks before the red light comes on. The timer and lights will be in plain view of both the speaker and the audience, and it will be in front of the member who is acting as secretary for the session.

2. Please be certain that your slides in the carousel (as you hand it to the projectionist) have been "run through" by you *at least once* in the *same* carousel: This will completely eliminate the problems of out-of-order, reversed, or upside-down slides.

3. Please read your paper ahead of time to someone: your spouse, your secretary, your colleague, etc. If you are a resident, be sure to "present" it to your chief exactly as you will present it at the meeting. Please be certain not to perform your first reading before the membership.

4. Please have your name on the outside side of the carousel in white one-inch adhesive tape with your name in black one-inch letters, so that the projectionist can easily identify your carousel not only for presentation, but also so that if you call for "my last slide in the first carousel," he can easily find it for you, even though he does not know you.

5. The Chesapeake Room at the Greenbrier is an excellent room for a scientific meeting. It will be set up to seat approximately 175 persons in "schooldesk" manner with long covered tables in front of rows of chairs. There will be smoking and nonsmoking sides. On the front row on the audience's left will be a short reserved table designated as the "bull pen" for the speakers for the next four papers (in the group designated for discussion). This will allow the next speaker to step to the speaker's stand without delay; the microphone will be adjusted by the secretary, and the speaker will be given any last-minute instructions or suggestions. Before the session each speaker should have already taken the opportunity to become familiar with the pointer (and its focus), the manner of changing slides, etc.

6. You will be introduced by the session chairman or the secretary. Any information other than that appearing in the program or in the paper abstract should be communicated to the chairman in writing, well in advance. It would be helpful if you would send a curriculum vitae to the chairman.

7. A pointer will be provided. As a tip from those of us who have learned the hard way, you may find it helpful to rest the pointer across your arm, bracing it to eliminate that tell-tale nervous tremor that is magnified by the long lever arm between yourself and the screen.

8. The speaker's desk will be on stage just to the audiences' left of the screen. There will thus be no obstruction (including the speaker) between the line of view of the audience and the screen. There will be a light on the reading desk. On a lower level, just above the level of the audience, there will be a table at which the chairman of the morning and the secretary for the session will be seated. If there is a panel, the members will be seated at this table, unless they desire to be seated on the stage (logistically difficult).

9. There will be microphones at the speaker's desk, at the chairman's table, and midway down in each of the three aisles in the audience (floor microphones). It is hoped that no one will attempt to address the session without using *one* of these microphones.

10. It is suggested that you make your reply to any discussion or questions only after all of the questions and discussion have been completed. This will allow you time to think about your reply and to weigh details with which you are most familiar or which you feel are most important.

11. Keep in mind that the genius of the Southeastern is the free and frank discussion that follows the excellent papers. Keep in mind also that these are your friends. Organize your replies and make them pertinent and brief so that the meeting can seem to proceed at a leisurely pace.

12. Please remember that there is nothing more disastrous than a slide with too much material on it, no matter how revealing or important the information. Most good slide makers agree that there should be only one good idea or point on each slide except when two things are being compared. If you try to put too much information on a slide, it will simply be missed or even ignored. Feel free to use cartoons, either relevant or irrelevant (or reverent or irreverent). Some of the best teaching occurs whenever a new and novel (and unforgettable) means is used to impress new truths upon an old audience or old truths on a new audience. Cull your slides carefully: A rapid progression from an overexposed to an underexposed slide and back again usually gets in the way of what you are trying to illustrate. Do not be afraid to read your slides to the audience. At any rate, look up frequently to see that the projector and you are synchronized.

13. All of the above suggestions are made in the interest of helping you to get a better hearing for your paper. We wish you the best and we look forward to sharing your presentation with you. Thank you for participating.

Sincerely yours,

Joel

for the Scientific Program Committee

Program variety

The enemy of any good program is fatigue. It is probably best combatted by variety and by remembering that fatigue is either a function of time or is time related. People will tire of even a good thing, but they will tire more quickly and surely as mediocrity is approached. You will need to be especially inventive if:

The program lasts three or more consecutive days, using half-day (or more) sessions

The program lasts more than two days of morning and afternoon sessions

The program lasts more than one and one half days of morning, afternoon, and evening sessions.

If any of these apply to your situation, it is particularly important to consider some of the following suggestions:

1. Limit any long sessions with a single speaker to about fifty minutes before having some form of break either in continuity of speaker or continuity of place or seating
2. When topics shorter than fifty minutes are used (ten minutes, for example), schedule a discussion after each two to four presentations (appropriately grouped) and a break every two hours
3. When the variations listed below are followed, begin with the didactic and progress to other forms, which require less effort to hold attention

Suggested methods to vary the program include:

Lecture

Panels

Movies

Videotape sessions

Special teaching sessions (classes with a limited curriculum on a particular subject)

Groups (including meals, cocktail parties, etc.)

Breakfast, luncheon, and dinner sessions

Role-playing

Laboratory experiences

Poster sessions

By interplaying these various approaches, you can increase the interest and attention of your audience.

SESSION CHAIRMAN AND SECRETARY

After the program has been laid out, you must select someone to preside over the sessions. This is usually best or most easily accomplished by two persons who are designated as chairman and secretary. The chairman is in charge and presides. He or she opens the session, announces the titles, and introduces the speakers. The chairman's most important duty is to keep order, to ensure that speakers adhere to time limits, and to moderate the discussions. This person must have an innate sense of timing and of humor, and must enjoy the respect of the group.

The secretary is no less important. He or she presides when the chairman is absent, and must be on the lookout for signals or feedback that the chairman may miss. The secretary must see that the speakers understand the lectern and know how to operate the light, pointer, slide changer, etc., and must see that the microphone is properly adjusted. Most of all, the secretary must see to it that speakers feel comfortable and encouraged.

Send a letter to the chairman and secretary outlining their duties (see box on p. 198 for an example).

THE PHYSICAL SETUP

Unless space is at a premium, the best way to set up a meeting is in schoolroom fashion. The seating is placed along one side of long cloth-covered tables, with registrants facing the front. This gives a writing surface, adequate space, and a place for water and ash trays. Be sure that you inquire whether there is an extra charge for pads and pencils. Most of your registrants will have writing instruments and can make notes in the program or abstract booklet.

Auditorium or theater style refers to uninterrupted rows of seating without the intervening tables. Unless there are foldaway desk surfaces, there is no place to write and it is difficult for latecomers to be seated. It is also difficult to reach the microphones for discussion. In general, there is a cramped feeling and the only advantage is that the room will hold more people.

Use the smallest room that will hold your audience. Most speakers feel better and therefore do better when speaking to a packed house. It has the same effect on the audience; they share a heightened enthusiasm and benefit from a better presentation from the speakers.

Consider having a smoking and nonsmoking section, clearly marked with legible signs.

All needed signs have to be available ahead of time, either from the hotel or brought along. The hotel will probably assist you by placing a sign in the lobby indicating the registration area.

A projection screen may be placed at either center stage or diagonally in the corner to the audience's right. The speaker's stand should be to the audience's left. If the screen is diagonally placed to the audience's right and the speaker's stand somewhere diagonally on the audience's left, this gives a good view of the screen from the speaker's stand, allowing speakers to see without having to consciously turn their heads. This constant turning to look at the screen results in interrupted thought and microphone fade-out. The more the speaker's stand approaches the mid-axis of the audience, the more difficult the delivery. Give your speakers a chance to make a good presentation. A suggested room arrangement is shown in Fig. 25-2.

No matter how carefully you have laid out these details on the drawing board, a final on-site personal check

TO PERSONS WHO WILL ACT AS CHAIRMEN AND SECRETARIES OF THE MORNINGS

The chairman is to introduce each speaker appropriately and briefly (with the exception of the Upchurch lecturer who will be introduced by the president of the society.) As chairman you are the person actually responsible for the morning; most of all you must keep things orderly and on schedule and decide when to encourage discussion and when to conclude it (you may rarely want to steal time from another discussion period if interest is overwhelming). You must keep order. Insisting that all floor discussion and questions be made through the floor microphones will make this much easier and almost automatic. All questions should be directed to the speaker through the chairman. The chairman should be good natured, humorous, and objective; and should make every attempt to avoid allowing a speaker, a discusser, a questioner, or the listeners to feel uncomfortable.

You must see that the session begins on time, even if you and the speaker are the only persons present. Use the bell to round up the talkers in the hall (both before 8:00 and at the end of the coffee break). In the event of too lively informal discussion, this could function as a gavel also.

You should feel free to leave the meeting in the hands of the secretary and may exchange positions with him or her for a portion of the session, if desired.

The secretary escorts speakers to the podium, adjusts the microphone (or places the lavalier mike) appropriately, sees to it that the light on the speaker's podium is on, and makes certain that the speaker understands how to change the slides. The pointer must be handy, in order, and its use understood. The secretary also starts the timer. A comforting word or smile may do much to make speakers feel at ease, no matter how experienced or expert they may be.

The general success of the day depends upon these two persons. Every one enjoys an orderly session more than otherwise, and everyone thus has a say. The membership's repeated response to questionnaires is that (1) more time is needed for discussion and (2) the afternoons should be for recreation and therefore free; it is hard to give them both.

You may make minor changes in the schedule; if someone needs to present earlier in order to catch a plane, try to be accommodating.

The last session each morning is likely to run overtime; use your judgment, but always stop it before it grinds down or lapses into nonproductivity.

Consider yourselves as the ranking officers of the society during time that the "gavel" is in your hands. The leadership during this time is your responsibility.

Certain speakers have suggested certain members to discuss their papers. You should be aware that certain members have been primed in case no spontaneous discussion arises.

Thank you.

Chairman & secretary
Screen
Lectern
Front row for next speakers
Smoking
Non smoking
#
Mike
#
Floor microphone
#
Mike
Projection

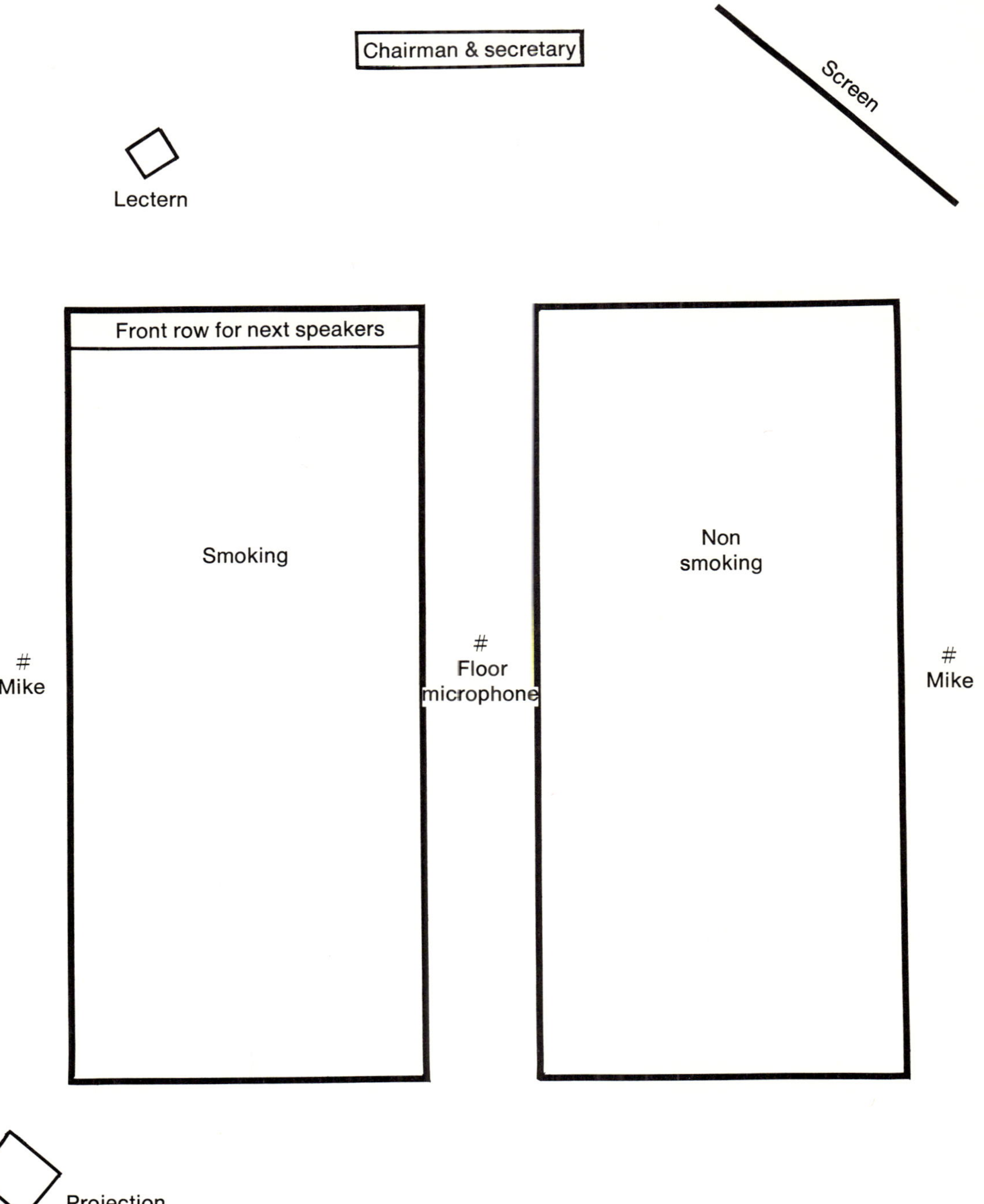

Fig. 25-2.

must be made. Plan to spend at least an hour in the main auditorium doing this before the meeting starts. If you do it the night before, there will be time to make those all-important last-minute changes that can make the difference between success and failure of your program.

The speaker's stand must be equipped with a microphone that picks up the speaker's voice even when his head is turned. If this is not available, then a lavalier microphone will have to be used, but this takes valuable time for placement and adjustment each time a new speaker comes to the stand. There must be a reading light, a pointer, and a slide changer (or signal to the projectionist).

The chairman's table should be equipped with at least two microphones and seating for the chairman and the secretary of the session. If you are having a panel during the session, be sure to have the required number of chairs and microphones to accommodate all the panel members. Keep rearrangements within each program segment to a minimum.

A timer is an absolute necessity. The best is one with a series of lights that warn when the time is nearly up and, more obviously, when the time has expired. A buzzer should sound also at the conclusion of the assigned time. If the lights can be easily seen by both the speaker and the audience, the temptation to go into overtime will be minimized. Good-humored references to this also help to reinforce the idea.

A handbell is also useful: it can be used to signal the starting of the sessions and the ending of the breaks. Nothing is more distracting than having latecomers interrupt a speaker while belatedly trying to get back to their seats. The secretary can simply ring the bell or have the lights blinked to signal the end of the break and to encourage everyone to return to the meeting room promptly so that the program can continue on time and without distraction.

There should be a floor microphone on each aisle in the audience. If all questions are directed through the microphones, order is almost automatic and the session is easier to moderate.

By now the task seems formidable, with many details and too much responsibility. Remember that there are two ways to guarantee a poor program: the first is to ignore the advice offered here; the second is to follow it as if it were *all* true and applicable. You must analyze your group and its individual needs and tailor a program to fit these needs. You must be determined to have a good program with the widest possible base and the widest possible involvement of the membership. You must strive to make this not your success, but your group's success. Only as it belongs to and comes from everyone will it be worthwhile. Your constant goal must be to help your colleagues have a worthwhile experience and a good time. As with any host, this involves some element of personal sacrifice, which must not be apparent to those attending.

CHAPTER 26

Audiovisual planning

Earl Bauer

When determining audiovisual requirements for a meeting, you must take a number of factors into consideration. These include:

Room size
Room setup
Speaker ready room
Determination of each speaker's requirements
Ordering equipment

ROOM SIZE

Just as a room has dimensions, so do people. This must be taken into consideration when you are selecting a room for a meeting in which audiovisuals are to be used (see also Appendix D-4).

1. The top of the head of an average adult seated in a straight chair will be 4½ feet above the floor.
2. When seated in a straight chair with feet extended, a person will require 3 feet, 2 inches from the back of the head to the toes.
3. While seated with arms folded, a person requires 22 inches on an armless chair or 28 inches on a chair with arms.
4. If a seated person raises his hand, the fingertips will be 5 feet, 4 inches above the floor.

From these figures you can determine that the average person will require a minimum of 7 square feet to be comfortable in a meeting room. These dimensions also tell us that in order to keep hands out of the projected image, the projector lens must be at least 5 feet, 4 inches above the floor and the bottom of the screen at least 3 feet, 6 inches. If the audience is to be coming and going during the meeting, the screen and projector must be raised even further.

A formula for selecting the proper size for a meeting room can be derived from the previous figures:

No. attending × 7 sq ft × 150% (aisle, stage) = Room size

There may be some exceptions to this in smaller meetings (25 to 150 people) where as much as 170% will be needed for screens, aisles, and risers. The chart below takes this into consideration and is a good general guideline:

Audience size	Total square feet
25	400
50	675
75	975
100	1,200
150	1,700
200	2,100
300	3,150
400	4,200
500	5,250
750	7,875
1000	10,500

Screen size

When choosing the screen size for a given room a simple formula is helpful:

Room length ÷ 6 = Suggested screen height

Ceiling height

To determine the minimal ceiling height necessary you can use this formula:

Room length (in feet) ÷ 6 + height screen off floor

In rooms up to 50 feet long allow 4 feet; 100 feet long, 5 feet; and over 150 feet long, 6 feet.

To apply the formula for a room 90 feet long:

90 ÷ 6 = 15 + 4 = 19 feet minimal ceiling height

Low ceilings. Unfortunately, many rooms may have adequate size for the anticipated attendance but have inadequate ceiling height. If you encounter this in your meeting planning, several alternatives are available. By increasing the light output of the projector, you can use a factor of 8 in determining the usable seating area of a meeting room. As an example, if you have usable ceiling height (no chandeliers) of 16 feet, deduct 4 feet (distance screen is off floor), which means you can use a 12-foot screen. Multiply this by 8 and you find everyone seated up to 96 feet away will be able to interpret the information presented on the screen. This is a gain of 24 feet of seating area, which is significant.

Some facilities will exaggerate room capacities in their brochures. Measurements are usually accurate, but you should apply our own formulas when calculating the actual room capacity. In planning, you must also keep in mind local fire regulations, which may specify the maximal number of chairs per row or minimal aisle widths.

Other factors. Other things you must consider when selecting a room for satisfactory audiovisual use are:

1. Sound system quality and location of speakers and controls
2. Dividing walls and their sound-dampening qualities
3. Light controls and dimmer locations
4. Screen placement
5. Location of projector platform
6. Selection of projector lenses
7. Seating arrangement and type

ROOM SETUP

Room setup and screen placement are as much a part of the projection system as is correct selection of lens, lamp, and screen size and type. Too often little thought is given to this aspect, with the result that a substantial part of the audience has a poor seat or is unable to see the screen. How often have we seen a room setup similar to that shown in (Fig. 26-1)? The screen is located in the center of the room and the projection table is right smack in the center of the audience. This places the screen in such a position that the presenter must turn away from the audience to view it and the projector and projectionist are in a position to be distracting to the audience. This is frequently encountered if the projector is supplied with only one lens and must be placed to fill the screen with the projected image. With proper planning such a setup is no longer necessary, nor should it be tolerated.

To set a room correctly requires a sizable investment by your audiovisual supplier in lenses and equipment, but should add little to your rental charges. When planning a meeting this small additional expense will be worth it to ensure that everyone in your audience has a good seat.

Fig. 26-2 shows a traditional setup. Note that area D is beyond the acceptable angle of view because of image distortion. An 8-foot screen at that angle is only 4 feet wide to a viewer and, believe it or not, only 2 feet wide to the presenter. Area C to the right front has unacceptable sight line, since the right side of the screen is blocked by the lectern and the presenter. Area D adjacent to area C has visibility loss of 100%. The audience seated here can see the presenter but not the screen

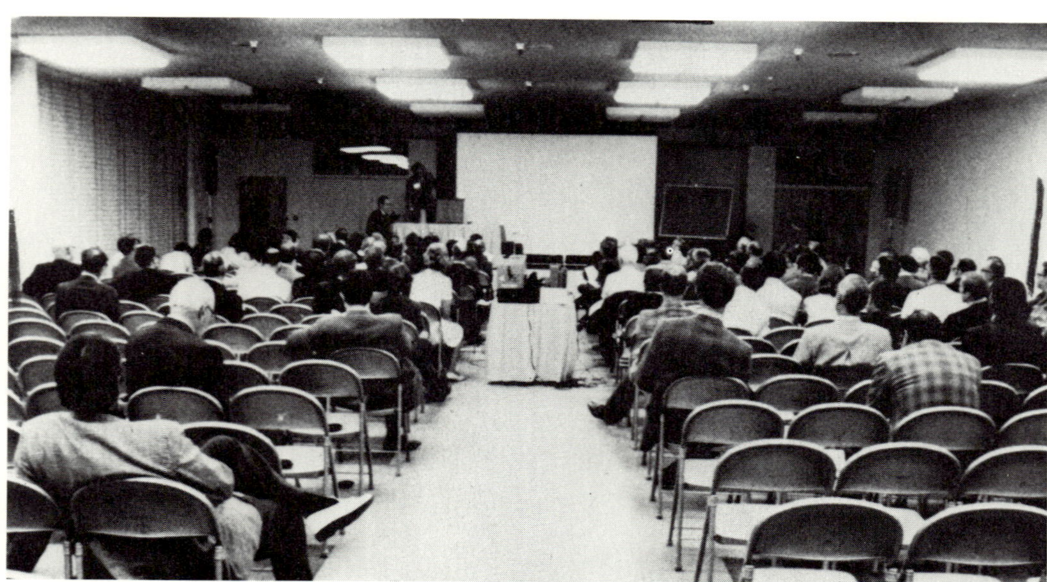

Fig. 26-1. The usual room setup. Note that the screen is in the center of the room and that the projection table is located in the middle of the audience. This makes it necessary for the speaker to turn away from the audience in order to see the screen. The placement of the projector is such that it is distracting or obstructive to much of the audience.

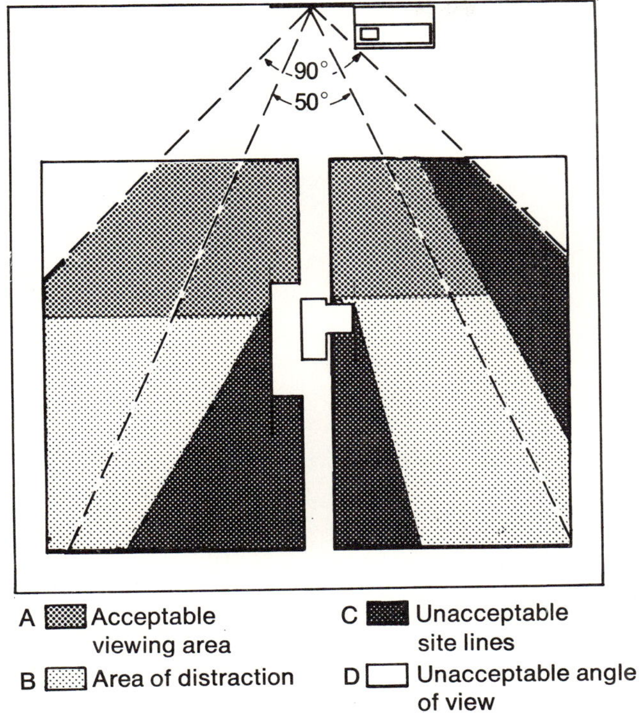

A — Acceptable viewing area
C — Unacceptable site lines
B — Area of distraction
D — Unacceptable angle of view

Fig. 26-2. Diagram of the traditional setup. With this arrangement only 30% of the audience has an unobstructed or undistracted view of the screen.

(Fig. 26-3). Area C to the rear also has sight line problems created by the projection platform and the projectionist. Area B, the area of distraction, contains that portion of the viewers who can see the screen and the presenter, but are distracted by the extraneous light, movement of the projectionist and projector, and by the noise and confusion of presenters bringing in or picking up their slides. Area A is the acceptable viewing area. This fraction of viewers, 30% to be exact, is the only group being treated fairly.

A better room setup is depicted in Fig. 26-4. This provides maximal viewing for not only the audience, but also the presenter (Fig. 26-5). Fig. 26-6 shows the ideal room setup, as follows:

1. The screen is placed in the corner of the room. It is a matte white screen with a 90-degree acceptable viewing angle. This means that the entire audience has good screen visibility.
2. Even the presenter, who is in the middle of the room, is on the edge of the acceptable viewing area.
3. The projection table is placed on a riser in the opposite corner of the room from the screen to project over the heads of the audience. This moves all the confusion, noise, and light to the rear of the room and gives the select seating areas to the audience instead of to the projection equipment.
4. All power cords and remote cables are taped to the wall instead of being located in the aisles. This keeps members of the audience from tripping over the wires and injuring themselves or disconnecting the power supply.

This type of room setup makes a lot of sense, as well as a lot of happy viewers.

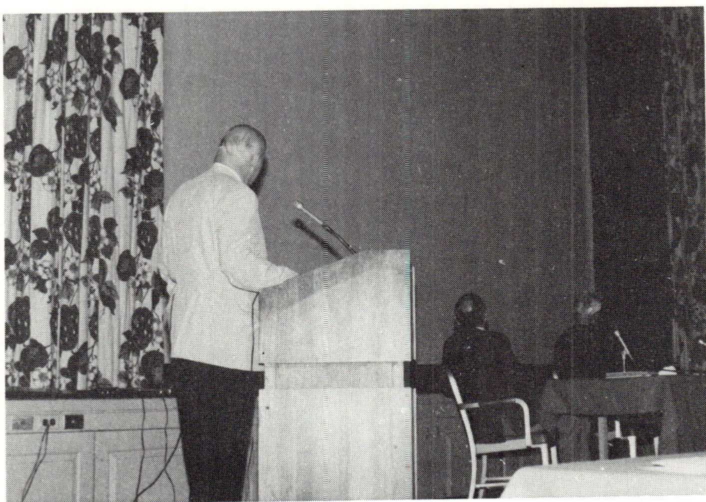

Fig. 26-3. Obstruction of the screen by the podium and presenter for a portion of the audience when the traditional room setup is used.

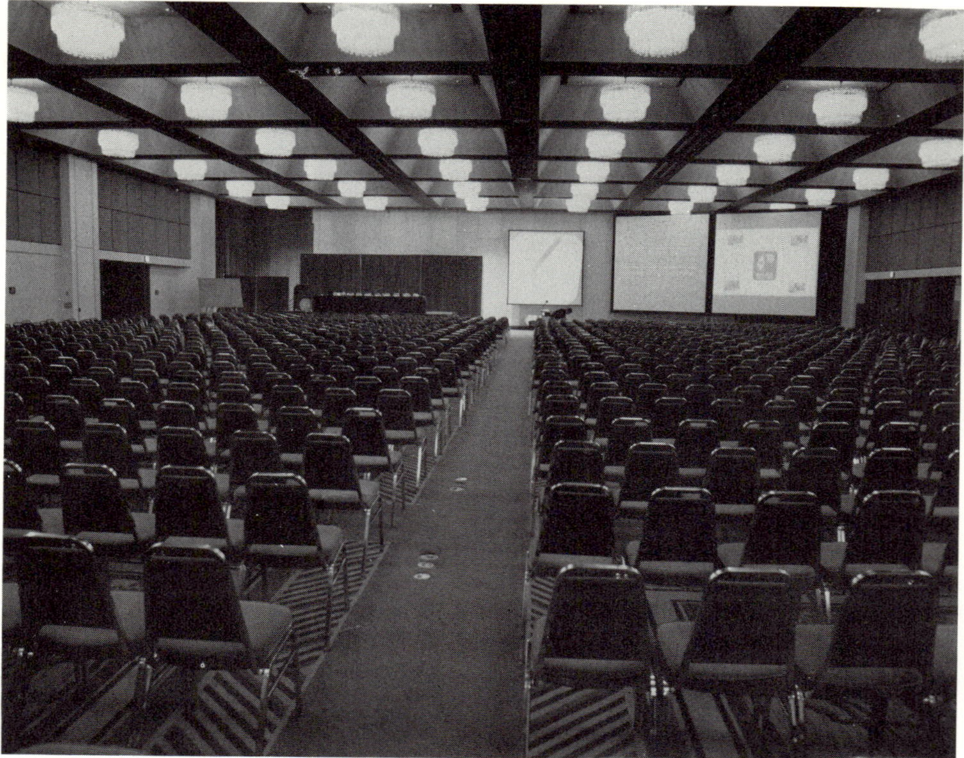

Fig. 26-4. A better room arrangement. The screen is placed in the front corner of the room where it is visible not only to the entire audience, but also to the speaker. An additional screen may be placed in the center or opposite front corner for use with an overhead projector or as a "silent pager."

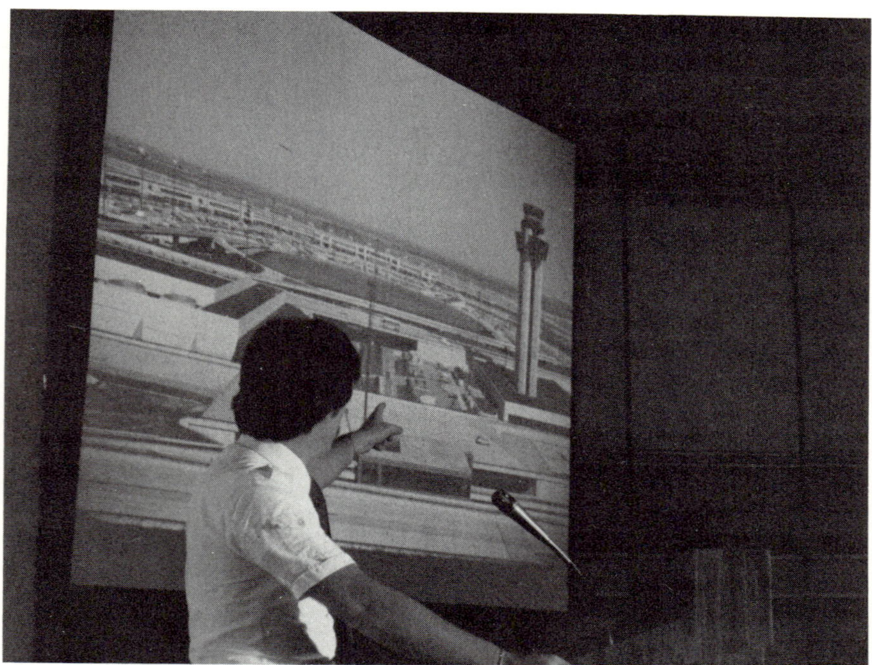

Fig. 26-5. The speaker's view of the screen when the recommended setup is used. Note that he may view the screen without turning away from the audience.

7. Dissolve systems are becoming increasingly popular with scientific speakers. Their use can add interest to a presentation, as well as increase audience retention. If a dissolve system is used, the supplier must be provided with the brand name and model of the equipment. Remember, also, that a dissolve presentation requires two projectors, thus increases costs.

8. Programmers are also being used more often. If you are going to allow your speakers to use this, it is essential that the supplier be provided with the exact manufacturer and model number. It is best to use the same unit for playback as was used for programming.

9. An electric pointer should be provided for any presentation that requires the speaker to explain visuals. It costs so little and does so much.

10. The screen is one of the most important parts of the projection system; it is the one piece of equipment that everyone sees. If budget is a problem, cut back on something else, but get the best screen available. For smaller audiences you can use a tripod type screen, but be sure it has a matte white rather than beaded surface.

Anytime you need a screen larger than 6 × 6 feet you are compromising to use anything but a fastfold type where the screen is snapped on an aluminum frame. This will give you a perfectly flat surface, and if you use matte white fabric you are assured of the finest reflecting surface available. Wall-mounted roller type screens, particularly those with the case mounted on the bottom, do not lie as flat as the snap-mounted type and tend to produce distortion of the projected image. The roller type usually rents for about 50% of the charge for the snap mounted, but the saving is not worth it in terms of quality of projected image.

11. The last major decision you must make before setting up your audiovisual guidelines is whether or not you will allow multi-image projection. If your speakers must frequently say, "If you will remember the last slide," you must seriously consider dual projection. Another circumstance that demands dual projection is when comparisons must be used, such as before and after photographs of patients. This will, of course, require two projectors and, in some cases, a larger screen.

To help you with your decisions regarding audiovisual equipment and as a guideline for preparing speaker audiovisual request forms, the following checklist should be helpful:

2 × 2 inch slide projector
    Standard 23 mm × 34 mm format
    Super slide
    Single frame
    126
    2 × 2 inch Kodachrome duplicate
Motion pictures
    16 mm optical sound
    16 mm magnetic sound
    16 mm silent
    16 mm stop action
    Super 8 sound
    Super 8 silent
Overhead projector
Opaque projector
3¼ × 4 inch projector
Dissolve system
Programmer
Electric pointer
Projection screen
    Single image
    Dual image
    Triple image
Videotape
    ¾ inch casette—color
    ½ inch casette—color Betamax or VHS
    Color monitor
Tape recorder
    Reel-to-reel
    Cassette

CHAPTER 27

Meeting planning

Linda Campbell

How do you plan a meeting? If you are like many persons, you "wing it" and learn through painful experience the need for improvement in your organization and planning. Meanwhile, you leave an exhausted and frustrated hotel staff in your wake; you have a printed program that is not quite correct in its listing of schedules and room names; the projection equipment that you ordered just does not quite do what you thought it would; and when it is all over, the bills are giving you a massive headache, particularly when you find out all the ways you could have saved some money!

I cannot offer all of the answers, but rather will outline a basic method of meeting planning, based upon practical experience and recommendations. These methods will not work for all meetings or every circumstance, but are designed as guidelines for you in your interaction with hotel employees, suppliers, and attendees. The points listed below are sequential, and will take you from your first thoughts of a meeting through its completion. These recommendations are for a meeting of less than 150 persons, although they can be adapted for larger groups.

1. DETERMINE YOUR REQUIREMENTS FOR THE MEETING (8 months prior to meeting)

When are you planning to hold the meeting? How long will it be? How many persons do you anticipate will attend? How many sleeping rooms will you need, including those for attendees and faculty? How many meeting rooms will you need, and how many persons will be in each room? Will you have any exhibits? Do you plan any breakfasts or luncheons? How about coffee breaks? Will there be a reception?

When will your attendees arrive—the night before it begins, or can they arrive in the morning prior to the first session? When will they depart?

How will your attendees arrive—by car or plane? What kind of plane connections are there, and how large is the airport? Is there limousine service from the airport to the hotel?

From all of these questions, you should be able to develop a profile of your meeting: its schedule, the number of persons attending, and a potential location. Obviously, if you have three breakout meetings plus a luncheon, it is going to be impossible to place the meeting in a hotel that has only two major rooms. Once you have a good idea of your projected requirements, you are in a position for the next step.

2. CONTACT THE HOTEL SALES OFFICE (8 months prior to meeting)

Telephone the sales office and advise them of your projected meeting dates and number of persons attending. You may wish to have alternative dates selected in the event that your first choice of dates is not available. You will also need to roughly outline your requirements, for example, one large meeting room, no workshops, two luncheons, one reception, etc. If the hotel advises you that they have the facilities available at a time agreeable to you, then you should schedule a visit to the hotel to discuss the arrangements for the meeting.

Plan to spend at least two hours at the hotel. You will want to begin your discussions with a sales representative, and you will then want to meet the catering manager (the person responsible for any food functions—breakfasts, luncheons, dinners, receptions, coffee breaks) and the convention service manager.

The convention service manager is your liaison with the hotel. This person's responsibility is to solve your problems and to fit your meeting into their hotel successfully. Some hotels give this function to their catering department. The convention service manager is the person who supplies the tables and blackboards when you need them, and is usually the person who gives meeting room assignments. In other words, the convention service manager is your key to a good meeting. This is the person with whom you should work closely throughout the planning stages and operation of your meeting.

When you go to the hotel for your appointment, look around you as you enter. Is the lobby attractive—but more importantly, is it clean? Are there unpleasant persons hanging around? Are there lines at the front desk check-in area? What about lines at the cashier windows? When you ask a bellman for the location of the sales office, is he courteous and polite or indifferent? Are the carpets and furnishings in good repair? Are there sufficient elevators, and are they in working order? Is the hotel staff busy doing their jobs, or are they carrying on extended personal discussions, ignoring the customers?

If you have a chance, try out the coffee shop. It has a different kitchen from the one that will serve your luncheons or other food functions, but you can look at the menu. Is it fairly standard, or are there some interesting entrees? Is the service pleasant and competent? Are tables cleared rapidly after the diners have gone? Are there long lines waiting to be seated? Is the food attractively served and of good quality? How long did you have to wait to order and for your food? Are the prices reasonable? If you pick up a house telephone inside the hotel, is the operator helpful?

None of these items is guaranteed to give you a good meeting, but you will get a good idea of the way the hotel is run—whether it is an efficient, professional organization, or an unorganized, inept group of unprofessional persons working for a hotel. Meetings usually reflect the characteristics of the hotel. A well-run hotel provides a well-run meeting, or at least one that is better than it would have been in a poorly managed hotel.

Now that you have an idea of the hotel's characteristics, begin your discussions with the sales representative. Outline the meeting requirements that you have previously determined. It is helpful if you have two copies of this, one for you and one for the hotel's files. Ask the hotel representative to give you a tour of the meeting rooms, and before you go, be sure you have a copy of the hotel brochure with floor plans and dimensions of the meeting rooms. Look carefully at the meeting rooms. Are there chandeliers that would interfere with audiovisual projections? How thick is the airwall dividing your room from the next? What is the ceiling height? Are there windows in the room? Do they have blackout drapes for projection? Is there a house sound system? If possible, look at a room that is set for a meeting. Is it set neatly? Are the tablecloths straight? Are there pads and pencils for the attendees? Is the ice water in place? How are the lights controlled in the meeting room? Ask any questions that you have. You will get a good idea of how knowledgeable the hotel staff is.

After you have toured the meeting space, ask to see some sample rooms—not the suites or deluxe rooms, but standard sleeping rooms. How large are the closets? Is there sufficient storage space? Is the vanity large enough? Are there sufficient towels and washcloths in the bathroom? Is the room clean and ready for occupancy? If you checked into the room, what should be there that is not? Is the bedspread in good condition? Are the drapes hung straight? Is there something in the room that needs to be repaired? Are there soft drink and ice machines on each floor? Are the rooms relatively soundproof?

If you are satisfied with your examinations thus far, it is now time to give your meeting requirements accurately and precisely to the convention manager. There are three basic meeting room setups: (1) theater style, (2) schoolroom style, and (3) conference style.

Theater style, also known as auditorium style, has rows and rows of straight-backed chairs facing the front of the room, much like a movie theater.

Schoolroom style has rows of tables and chairs facing the front of the room. It is also known as classroom style, and is excellent for taking notes since each person is seated at a table.

In conference style there is one long rectangular table, with chairs around it. This style is often used for committee meetings.

Which of these setups will best meet the needs for your meeting? Conference is good for no more than about twenty persons. Schoolroom style is excellent for extended educational programming. Theater is best used when you have little need for note-taking, and is also used to fit the maximum number of persons into a room, since it requires less space than schoolroom style.

Tell the hotel representative your room setup preference so that an appropriately sized meeting room can be arranged for the size of your group. However, watch out at this point.

All hotels have attractive brochures, with all sorts of pictures and floor plans, along with room dimensions and capacities for theater, banquet, and schoolroom seating. *Do not believe* the room capacities listed in the hotel brochure. If you do, you are liable to end up with that many persons in the room, but no aisles and no head table—just rows and rows of chairs as close together as possible.

It is very easy to figure the capacities of rooms if you have the dimensions of the room (which are usually correct in brochures). All you need are some basic square footages per person for each style of seating, and you can calculate the actual seating capacity of the room.

Schoolroom seating capacity

If the room is 700 square feet or larger, divide the total square footage by 14 square feet per person.

If the room is less than 700 square feet, divide the total square footage by 17 square feet per person.

EXAMPLE: The Sayonara Ballroom is 60 feet wide by 65 feet long. The total square footage is 3,900 square feet: $3,900 \div 14 = 279$ persons

Theater seating capacity

Divide the total square footage by 10 square feet per person. (When you are really tight on space, you can use the figure of 8 square feet per person, but this is better for extremely large sessions when maximal seating to capacity is required.)

EXAMPLE: The Chicago Ballroom is 40 feet wide by 50 feet long. Total square footage is 2,000 square feet: $2000 \div 10 = 200$ persons

The above capacities are for a meeting requiring a stage and head table, plus audiovisual equipment. These are good yardsticks for most meetings, and will give you a comfortable set for the appropriate number of persons.

If you will be using audiovisual equipment for your meeting, *determine the ceiling height of the meeting room.* This is critical in calculating the size of screen to use for audiovisual presentations. To determine the necessary screen size divide the length of the meeting room by 6. For instance, if a meeting room is 60 feet long, a 10 foot screen is required for that room ($60 \div 6$). The bottom 4 feet of the ceiling height is unusable, since the seated audience occupies that space. Therefore, for a 10 foot screen, we need at least a 14 foot ceiling height (see also Chapter 26).

For food functions there are additional square footages to consider. Most luncheons and other events are set in round tables of either eight or ten persons. Once you have the square footage of the room, you can figure ten square feet per person for a banquet table setup capacity.

For receptions, you will need between 5 and 10 square feet per person. Ten square feet will give you a lot of room for a more formal reception, while five square feet will be very cozy. You should also consider how much space will be taken by buffet tables and bars, but most persons use 7.5 square feet as the recommended amount for receptions.

Work with the hotel personnel to get your meeting space assigned, based on these figures. It will also be necessary to discuss housing requirements. You will need to give the hotel the arrival and check-out dates of your attendees. Indicate whether most persons will stay for the duration of the meeting, or if some of them will check out earlier. Give the hotel your very best estimate of the number of rooms you will require, including those for faculty. Ask the hotel what the rates for the rooms will be and how that differs from the rack rate. (The rack rate is the one you would get if you just walked up to the desk and asked for a room.) Most hotels will give a convention rate to groups.

Determine how you are going to handle reservations. Do you want to send in a list of everyone attending with their address, arrival, departure, and type of accommodations? Would you rather send out a rate card to each person and then have them return their individual reservation to the hotel? All hotels will print up rate cards for conventions. They will give you a certain number free (such as three hundred of them when you block one hundred sleeping rooms), which are imprinted with the name of the meeting and the room rates for it. If you decide to use rate cards, be sure that you give the hotel ample time to print the cards; it usually takes about four weeks to get them.

Based upon your block of sleeping rooms, the hotel will give you a complimentary room. In most cities, if you sell fifty rooms, you will receive one room free. If you sell one hundred rooms, you will receive two complimentary rooms (or one one-bedroom suite). Confirm the hotel's complimentary policy with the sales representative.

Before you leave the hotel, you will want to pick up a set of sample menus and find out whether the printed prices will be in effect during your meeting. If they will not be, determine the estimated increase. Also, you will need to check the amount of hotel gratuity and tax. Gratuities are service charges added to the bill for any food function, and are usually between 15% and 17% of the total food bill. With the addition of taxes from 5% to 7%, the tax and gratuity for a function can easily add another 25% to the cost of the bill.

Hopefully, your meeting with the hotel sales personnel has gone well, and everyone is ready for an excellent relationship during the remainder of the planning stages. Do be sure that the hotel confirms its agreement with you in writing—the number of sleeping rooms blocked, the rates, the number of meeting rooms blocked, any special charges, their complimentary room policy, and any other agreements made by you in your discussions.

If your discussions have not gone well, then you may wish to consider an alternate facility in the same area that has adequate meeting space and sleeping rooms. You will then have an opportunity to compare the attitudes of the two hotels and form an opinion about which one is more service oriented.

3. BUDGETING, PROGRAMMING, SELECTION OF SUPPLIERS (6 to 7 months prior to meeting)

How you complete these steps is vital to the success of the meeting. Obviously, your selection of outstanding speakers will determine how many persons attend the meeting. But how you use those speakers will help you determine the financial success of the meeting. Is it practical to hold a meeting in Phoenix and have a guest speaker imported from New York who speaks for only five minutes? This is a qualitative judgment that only you can make. Perhaps two speakers from the West Coast would be better contributors to the program content. Do not forget: audiences like discussion periods, and they help provide a change in the meeting format.

If you will require audiovisuals, it would be wise to select your supplier at this time, so that you will have budgeting input. When you select a company to handle your needs, you may wish to talk to others in the area who have held meetings and see whom they recommend. You may want to ask the convention service manager of the hotel if there is an in-house audiovisual supplier. You may wish to contact a company who has handled a meeting that you attended. Ask the company for a proposal to handle your meeting based on the type of equipment and requirements that you have. You may wish to get additional proposals to compare companies. If you are not familiar with the company's work, ask if they have another meeting scheduled in your area that you could observe. If all presentations at your meeting will require audiovisuals, the quality of performance from the supplier is critical. Therefore, you may not be better off with the cheapest proposal, but with the company that has the equipment and the manpower to do the job. Once you have selected the company, be sure that you keep them fully advised as to the programming schedule, the meeting rooms, and so forth. They can also offer their expertise to you on such items as in meeting room setups, hotel services, and equipment required.

When you begin budgeting, you will need to figure major costs—faculty, printing and mailing, audiovisuals, food functions, etc. Be sure that you make up a detailed budget for the meeting, based upon the information that you have received from the hotel, your selection of faculty, and the audiovisual supplier. Some basic figures are:

Coffee breaks
One gallon of coffee will serve 20 cups.
Receptions
The average drink consumption per person is two to three drinks per hour.
The average person consumes six to eight hors d'oeuvres per hour.
One bartender is needed for each 100 persons.
You will probably have to pay a bartender charge, unless the bartender sells a minimum amount of liquor (usually $150 to $250 per bartender). This is a labor charge.
Labor
In many hotels, you will be required to use union projectionists. They usually have a four-hour minimum call. If you use them for only two hours, you will pay for four regardless. They are on straight time ($15 to $18 per hour) during weekday hours of 8:00 AM to 5:00 PM. They go into time and one-half after 5:00 PM and on Saturdays. From 12:00 midnight to 8:00 AM and on Sundays, they will

either be time and one-half or double time ($30 to $36 per hour). Watch the scheduling of your meeting, so that you can avoid overtime charges for labor.

In determining the expenses for the meeting, the following areas should be considered:

Brochure printing and mailing
Honoraria and faculty expense
Program printing
Food function expense (breakfasts, luncheons, dinners, receptions, coffee breaks, tax and gratuity)
Ticket printing
Gratuities/tips to outstanding hotel personnel
Bulletin typewriters
Badges/badgeholders
Audiovisual equipment and projectionists
Sound equipment and personnel
Telephone
Busing
Signs
Security
Office expenses (postage, photocopying, etc.)

Once you have determined your expenses, you can figure the income necessary to offset the expenses and/or provide excess income, and can set the registration fees accordingly. If you have determined that 100 persons will attend your meeting, and you have estimated $10,000 expenses, then you had better set a registration fee higher than $50 per person.

4. SOLICITATION MAILINGS AND REGISTRATION (3 to 6 months prior to meeting)

Once you have determined the faculty and the program scheduling, it is relatively easy to send out an announcement concerning the dates, location, hotel selected, and so forth. Mailing labels for all members of the American Society of Plastic and Reconstructive Surgeons, applicants for membership, and plastic surgery residents for example, are available from the Society office, at a nominal cost. This provides a listing of 3,500 persons. Labels are also available based on geographic location, for instance, labels for the states of California, Washington, Oregon, and Nevada. Through an outside supplier you can have access to the entire mailing list of the American Medical Association, with specialty breakdown, plus geographic breakdowns. These labels are also categorized by type of practice, age, primary specialty, secondary specialty, etc.

When you design your registration form, be sure that all pertinent information is included and correct. This should include the following:

Dates of meeting
Name of meeting
Location of meeting
Registration fees
Schedule of events

List of speakers
Refund policies
Where to send registration
Housing information
Transportation information (if appropriate)

The form should be clear and concise, easy to read, and easy to complete.

When the registration forms begin coming in, you should acknowledge receipt of each one with some kind of simple form acknowledging the amount of money, the person who registered, and the name of the meeting. To keep track of the registrants, you may wish to set up an alphabetical card file, with an index card for each registrant, indicating the person's registration category and the amount of fees paid. This alleviates the need for lists, which are constantly outdated and changed. The index card also provides space for any necessary notes. The alphabetical card file is also easily utilized for on-site registration, and pretyped badges can be placed in front of each index card to be picked up by the registrants. Attendance verification can be indicated on the index card, so that you have an accurate listing of the final registrants.

5. CONTINUE TO WORK WITH HOTEL PERSONNEL (3 months prior to the meeting)

Since your initial meeting and correspondence with the hotel convention manager there have probably been some changes in your scheduling. Be sure that you contact the convention service manager to review these. If you will be using audiovisuals for your meeting, you will need to be sure that you have the meeting space on a twenty-four hour hold—in other words, the hotel cannot use your meeting room for an evening dinner and make you tear down all the equipment and put it back up again at midnight. The twenty-four hour hold is necessary not only to avoid labor charges but also because you should check the room the afternoon prior to the beginning of the meeting. In this way, you will have an opportunity for a relatively relaxed setup and testing time of the equipment, rather than rushing around before the 8:00 AM session begins. The hotel should provide you with the names of the rooms to be used for your meetings by the time you make this follow-up call.

Be sure to keep the audiovisual supplier abreast of any changes in meeting times or dates, since this could affect your budgetary figures.

6. PLAN THE MISCELLANEOUS (2 months prior to meeting)

This is the stage of meeting planning where you seemingly have millions of details to handle. None of them is difficult, but they must all be arranged. The activities to be done include:

Ordering signs
Ordering badges and badgeholders
Ordering a bulletin typewriter
Ordering registration personnel
Printing a final program
Handling the faculty or VIP housing
Determining your final room setups for the meeting rooms
   to be used
Ordering security
Obtaining necessary supplies
Finalizing audiovisual requirements
Printing tickets
Ordering handouts and brochures from the convention bureau

Signs. Signs fall into two classifications: directional and labeling. A directional sign is placed in a location to point the way toward a meeting room, a luncheon, or a registration area. It usually has an arrow on it, so that the attendees can follow the signs to your function. A labeling sign is the one that you put outside the door to your meeting, for example:

```
GENERAL SESSION
GRAND BALLROOM
```

```
PLASTIC SURGEONS
LUNCHEON
```

A standard sign size is 22×28 inch, which is easily visible. Keep sign copy simple and use large lettering. Signs are placed on easels, and you will need to check with the hotel to see that they have a few available for your use. The key signs that you will need are for registration, general session, and luncheons or receptions.

Badges. Name badges are a must for meetings. If you have a one-day meeting, then you can easily use the stick-on badges. However, if your meeting is longer, you will need to obtain badges and badgeholders. Badges can be purchased or specially printed for you. There are two basic sizes: $2\frac{1}{4} \times 3\frac{1}{2}$ inches, or the larger size of 3×4 inches. Obviously, you must obtain badgeholders to match the size of the badges, and the larger ones are more expensive.

Badgeholders come in three styles: pin, pocket, and clip-on. Most women prefer pin badges. Most men prefer pocket badges, unless it is an informal meeting where they will not be wearing jackets. Clip-on badgeholders are very nice, but are the most expensive of the three.

Bulletin typewriter. A bulletin typewriter has large type and is used for most meetings. These can be obtained from a typewriter rental agency. In some cases, the hotel will supply them, or the convention bureau may provide them if you request registration personnel from them. Check whether it is a manual or electric typewriter, so that you have the outlets available in the registration area if necessary.

Most cities have an active convention bureau or chamber of commerce, whose job it is to attract meetings to the city. They usually can provide you with a great deal of assistance and information concerning the city and local attractions. They also can provide you with inexpensive, experienced registration help. They will have a list of suppliers available who support the bureau. From this list you can easily find badge and badgeholder suppliers, bulletin typewriters, and so forth.

Final program. The final program is the one that is given out at registration. It needs to include the dates of the meeting, location, final schedule of events, final program, and meeting room names. It may also include a listing of faculty members and any other information pertinent to the meeting. Be sure that the room names are correct as listed, otherwise you will spend a great deal of time correcting that mistake during the meeting. You can have the program typeset by a printer, which means that you will need to go through two proofreadings and correction stages. You can also have the program typewritten on a piece of plain white paper and have it multilithed, which is much less expensive than typesetting. Multilithing is also much faster than typesetting.

VIP housing. Normally, a hotel will hold a block of sleeping rooms until three or four weeks prior to the first day of the meeting. At that time, all unused rooms are returned to the hotel for sale on a first-come, first-served basis. Your late attendees may or may not be able to obtain a room at the hotel, depending upon how busy they are over the time of your meeting. Because of this, you will want to handle your faculty or VIP housing with a special mailing to them. You can send them rate cards to be completed and sent to the hotel, but a letter needs to be sent spelling out the expected arrival date and any other special information. You can also have them send their arrival and departure dates to you, and you submit their requirements to the hotel. This way is easier if you plan to pay for their rooms during the meeting. The hotel has a complete listing of all persons who are to be on the master account, and there are fewer errors. Also, you are assured that faculty/VIP persons are handled correctly, and that rooms will be awaiting them. You may wish to guarantee the rooms for late arrival, so that they will be held past 6:00 PM, in the event that the faculty member is not arriving until late evening. The only problem is that you must pay for the room, regardless of whether it is occupied, so be sure that you have accurate arrival dates for faculty members.

Final room setup. Now is the time to finalize plans for your meeting setup. Do you want a stage? If so, will you need a podium? A head table? For how many? Any microphones on stage? Where are the aisles in the room going to be? Are standing microphones required in the aisles? A hotel will normally provide small (3 × 4 inch) pads of paper on a complimentary basis. They will also give you small pencils, and will set the room with ice water and ashtrays. They will not usually supply 8½ × 11 inch pads of paper. Suppose you planned the room set up in schoolroom style when you booked the meeting with the hotel, and now you have had an overwhelming response to your meeting. You have insufficient seating planned for the number of attendees, and no alternate room is available in the hotel. A good alternative is to set half the room schoolroom style (the front portion), with the rear section set theater style. This will give you ample seating, and will still provide convenience for note taking.

What kind of requirements does the audiovisual supplier have for the meeting room? A projection platform? What size—length, width, and height? What size stage is recommended? Where should the screen and projection platform be placed? All of these items go into a room setup and must be determined in advance.

Security. Security may be needed for your meeting and can usually be obtained through the hotel. Companies may also be listed in the convention bureau service guide. If you need to guard something, remember that more things disappear *after* a meeting is over than during the daytime sessions.

Supplies. Now is the time to gather your meeting supplies—all the pens, pencils, scissors, scotch tape, masking tape, filament tape, glue, paper clips, thumbtacks, staples, staplers, staple removers, paper, envelopes, blackboard erasers, chalk, extension cords, Band-aids, sewing kit, aspirin, liquid paper, receipt forms, bulldog clips, file folders, and any other thing you can think of that will make your meeting run well. Be aware that certain things disappear easily and you will need more than one of them. These include scissors and staplers, as well as Scotch tape dispensers.

Audiovisual equipment. Contact the faculty/speakers to see what their audiovisual requirements are. Discuss with the audiovisual supplier his recommendations as to screen size, type of projector, and other audiovisual equipment requirements. Use his expertise and recommendations to give you the best possible meeting.

Tickets. Any tickets that will be required should be printed at this time. Be sure you have the name of the function and the correct date, time, and room name. You may also wish to include the price. Be sure that the tickets are numbered consecutively, so you will have an accurate count of how many have been given out. If you need tickets for more than one function, be sure that they are in different colors. Tickets are good for maintaining control of your numbers for a luncheon or other function of that type. If each person attending is required to present a ticket to the waiter, then you know that all persons attending your luncheon are those who have paid the necessary fees.

Handouts and brochures. Arrange for free maps, restaurant listings, and other city attractions brochures from the convention bureau. These can be delivered to the hotel the day prior to registration, and are a nice method of welcoming attendees and providing local information.

7. SUBMIT FINAL REQUIREMENTS TO THE HOTEL (1 month prior to meeting)

No later than three weeks prior to your meeting, it is necessary to give the hotel convention coordinator all requirements for your meeting. This means a schedule of events, by day and by time, all room setup requirements, all menu selections, all coffee breaks, hotel posting instructions, and billing instructions. It will help if you submit floor plans of the way you want the rooms set. These do not have to be professional floor plans, but a sketch of where you want the head table, where you want the microphones, where the projection platform will be, and so forth. A simple and basic format for this is as follows:

This format can be used for all functions during the meeting, and should be submitted by day, in time order. In other words, the breakfast at 7:30 AM would be the first listing for the day, followed by the meeting from 9:00 AM to 12:00 PM, followed by the coffee break from 10:30 AM to 11:00 AM, followed by the luncheon from 12:00 to 1:00 PM.

These instructions should be submitted directly to the convention service manager of the hotel, with copies to the sales representative, catering department, and the audiovisual supplier. Keep a good, clean copy for yourself, and use it as your master copy, with any notes indicated in red.

All hotels have a board somewhere in the hotel listing the functions that are taking place that day. At the end of your letter of instructions, it would be a good idea to indicate how you want your functions posted. For example, it might be posted "Chicago Society of Plastic Surgeons Meeting." If you do not want your meeting posted, this should also be indicated.

It is a good idea to recap the billing instructions at the end of the letter of instruction. You will need to indicate who is authorized to sign the charges for food functions, who can sign room charges to the master account, and where the bill should be sent.

8. SUBMIT FINAL AUDIOVISUAL REQUIREMENTS TO SUPPLIER (1 month prior to meeting)

No less than two weeks prior to the meeting (one month is better), you should submit all requirements to the audiovisual supplier, along with a copy of the final program. If you have been working together during the planning stages of the meeting, this should be relatively easy, since he or she will know and understand your

---

DATE

NAME OF FUNCTION   TIME SCHEDULED   ROOM ASSIGNED

Insert instructions on room setup, head table requirements, microphone and sound requirements, how many persons will be seated in the room, and special requirements.

NAME OF FUNCTION   TIME SCHEDULED   ROOM ASSIGNED

If it is a food function, indicate the number of persons to be served, the room setup (e.g., round tables of eight or ten), whether tickets are to be collected, the menu selected, price, and appropriate taxes and gratuities.

NAME OF FUNCTION   TIME SCHEDULED   ROOM ASSIGNED

List coffee breaks, indicating the number of persons to be served, the time of service, the time the coffee break is to be ready to serve, if you also require hot tea, decaffeinated coffee, or soft drinks, and any food you may need.

meeting requirements, and will have been able to suggest equipment to you. If you have not been communicating, then you should think about the following equipment:

Carousel projectors (35 mm)
    How many?
    Do you need high-intensity equipment?
    What lens size?
    Do you want the projection "remoted" to the podium?
    How many extra slide trays are needed?
Film projectors (16 mm)
    Are the films optical (preferable) or magnetic?
    What happens with a super 8 film?
Screens
    Size of screen for audience and room (horizontal format preferred, since it makes better use of the ceiling height)
    Number of screens required
Overhead projector
    Number required
    Time of presentation
    Acetate rolls or sheets for writing
    Marking pens
Electric pointer
Speaker timer and warning light system
Tape recording
    Cassette recorder
    Blank cassettes
    Labels for the cassettes
Professional projectionist
Microphone and sound requirements
    Number of microphones required
    Preferred type of microphones to be used (lavaliere, podium, table, standing)
    Location of microphones

9. LAST MINUTE DETAILS

Forty-eight hours prior to each food function (sometimes twenty-four hours), you will need to give the final guarantee to the hotel. Once this guarantee (estimated number of persons attending) is given, you have committed yourself to pay for that number of servings. The number of servings can be increased up to a point, but it is almost impossible to advise the catering service at 10:00 AM that you need an additional twenty-five servings when you have a luncheon for forty people planned. They just do not have the quantity of food available to do it. If you do end up serving the extra people, then twenty-five plates will probably be of some food other than what you ordered for the luncheon. The guarantee is critical, since you want to be close enough to take care of all persons attending, but not to lose money on it. The hotel will also overset your guaranteed number, usually by 5% to give you an additional margin of safety. You are not required to pay for the overset, unless, obviously, the food is consumed by those attending.

You may also want to check with your typewriter supplier to make sure the delivery will take place as scheduled, with the convention bureau about the free brochures, and with any other person who is scheduled to provide something for you at the meeting.

10. THE MEETING

At long last, you have arrived at the hotel for your meeting. You will need to meet with the convention service manager to review the specifications for your meeting. The service manager has taken the instructions you provided and has put them into hotel language for their internal use. You should ask for a set of "specs," so that you can review them and make sure there are no errors. You also should review the billing and posting instructions. Check with the reservations manager about faculty arrival and see that they have all changes that you have, and that the necessary rooms are guaranteed. You will also need to meet with the catering department to review the arrangements for your food and beverage functions.

Set up your office or headquarters area with the supplies you purchased. Have all deliveries of typewriters, brochures, signs, etc., made, and put them around in such a manner that you can find them easily. Be sure you have received ample wastebaskets from the hotel. Set up the registration area and be sure you have some alphabetical dividers to keep your registration forms divided correctly. You will need a list or file of attendees, receipt forms, programs, handouts, badges, and badgeholders, plus the bulletin typewriter. It helps greatly to have written registration instructions for the temporary registration personnel that will be helping with the meeting. When these persons appear, you will need to take time to brief them thoroughly, show them where the supplies are, and be available as they register the first few persons so that any questions or confusion can be handled at that time.

You are now free to oversee the setup of your main session room and the audiovisual equipment. Here is where a floor plan can be so helpful. Usually there will be a crew of people setting up the room, under one supervisor. If they have several copies of your floor plan spread around the room, there will be few questions, and the room will usually be set correctly. The convention service manager will check with you periodically to see if you have any problems, but will not be with you constantly. Be sure that you know who else can help you if the service manager is not available—an assistant or someone from the catering department, for example.

Put your signs in place outside the main meeting room and in the registration area, but do not put them up before you are ready to register people.

After the meeting begins, you can breathe a sigh of relief. Your primary concerns now are whether or not coffee breaks are served on time, luncheons are set, signs are in appropriate places at the correct time, and messages are received correctly. All of your preparation has given you an opportunity to actually enjoy the meeting. Since you handled so much in advance, there are relatively few items to handle at the time of the meeting, and it runs successfully.

Once the meeting is completed, your major concern is the payment of the master account, writing any necessary reports and recommendations, and sending a thank-you letter to the hotel.

FINAL THOUGHTS

In summary, there are four basic recommendations that will help you have a successful meeting:

1. Know what you want—the kind of meeting, the type of meeting, its purpose, etc.
2. Use the expertise of suppliers and hotel staffs. They are professionals in their areas.
3. Keep calm.
4. Anticipate the worst. It usually will not happen, but in case it does, you are prepared to cope with it.

Appendixes

Journal writing

AI □ Searching the literature

Guide for searches of printed and other types of material*

Current search of journal literature
  Medline search (if suitable)
  Abridged Index Medicus (AIM)
Review of the literature
  Since 1960
    Medical Subject Headings (MeSH)
    Index Medicus
    Cumulated Index Medicus
  Before 1960
    Current List of Medical Literature
    Quarterly Cumulative Index Medicus
    Index-Catalogue of the Library of the Surgeon General's Office, U.S. Army
    Excerpta Medica
  A possible shortcut
    Bibliography of Medical Reviews (BMR)
  Modifications of earlier work
    Science Citation Index

Fields related to medicine
  Biological Abstracts
  BioResearch Index
  Chemical Abstracts
"More current than current"
  Most recent issues of known productive journals
  Current Contents
Foreign languages
  English abstracts in foreign journals
  English abstracting journals
  Translation
Books
  NLM Current Catalog
  Bowker's Medical Books in Print
Tapes and other computerized systems
  Medline system
  Chemical Abstracts Services
  BioSciences Information Service
  Institute for Scientific Information
  Excerpta Medica System
  Science Information Exchange

*From Beatty, W. K.: Searching the literature comes before writing the literature, Annals of Internal Medicine 79(6): 917, 1973.

A2 □ Basic elements of investigative papers

INVESTIGATIVE PAPER OR ORIGINAL CONTRIBUTION

Length: Depends upon whether it is new or a modification, and journal to which submitted.

Content

Title: Informative and brief. This is important in indexing, storage, and retrieval.

Bylines

According to Southgate: Not more than six authors.

According to DeBakey: Should contain the names of those who have contributed materially to the work and its report. Those who have participated only in an advisory or supporting capacity should be thanked in the acknowledgements at the end of the paper.

Abstract (if required by journal to which submitted): Present essential points made in paper, including purpose, methods, results, and conclusions.

Table of contents

Introduction

Length: Depends on style of journal and audience you are addressing.

Literature review

Length: Depends on audience to be addressed. Should limit and refer to previous cumulative reviews.

Methods and materials

Present in logical order.

Include enough detail that a competent worker could repeat the experiment or clinical observations.

Be concise:

Do not include negative and normal results.

Time relationship: Use a single baseline.

Avoid abbreviations, cliches, and jargon.

Results

Record data in an attempt to form general scientific principles.

Tables and figures should complement rather than duplicate text.

Discussion

Discuss results in relation to method.

Relate to original problem.

Relate to existing knowledge; interpret and consider the implications.

Conclusions

Conclusions are of three types. Use one or part of all three:

1. Establish, confirm, or contradict hypothesis.
2. Factual—simple statement.
3. Advocative—make recommendations.

Summary

Length: 150 to 200 words.

Content: Recapitulation; factual statement of problem, method of study, results, and conclusions.

Do not introduce new material.

Usually journals do not require both abstract and summary.

Variations (in arrangements of methods, results, discussion, and conclusions)

Methods and results combined in following situations according to Shepard:

Methods and Results, combined—Three situations can be managed appropriately by combining the Methods and Results sections: (a) when the methods and results of each of a number of experiments, more or less related, are best discussed together as a set; (b) when a number of experiments are reported, the first of which raises questions answered by the second, and so on; and (c) when the methods and results of a number of experiments are best described in relation to each other (rather than the methods in the Methods section and the results of all experiments in the Results section) to avoid back-and-forth reference to Methods and Results, should these sections be separate.

Results and Discussion, combined—Four situations can be dealt with by combining the Results and Discussion sections: (a) when the results of a number of experiments are related closely enough to merit discussion together; (b) when the results of each of a group of experiments require discussion as a set, perhaps in preparation for a general discussion later; (c) when, otherwise, it would be necessary to restate the results in the Discussion section; and (d) when specific results of experiments or description of clinical findings, in being reported at that point, lead to mention of generalizations.

Results and Conclusions, combined—Sometimes discussion of results is unnecessary. Thus, an experimental investigation or a description of a technique may call simply for a conclusion rather than a discussion, in which case the Results and Conclusions may be combined.*

Appendix: Detailed description of method and analysis that are not essential to understanding of paper: e.g., statistical methods and analysis, chemical materials, etc.

Addendum: Information that comes to light at late stage in preparation of text.

References: Some journals include only citations of work mentioned in content of paper. Thus it differs from Bibliography. Others separate Bibliography from Additional References. Check with the author's guide of journal selected.

---

*Shepard, D. A. E.: Parts of a scientific paper: II, Medical Communication 3(4):22, 1975.

Bibliography

Consult the guide to authors of publication to which submitted.

Locate correct journal abbreviations in front of *Index Medicus*.

Alphabetical order most generally accepted.

General rules according to DeBakey:

If an article is cited in a foreign language not using the Roman alphabet, translation is indicated.

Manuscripts in preparation should be given as "data to be published."

"In press" indicates paper has been accepted for publication.

Permission of the individual who is being quoted or whose work is referred to is necessary if an unpublished "personal communication" must be used.

Accuracy is essential, including punctuation.

CASE REPORT

Length: 1,000 to 1,500 words.

Content

Ascertain after reviewing literature that it is sufficiently unique to be worth reporting.

Include pertinent data only.

Precisely define terms so that they are scientifically comparable at later date by another.

Discussion and conclusions must be relevant.

NEGATIVE RESULTS

Length: 500 to 600 words of text, one to two short tables, four to five references.

Content

Experimental data as basis for conclusions.

Description of materials and methods.

Diagnostic signs.

Laboratory determinations.

Explanation of procedure.

Brief comments.

Conclusions or summary.

Purpose is to inform others who plan to undertake similar studies.

REVIEW ARTICLES

Length: Depends on journal's policy.

Content

Current appraisal of "the state of the art" in pathogenesis, diagnosis, or therapy.

Identify opposing theories and evaluate.

Recognize that further study may provide answers to some current question.

Prerequisite: Review all material.

BOOK REVIEW

Length: 250 to 5,000 words.

Content

Scope—To what group of readers would it be useful?

Completeness.

Appropriateness of contents (bibliography, illustrations, index).

Format—Typography and physical characteristics.

Evaluative—Reviewer must know field to make judgment, appreciate validity of points, and distinguish the new and original.

Adequacy of coverage.

Relate to broader context of medicine.

Judge style—Reviewer must write with style.

Be critical—If book is inferior, so state, but judge book not author.

EDITORIAL (according to DeBakey)

Length: Usually not to exceed 1,000 words, rarely more than 2,000.

Content

May be an opinion, a proposal, or summary of the literature concerning a subject of interest to the readers.

Information is provided but used to a variable degree as basis for interpretation, extrapolation, evaluation, or advice or persuasion.

Implies authorative source and style is important.

Less need for documentation than for conventional stanardized communication.

An informative or catchy title may be used.

LETTERS TO THE EDITOR:

Length: Usually not to exceed 250 words.

Content

Explains, amplifies, corrects, or otherwise comments substantially upon an article recently published in the journal.

Correct errors—work improperly cited, interpreted, or neglected.

To make public reservations about an article.

USE OF STATISTICS

S. Shindell in a series of publications in J.A.M.A. under the title of Statistics, Science, and Sense, discusses:

Designing an investigation

Defining a population

Drawing the sample

Recording and summarizing data

The average

Dispersion

Probability

The standard deviation

The degree of variability

Examining attribute to different groups
Measure of association
Regression and correlation
Common fallacies to be looked for
Arguing a particular proposition without support of
data
The logic of investigation

The time to be concerned with statistics is before one starts a study. At that point one can determine the essential question he wishes to investigate, not only in terms of specific experimental hypothesis or logical proposition he wishes to examine, but also the specific statistical question, "Is change operative?" which the mathematical manipulations can answer.*

---

*Shindell, S.: Statistics, science, and sense, J.A.M.A. **186**:852, 1963.

He also warns:

The major problem, however, in viewing results consists not simply in those observations produced by chance but in those produced by fallacies in reasoning. No amount of statistics can affect faulty logic.*

According to Shuster any article containing even the most elementary statistical procedures should be reviewed by a competent statistician. The simplest techniques, such as tests and contingency tables, are often misused.

---

*Shindell, S.: Statistics, science, and sense, J.A.M.A. **186**:784, 1963.

A3 □ The abstract

The present day abstract that accompanies a scientific paper is a relatively new concept. Since the beginning of expository writing, there have been attempts to pull things together at the end, but there has been no standard. In the heyday of German medicine in the last century, the *Zusammenfassung* ("seizing together") came into being, but it was variable in length and content in conformance with the whim of the writer.

The following advice given by Sir Clifford Allbutt, as recently as 1923, shows the expressed need for such a summary in certain articles.

On the completion of a long thesis, or important scientific essay, it is well to draw up a syllabus of the argument and to place it at the beginning: in any case let the conclusions be set out succinctly at the end: it is not for the author to compel the reader to peruse his essay.[1]

Morris Fishbein's concept of the summary was, as recently as 1938, still unfocused, unsure, and unstandardized.

The summary—a brief abstract of the article—may appear at the beginning or at the close. Not every article should be summarized. Those of more than average length (more than 1,500 words), those which involve much description of detail and technique and those which aim at a complete survey of literature on the particular subject demand a summary. A brief digest of a long article in the introductory paragraph often will stimulate someone to read the article who otherwise would not.[2]

The pressures to organize the abstract into a standard form have never been as compelling as they are today.

Reprinted from Warren, R.: The abstract, Arch. Surg. **111**:635-636, June, 1976. Copyright 1976, American Medical Association.

Since World War II the proliferation of medical literature has accelerated. The *Index Medicus* now covers 2,400 journals, as opposed to 1,200 before the war, and the abstract has taken on a new meaning that derives from a clearer view of its two practical purposes. These are (1) to give, in a limited number of words, the content and message of the article so as to satisfy the need for selectivity in reading that shortage of time forces on us; and (2) to permit distribution of the salient points of the article to a wider audience than the readers of the journal in which it is published. Abstract journals often reprint that component of the published article verbatim.

What, then, exactly is the modern abstract? If one peruses the *Oxford English Dictionary*, one finds "summary," "synopsis," "conspectus," "précis," "epitome," even "abridgement" and "syllabus," in varying degrees of overlapping synonymity with "abstract." Should each of us try to decide for himself whether he prefers "an adding up," "a seeing together," "an overview," "a precise stipulation," "a cutting across," "an abbreviation," "a verbal synthesis," or "a selective taking out or sampling"? No. We must not let the dead languages behind the words divert us from our purpose. If I were to say that I prefer "abstract" because it is the only one of the eight in the *Oxford English Dictionary* after which the definition "essence" appears, I would immediately invite the counterargument that "abstract" also implies "the removal of only part of something, not necessarily the whole." So be it. Essence is what we are after.

What rules should govern? The following outline was conceived for a recent course in medical writing.

Guidelines for preparation of the abstract

1. Restrict length to . . . words. The maximum number varies among journals. Most have agreed on 150. You will write a better abstract if you discipline yourself to limit your abstract to an actual word count that you will not exceed, although you may well stay below it.
2. Set down the substance of the article factually. Use the following format, but do not include the subheadings:
   a. Problem
   b. Methods
   c. Results
   d. Conclusions
   The order of importance, and hence the priority of space devoted, runs c, b, d, a. No more than one sentence should be devoted to d or to a, either of which can often be omitted. The results selected to be reproduced in the abstract should be expressed in numbers. Use the past tense (the present can rarely be used for a and d if the assumption therein can be stated as established, universally accepted facts).
3. Avoid:
   a. Contents alone, that is, merely listing or describing the contents: "Ten cases are analyzed, and the results presented."
   b. Convictions without supporting evidence (author's prejudices).
   d. Conclusions alone, without the evidence on which they were based.
4. Suggestion: read several abstracts from your office journals and see which type best provides you with the actual substance of the article.

As an exercise, let us take an abstract from one of the articles in this issue and randomly pick that on page 716 by Karakousis et al. First, see if it passes muster according to our requirements, and then let us prepare some samples based on the same article arranged in the three unsatisfactory categories mentioned. These will be examples of forms that are only too often submitted with articles for publication.

Abstract

Twenty-one patients with malignant melanoma received immunotherapy with BCG. Thirteen patients had adjuvant immunotherapy on a monthly schedule. Of these, eight with regional lymph node metastases (stage III) had been treated by lymphadenectomy. Two of the stage III patients had tumor recurrences within one year, while six are alive and free of melanoma at a median interval of 22 months. The remaining five patients (stage I and II) had level 4 or 5 (Clark classification) primary lesions. Their average tumor-free survival has been 18 months, but there was one regional recurrence in six months.

Eight patients received intralesional treatment with BCG. The extent of local response correlated inversely to the stage of their disease. Higher doses of BCG or multiple simultaneous injections into the same lesion did not produce complete resolution of nodules in patients with far-advanced melanoma. In none was the course altered by intralesional therapy.

The abstract, as it stands, gives, in approximately 135 words (the prescribed limit in the ARCHIVES OF SURGERY), succinct information on methods and results. Although no introductory statement is made concerning the problem addressed, this does not bother the reader excessively, because the need for such a study is implied by the authors having undertaken it at all. This omission is indicative of the lower importance of this element of the abstract. Conclusions are mentioned in the last sentence of this example, but they apply only to the eight patients receiving intralesional injections of BCG. A sentence expressing the author's conclusion as to the meaning of the results in the 13 patients treated intradermally with BCG would have improved the abstract. To keep within the prescribed length, this would have required the removal of some words, which might have been done by deleting the part of the third sentence that mentions lymphadenectomy. Information that this was performed does not, against the background of the rest of the abstract, give additional insight to the reader.

When the above article was submitted, the demonstrated satisfactory abstract came with it. If it had not been satisfactory, either the Editors would have rewritten it or requested that the author do so. Here are some examples I have prepared of the three categories of unsatisfactory types of abstracts that editors so frequently receive.

"Contents"

Twenty-one patients with malignant melanoma received immunotherapy with BCG. Thirteen patients had adjuvant immunotherapy on a monthly schedule. Eight had stage III lesions, and five had stage I or stage II.

Eight patients received intralesional injections of BCG. All 21 patients were followed up carefully. The group was analyzed for recurrence and survival rates, and conclusions drawn and recommendations made.

"Convictions"

The authors studied 21 patients with malignant melanoma receiving immunotherapy with BCG. Thirteen had adjuvant immunotherapy on a monthly schedule (eight stage III and five stage I or II). Eight patients received intralesional injections of BCG. All patients were carefully followed up.

It is the author's present practice, on the basis of the information derived from this study, to treat patients intradermally with BCG on a monthly schedule, but not to use the intralesional method.

"Conclusions"

Twenty-one patients with malignant melanoma received immunotherapy with BCG. Thirteen patients had adjuvant immunotherapy on a monthly schedule, eight stage III and five stage I or II. Eight patients received intralesional injections of BCG. The patients were carefully observed for recurrence and survival.

On the basis of this work, it is concluded that the intradermal method of BCG administration on a monthly basis, as described, holds promise, but that the intralesional method is ineffective.

The differences between the examples on the one hand and the proper type of abstract on the other seem obvious as one compares them. The one entitled "Conclusions" is stronger than the other two, but still does not give the supporting data that a careful reader would wish. In conclusion, let me list three "don'ts."

1. Don't place information in the abstract that is not in the paper. For instance, it upsets a reader's confidence if, when the paper has not been more precise than to say, "follow-up was several weeks," the abstract suddenly says, "follow-up was six weeks."

2. Don't necessarily use the same abstract that is submitted to a program committee for presentation of a paper at a meeting. In that form, explanation is frequently given more room and actual data less. Often, in any case, some of the data change between the time of the submission of the abstract and the presentation of the paper.

3. Don't publish a summary in addition. The abstract should replace it completely. A list of conclusions at the end of the article, however, is most helpful.

We writers of scientific articles find it difficult to appreciate that the majority of readers will not wish to bask in the warmth of our felicitous prose. They want the essence of our message in the shortest time and with the least effort possible—and they want facts, not topics.

Richard Warren, MD
Boston

REFERENCES

1. Alibutt T: *Notes on the Composition of Scientific Papers*. London, Macmillan & Co Ltd, 1923, p 22.
2. Fishbein M: *Medical Writing: The Technique and the Art*. Chicago American Medical Association Press, 1938, p 33.

A4 □ Editorial information for authors

PLASTIC AND RECONSTRUCTIVE SURGERY

Information for Authors

The goal of *Plastic and Reconstructive Surgery* is to inform its readers of advancements in clinical medicine, significant research, and new developments in areas related to plastic and reconstructive surgery. This Journal provides a forum for responsible discussion among identified individuals. Unless otherwise clearly specified, the views expressed in articles, editorials, book reviews, and letters published by *Plastic and Reconstructive Surgery* represent the opinion of the author and do not reflect the official policy of the institution with which the author is affiliated, or the American Society of Plastic and Reconstructive Surgeons, Inc., the American Association of Plastic Surgeons, or the American Society for Aesthetic Plastic Surgery. Acceptance by this Journal of advertisements for products or services does not imply endorsement or preference over other similar products or services.

Papers on any aspect of plastic surgery—operative procedures, clinical or laboratory research, and case reports—are invited for publication if they contribute significantly to the literature.

The prose used in manuscripts must conform to acceptable English usage and syntax; and the contents must be clear, accurate, coherent, and logical. In accepting or rejecting a manuscript, the editors will also consider its originality, teaching value, and validity.

Manuscripts should not exceed approximately 4,000 words, with a maximum of ten diagrams, illustrations, or both. Occasional exceptions will be made for prize-winning essays, collective reviews, solicited material, or special works.

All manuscripts must be sent to:

Robert M. Goldwyn, M.D., Editor
Plastic and Reconstructive Surgery
1101 Beacon Street
Brookline, Massachusetts 02146, U.S.A.

The author should submit the original manuscript and two copies, with three sets of illustrations, and should retain one complete copy. The Journal is not responsible for losses in the mail.

Requirements of this Journal for Considering Manuscripts, and the Agreement of Author(s) to These Conditions

Decisions concerning editing, revisions, acceptances, and rejections will be made by the editors; editing may include shortening of the article and reducing the number of illustrations and tables, as well as other changes in format. An accepted article may be published with an accompanying discussion if the editors so desire.

Articles are received only for exclusive publication in this Journal, with the understanding that they have not been published elsewhere (in part or in full, in other words, or in the same words) and will not be submitted elsewhere unless rejected by the Journal.

Published manuscripts become the sole property of the Journal and will be copyrighted by the American Society of Plastic and Reconstructive Surgeons.

By submitting an article to the Journal, the author (or authors) agrees to each of the above conditions. In addition, the author (or authors) explicitly assigns any copyrighted ownership he (or they) may have in such article to said Society if the article is published in the Journal.

Preparation of Manuscripts

Copy must be typewritten, double-spaced, on one side only, on 8½ x 11 inch (22 x 28 cm) white bond paper, with 1½ inch (4 cm) margins at the left, top, and bottom and a 1 inch (2.5 cm) margin at the right. All copy must be double-spaced, including text, footnotes, bibliographies, legends, tables, and headings (i.e., all material that is to be set in type, large or small). Text references must be supplied for all tables and figures in order in the text, which will determine placement on the printed page.

The title page carries the full title of the article, followed by the authors' names, degrees,

Continued.

Fig. A4-1. Information for authors for *Plastic and Reconstructive Surgery.*

and city. Footnotes giving the principal affiliation of each author and where and when the paper was presented must appear at the bottom of the title page. Each page of the manuscript after the title page should carry a running head, which is a shortened form of the title. The first text page is numbered one.

At the conclusion of the text, the name and complete address of the principal author should appear. At the bottom of that page, list three to five nouns that are appropriate key words for indexing.

The references must be typed on separate pages following the text. All references must be cited in the text in numerical order, not alphabetically. References to journal articles should include (1) author(s), (2) title, (3) journal name (as abbreviated in *Index Medicus*), (4) volume number, (5) the first page number, and (6) year, in that order. References to books should include (1) author(s), (2) chapter title (if any), (3) editor (if any), (4) title of book, (5) city of publication, (6) publisher, and (7) year. Volume and edition numbers, specific pages, and name of translator should be included when appropriate. *The author is responsible for the accuracy and completeness of the references.*

Legends

Legends are required for illustrations and should be typed on separate pages following the bibliography. They should be brief and pertinent and need not be full sentences.

Illustrations and Tables

Consider the size and shape of the Journal page when planning your illustrations, and arrange them to conserve vertical space.

Photographs must be selected and prepared with great care. They must be in sharp focus and have good contrast. Glossy prints are preferable, and they should be larger than they will appear in the published article. If the exact arrangements of photographs into groups is important and unusual, the author should so indicate on a separate sheet of paper. Before-and-after photographs of patients must be identical in terms of size, position, and lighting. Backgrounds should be clean and uncluttered (retouching is permitted on backgrounds). Color photographs that significantly enhance the presentation will be considered for publication. If approved by the Editorial Board, a color page containing up to 6 photographs (or occasionally two such pages) may be allowed at a charge to the author of $350.00 per page.

Drawings should be rendered in black india ink on white illustration board. The size of any lettering must be large enough so it wil lbe legible after it has been reduced to the size in which it will be printed. Send originals on pieces of illustration board, along with two photostats, no larger than 9 x 13 inches (23 x 33 cm).

Acknowledgments

Illustrations taken from other publications must be acknowledged. Include the following information in the figure legend when applicable: author(s), title of article, title of journal or book, volume number, page(s), month, and year. The publisher's letter of permission should be submitted to *Plastic and Reconstructive Surgery.*

Correspondence and brief communications will be published as space permits at the discretion of the editors. They should be typewritten, double-spaced (including references, if any), and must not exceed 500 words in length; they will be subject to editing.

Galley Proofs are sent directly to the author from the typesetter. They should be read carefully and returned promptly to the editor with the author's approval indicated by initialing.

Reprints may be ordered when galley proofs are received. A table showing the cost will be enclosed with the proofs. The number of reprints will be limited if it is contrary to the interests of the Journal.

Fig. A4-1, cont'd. Information for authors for *Plastic and Reconstructive Surgery.*

THE JOURNAL OF

HAND
SURGERY

Official journal
AMERICAN SOCIETY FOR SURGERY OF THE HAND

Editor in Chief
Joseph H. Boyes, M.D.
P. O. Box 1374
La Jolla, California 92038
Telephone: (714) 459-8997

INFORMATION FOR AUTHORS

This JOURNAL welcomes original articles, in English, relating to any aspect of surgery of the hand.

Send manuscripts and all correspondence relating to the editorial management of the JOURNAL to the Editor in Chief, Joseph H. Boyes, M.D., P. O. Box 1374, La Jolla, CA 92038, telephone: (714) 459-8997. Statements and opinions expressed in the articles and communications herein are those of the author(s) and not necessarily those of the Editor, the Publisher, or the Society, who disclaim any responsibility or liability for such material. Neither the Editor, the Publisher, nor the Society guarantees, warrants, or endorses any product or service advertised in this publication, nor do they guarantee any claim made by the manufacturer of such product or service.

It is assumed by the Editor that articles emanating from a particular institution are submitted with the approval of the requisite authority *including all matter pertaining to human studies. Articles dealing with human experimentation cannot be accepted unless the experiment was approved by the author's local Human Experimentation Committee.*

Most of the provisions of the Copyright Act of 1976 became effective on January 1, 1978. Therefore, all transmittal letters must be accompanied by the following statement, signed by each author: "The undersigned author(s) transfers all copyright ownership of the manuscript entitled (title of article) to the American Society for Surgery of the Hand in the event the work is published. The author(s) warrants that the article is original, is not under consideration by another journal, and has not been previously published." Authors will be consulted, when possible, regarding republication of their material.

Manuscripts

Manuscripts. All typewritten material should be typed with double spacing and liberal margins.

Title page. Type a separate page with a clear and specific title as short as possible. Include the first name and highest academic degree for each author. Insert name and address of institution from which the work originated and include all information about grants. Designate one author as correspondent and supply his complete mailing address and telephone number.

Abstract. On a separate page supply a factual abstract of not more than 150 words, stating the problem, describing the methods of experiment and the results, and stating the principal conclusion. Make it clear and concise.

Text. Type manuscripts on one side of 21.7 × 28 cm (8½ × 11 inches) white bond paper only, with double spacing and liberal margins, and number the pages consecutively from one. Do not staple or bind. At the top of each page type title of work. Do *not* put author's name on text pages. Submit the *original* and three copies of all material including illustrations and retain one copy.

References. Restrict the bibliography to pertinent references. Refer to them in the text by number only; list and number them at the end of the manuscript in the order of their mention. Follow the style of the *Cumulated Index Medicus* for periodical references (authors, title, journal, volume, inclusive pages, year). For book references, give author, title, edition, city, year, publisher, and specific page if necessary.

Tables. Type each on a separate sheet of paper. Number them in sequence, refer to them in order in the text, and supply appropriate captions.

Illustrations. Number figures consecutively and refer to them in the order they appear in the text. Mark *lightly in pencil* on the back: figure number, author's name, and indicate the top. Do not mount them; supply a sketch indicating desired grouping if necessary. Original drawings or graphs should be drawn with black India ink on white bord. *Typewritten or freehand lettering is not acceptable.* All lettering must be done professionally and be large to allow for clarity when reduced. Do not send original art work or x-ray films. Glossy print photographs (5 × 7 inches) are preferred, for good black and white contrast is essential. Special arrangements must be made with the Editor for color plates or excessive illustrations. Type legends on a separate sheet of paper.

Abbreviations and measurements. Use standard abbreviations; supply an explanation for any unusual ones used. Give all measurements in metric units: For anatomical terms use the *Nomina Anatomica (N.A.)* (1960) or refer to the *Terminology for Hand Surgery* (1970).

Copyrighted material. Direct quotations, tables, or illustrations that have appeared in copyrighted material *must be* accompanied by written permission for their use from the copyright owner along with complete data as to their source. Photographs of identifiable living persons *must be* accompanied by signed releases.

Reprints. Reprints of articles must be ordered directly from the Publisher, The C. V. Mosby Company, 11830 Westline Industrial Drive, St. Louis, MO 63141, telephone: (314) 872-8370, who will send their schedule of prices. Individual reprints of an article must be obtained through the author.

Books. Books will be reviewed depending on their interest and value to readers. Books should be sent to the Editor in Chief. No books are returned and no acknowledgement of books received will be made.

Letters to the Editor. Letters to the Editor are invited. If related to published articles, a copy will be sent to the author(s) for comment before publication. Letters are subject to critical review and to current editorial policy in respect to publication in part or in full. Letters submitted for publication should be typed with double spacing and should include complete references and the complete mailing address of the writer.

Fig. A4-2. Information for authors for *The Journal of Hand Surgery.*

JOURNAL of the
AMERICAN ACADEMY OF
DERMATOLOGY

EDITOR

J. Graham Smith, Jr., M.D.

Department of Dermatology
Medical College of Georgia
Augusta, Georgia 30912
404-828-4684

INFORMATION FOR AUTHORS.

Editorial policies. The *Journal of the American Academy of Dermatology* is a refereed journal designed to meet the continuing education needs of the Academy members and the international dermatologic community.

Statements and opinions expressed in the articles and communications herein are those of the author(s) and not necessarily those of the Editor(s), publisher, or Academy. The Editor(s), publisher, and Academy disclaim any responsibility or liability for such material and do not guarantee, warrant, or endorse any product or service advertised in this publication nor do they guarantee any claim made by the manufacturer of such product or service.

As a result of the Copyright Act of 1976, which became effective Jan. 1, 1978, the following statement signed by the senior or corresponding author must accompany each manuscript submitted: "The undersigned author transfers all copyright ownership of the manuscript entitled [title of article] to the American Academy of Dermatology in the event the work is published. The undersigned author warrants that the article is original, is not under consideration by another journal, and has not been previously published. I sign for and accept responsibility for releasing this material on behalf of any and all co-authors."

Author(s) will be consulted, whenever possible, regarding republication of material.

The following sections will be features of the Journal:

Continuing Medical Education: In-depth, substantiated, educational articles presenting core information for the continuing medical education of the practicing dermatologist. Answers to accompanying questions may be submitted to the American Academy of Dermatology office for CME credit.

Therapy: In-depth critical reviews of a therapeutic modality or treatment procedure.

Clinical and Laboratory Studies: Original, in-depth clinical and investigative laboratory research articles. (See "Preparation of Manuscripts.)

Current Issues: Brief, provocative, opinionated communications, not necessarily documented, on one limited subject.

Clinical Review: A review of several clinical studies or a pattern appearing in several cases.

Gross and Microscopic Symposium: Selected presentations from the Symposium on Gross and Microscopic Dermatology held at the annual meeting of the American Academy of Dermatology.

Editorials: Brief, substantiated commentary on limited subjects.

Correspondence: Brief letters or notes to the editor. Individual case reports, unless of unusual interest, are discouraged.

Special Reports: This section includes items of special interest.

Meeting Reports: Concise statements summarizing important material for dermatologists presented at major dermatology meetings and seminars.

Reports From Other Fields: Research and clinical observations from other medical specialties that may have particular bearing on the field of dermatology.

Book Reviews: Books and monographs (domestic and foreign) will be reviewed depending on their interest and value to subscribers. Send books to the Editor, Dr. J. Graham Smith, Jr. No books will be returned.

Bulletin: Council reports, governmental issues, news, notices, meetings, socioeconomic issues, etc. as space permits. Items for this section should be directed to Mr. Bradford W. Claxton, Executive Director, American Academy of Dermatology, 820 Davis St., Evanston, IL 60201.

Preparation of manuscripts. Original manuscripts will be considered for publication.

Correct preparation of the manuscript by the author will expedite the reviewing and publication procedures. Please note the following requirements.

The original copy of the manuscript and all supporting material plus two xerographic (not carbon) copies must be submitted to the Editor. The article must be typewritten (one side only), double-spaced, on 22×28 cm (8½×11 inch) paper with adequate margins.

Style. Manuscripts must conform to acceptable English usage. Standard abbreviations should be used consistently throughout the article. Unusual or "coined" abbreviations should be spelled out the first time they appear in the text and followed in parentheses by the abbreviation. Consult the latest editions of the *Council of Biology Editors Style Manual, A Manual of Style* by The University of Chicago Press, or the *Stylebook/Editorial Manual of the AMA* for current usage.

Generic names of drugs should be used; however, proprietary names may be inserted parenthetically or listed at the end of the manuscript if relevant. (Refer to current edition of the *American Drug Index*.)

Fig. A4-3. Information for authors for *Journal of the American Academy of Dermatology.*

Weights and measurements should be expressed in metric units. Temperatures should be expressed in degrees centigrade.

Title page. The title page should include the title, authors' full names, highest earned academic degrees, and institutional affiliations and location. If the title is exceedingly long, a shortened title (no longer than 42 characters) should be included. Designate one author as correspondent (provide address and telephone number) to receive galley proofs and reprint requests.

Abstract. Each article should be accompanied by an abstract not exceeding 150 words typed double-spaced on a separate sheet of paper.

References. Number references numerically in order of their mention in the text. References should follow the style used in *Cumulated Index Medicus*. References should be listed with inclusive page numbers. Only those references mentioned in the text should be cited.

Illustrations and tables. Tables, figures, and legends should supplement, not duplicate, the text. A reasonable number of halftone photographs and line drawings will be published at no extra charge to the author. Special arrangements for four-color illustrations must be made with the Editor at a cost to the author of $300 per page (one side). For color photographs, submit original transparencies and two sets of unmounted prints on glossy (smooth surface) paper 10×13 cm (4×5 in) in size. Preferred size for transparencies is 5×5 cm (2×2 in). Please note that 35-mm transparencies are normally enlarged to twice their original size. If it is important to deviate from this standard, please indicate when the material is submitted. *Top* for each print (or transparency) must be indicated. For black and white illustrations, send three sets of glossy prints. Preferred size is 13×18 cm (5×7 in). Black and white photographs should not be made from color slides since they do not reproduce well. Drawings should be professionally prepared and transferotype used for any lettering or labels. Careful attention should be paid to sizing of illustrations with special instructions clearly noted. Photographic consent must accompany recognizable photographs of patients. Do not send original artwork; glossy photographs are preferred as black and white contrast is essential.

Illustrations should be numbered in Arabic numerals according to their mention in the text. Indicate (lightly in pencil) the author's name, figure number, and top or bottom on back of each illustration. Type legends double-spaced on a separate sheet of paper and insert at end of manuscript.

Tables should be self-explanatory and numbered in Roman numerals according to their mention in the text. Provide a brief title for each.

Permissions and patient consent forms. Author and publisher permission for use of previously published material (quotes, tables, or figures) and patient consent forms must accompany manuscript. Patients must be identified by numbers and/or letters, not by name. Institutional consent must also be available.

Reprints. Single reprints must be obtained from the author. Reprint order forms will be sent to authors after articles are published. Reprints in quantity must be purchased from The C. V. Mosby Company. Reprints may not be purchased without the author's permission, and they may not be used for any purposes other than those specified by the author.

Procedure for review. Some degree of manuscript revision should be expected and regarded as constructive. The author should suggest several reviewers for his manuscript. Every attempt will be made to use at least one suggested reviewer. Authors will be notified upon initial receipt of the manuscript. The editorial staff will examine the manuscript and send it to at least two reviewers. Reviewers will pay particular attention to scientific accuracy, relevance, appropriateness of style, and sizing of illustrations. Six to eight weeks is the usual length of time before an author is notified regarding acceptance. Longer delays are possible.

Editorial communications. Communications regarding original articles and editorial management should be addressed to: J. Graham Smith, Jr., M.D., Editor, Journal of the American Academy of Dermatology, Medical College of Georgia, Augusta, GA 30912/404-828-4684.

Communications regarding the Bulletin section of the Journal should be addressed to: Bradford W. Claxton, Executive Director, American Academy of Dermatology, 820 Davis St., Evanston, IL 60201/312-869-3954.

Communications of a business nature and all advertising communications should be addressed to: Journal Publisher, The C. V. Mosby Company, 11830 Westline Industrial Dr., St. Louis, MO 63141.

Checklist for authors of Clinical and Laboratory Studies:
—Submission letter (including suggested reviewers)
—Signed copyright transfer statement
—Original and two copies of articles
—Title page
—Abstract
—Article proper
—References (double-spaced on a separate sheet)
—Tables
—Legends (double-spaced on a separate sheet)
—Illustrations, properly labeled (original and two copies)
—Patient consent letters (photographic and informed consent) and permission letters to reproduce previously published material

Fig. A4-3, cont'd. Information for authors for *Journal of the American Academy of Dermatology.*

THE JOURNAL OF
PEDIATRICS

Editor

Joseph M. Garfunkel, M.D.
Box 3307
Springfield, IL 62708
(217) 789-4204

Publisher

The C. V. Mosby Company
11830 Westline Industrial Drive
St. Louis, MO 63141

Preparation of manuscripts

THE JOURNAL OF PEDIATRICS publishes articles on original research, clinical observations, and reviews of pediatric subjects and related fields.

Articles are accepted for publication with the stipulation that they are submitted solely to THE JOURNAL OF PEDIATRICS and are subject to editorial revision. Statements and opinions expressed in the articles and communications herein are those of the author(s) and not necessarily those of the Editor(s) or publisher; the Editor(s) and publisher disclaim any responsibility or liability for such material. Neither the Editor(s) nor the publisher guarantee, warrant, or endorse any product or service advertised in this publication, nor do they guarantee any claim made by the manufacturer of such product or service.

Most of the provisions of the Copyright Act of 1976 became effective on January 1, 1978. Therefore, all manuscripts must be accompanied by the following written statement, signed by one author: "The undersigned author transfers all copyright ownership of the manuscript (title of article) to The C. V. Mosby Company in the event the work is published. The undersigned author warrants that the article is original, is not under consideration by another journal, and has not been previously published. I sign for and accept responsibility for releasing this material on behalf of any and all co-authors." Authors will be consulted, when possible, regarding republication of their material.

Papers describing research involving human subjects are acceptable, but such papers should indicate that informed consent was obtained from the parents or guardians of the children who served as subjects of the investigation and, when appropriate, from the subjects themselves. In the event either editors or referees question the propriety of the human investigation with respect to the risk to the subjects or to the means of obtaining informed consent, THE JOURNAL may request of the author more detailed information about the safeguards employed and the procedures used to obtain informed consent. Copies of the minutes of the committees which have reviewed and approved the research may also be requested.

Brief instructions for preparation of manuscripts

All manuscripts and editorial correspondence should be submitted by first-class (*not* registered) mail to the Editor.

Format. Two copies (high quality xerox accepted) typewritten on one side of white 8½ × 11 (22 × 28 cm) paper, sequentially numbered, doubled spaced (including references) with liberal margins, 25 lines to a page, 70 character spaces to a line. Title page. Authors' names, degrees, academic titles. Designate one author as correspondent and provide address and telephone number. Galley proofs will be sent to corresponding author as will order forms for reprints at a later date.

Illustrations. Two sets (glossy photographs preferred for good black and white contrast or original drawings done with black India ink), professional lettering (typewritten or freehand lettering not acceptable), unmounted, numbered, marked lightly on back with authors' names, top designated. Legends on a single, separate sheet. Recognizable likenesses of living persons will routinely have eyes and bridge of nose covered. Permission from the subject, or from parent or guardian of a minor child, is required for publication of recognizable likenesses.

Written permission from the copyright-holding publisher must accompany previously published illustrations.

A reasonable number of illustrations will be reproduced at no cost to the author, but the Editor's approval must be obtained for color plates, elaborate tables, or an unusually large number of illustrations.

References. Numbered according to order of their appearance in the text, listed in Cumulated Index Medicus style; *verified* in standard medical bibliography or from the source.

Abstract. On separate sheet, a brief summation of 200 words or less, to appear at the head of the article.

Brief clinical and laboratory observations

Articles in this section should require three JOURNAL pages or less; the text 1,000 words or less. A combined total of two illustrations or tables with up to ten references will be accepted. An abstract is not necessary. At the discretion of the Editors, it may be necessary to limit some manuscripts even more; these limitations may apply to length, tables, figures, or references and will be communicated directly to each corresponding author.

Editorial correspondence

Letters pertaining to articles published in THE JOURNAL or to topics of current interest. Such letters are subject to critical review and to current editorial policy in respect to publication in part or in full and should be prepared in the same style as other manuscripts.

News items

Announcements of scheduled meetings, symposia, or postgraduate courses of regional or national interest and news items of general interest to pediatricians and related specialists may be sent for consideration to the publisher at least three months in advance of the date of publication desired.

Books for review. Books and monographs, domestic and foreign, will be reviewed depending on their interest and value to subscribers. Books should be sent to the Editor of The Book Shelf, Angelo M. DiGeorge, M.D., 2600 N. Lawrence, Philadelphia, Pa. 19133. *No books are returned* and no acknowledgment will be made of books received.

Fig. A4-4. Information for authors for *The Journal of Pediatrics.*

SURGERY

Editors in Chief

Walter F. Ballinger, M.D.
Department of Surgery
Washington University School of Medicine
4960 Audubon Ave.
St. Louis, MO 63110
USA

George D. Zuidema, M.D.
Department of Surgery
Johns Hopkins Hospital
601 N. Broadway
Baltimore, MD 21205
USA

Information for authors

Original communications. This journal invites concise, original articles of new matter in the broad field of clinical and experimental surgery as well as surgical education. Manuscripts should be submitted to either of the editors, at the above addresses. Statements and opinions expressed in the articles and communications therein are those of the author(s) and not necessarily those of the editor(s) or publisher, and the editor(s) and publisher disclaim any responsibility or liability for such material. Papers describing research involving human subjects should indicate that informed consent was obtained from patients who served as subjects of the investigation. In the event either editors or referees question the propriety of the human investigation with respect to the risk to the subjects or to the means of obtaining informed consent, SURGERY may request more detailed information about the safeguards employed and the procedures used to obtain consent. Minutes of the local human experimentation committees which reviewed and approved the research may also be requested. Neither the editor(s) nor the publisher guarantees, warrants, or endorses any product or service advertised in this publication, nor does either guarantee any claim made by the manufacturer of such product or service.

Manuscript checklist. The following guidelines are offered for manuscript preparation, and a checklist is provided for the author's convenience:

____ *Three complete sets of manuscript* should be submitted, typed on one side of the paper and double spaced (carbon copies are unacceptable).

____ *The title page* should include the name and highest achieved degree of each author, the institution from which the work originated, sources of financial support, and the exact and complete address of the one author who will be responsible for correspondence, galley proofs, and reprint requests.

____ *A synopsis or abstract* of no more than 200 words should be included, which concisely states the objectives, findings, and conclusions of the study.

____ *Standard abbreviations* should be used consistently throughout the article. Unusual or "coined" abbreviations should be spelled out the first time they appear in the text, with the abbreviation following in parentheses. Consult the *Stylebook/Editorial Manual of the AMA, Council of Biology (CBE) Style Manual,* and *A Manual of Style* by the University of Chicago Press for currently accepted usage.

____ *Illustrations* should be submitted in the form of three glossy prints and numbered in the order in which they appear in the text. Each should be marked lightly on the back in pencil with the figure number and author's name; the top should also be indicated. *Separate typewritten legends* should accompany the manuscript, and the approximate position of the figures in the text should be indicated. A reasonable number of illustrations will be produced free, but special arrangements must be made with the editors and publisher for color plates or more than six illustrations. Original drawings or graphs should be drawn in black India ink. Typewritten or freehand lettering is not acceptable; all lettering must be done professionally. Do not send original art work, x-rays, or electrocardiogram tracings; glossy prints of these should be submitted, for good black and white contrast is essential.

____ *Tables* should each be typewritten on a separate page, numbered in the order in which it was mentioned in the text, and given a brief descriptive title. All acronyms, abbreviations, and unusual units of measurement used in the title, headings, or body of the table should be fully explained in a legend. Omit all internal horizontal or vertical rules. For footnotes, use these symbols in sequence: *, †, ‡, §, ||, ¶, **, ††. Glossy prints and reduced versions of typewritten tables are unacceptable.

____ *The reference list* should be typewritten with double spacing and restricted to cited works listed **alphabetically** in the minimal punctuation style of *Index Medicus*. For periodical references, give all authors, title, journal, volume, inclusive pages, year; e.g.,

> 1. Blaisdell WF, Clauss RH, Galbraith JG, Smith JA Jr: Joint study of extracranial arterial occlusion. IV. A review of surgical considerations. JAMA 209:1889-95, 1969

For book references give all authors, title, edition, city and year in which published, complete name of publisher, and specific inclusive pages, if necessary, also in the minimal punctuation style; e.g.,

> 2. Sagawa K: The use of control theory and systems analysis, *in* Bergel DH, editor: Cardiovascular dynamics, ed 2. London, 1974, Academic Press, Inc, pp 115-9

____ *Copyright ownership* is to be transferred by the following written statement, which must accompany all manuscripts and be signed by one author: "The undersigned author transfers all copyright ownership of the manuscript [title of article] to The C. V. Mosby Company in the event the work is published. The undersigned author warrants that the article is original, is not under consideration by another journal, and has not been published previously. I sign for and accept responsibility for releasing this material on behalf of any and all co-authors." Authors will be consulted when possible regarding republication of their material.

____ *A shortened title* of no more than 50 characters or spaces may be supplied by the authors, if preferred, for the running heading.

Editorials. Editorials should be concise and brief (not to exceed 1,000 words, except under unusual circumstances) and should express the personal opinion of the author and contain a minimum of references, if any. Editorial material to be considered by the editors may include not only timely subjects of clinical interest, but also material of general interest to the surgical community, including topics of social significance. Following the guidelines for original manuscripts, three copies of each editorial should be sent.

Letters to the editors. The editors invite comments in the form of letters which express differences of opinion or supporting views of prior editorials or recently published papers in SURGERY. Each letter must not exceed 500 words, should be typed with double spacing, must include complete references, and should be submitted in triplicate. The editorial board reserves the right to accept, reject, or excerpt letters without changing the views expressed by the author. No anonymous correspondence will be published, and therefore each author should include his complete address.

Reprints. Reprints of articles must be ordered directly from the publisher who will send a schedule of prices at the time of publication of the article. Individual reprints of an article must be obtained directly from the author of correspondence.

Book reviews. Books shall be reviewed only at the discretion of the editors.

Fig. A4-5. Information for authors for *Surgery*.

INFORMATION FOR AUTHORS

The Editors of POSTGRADUATE MEDICINE are pleased to consider original, unpublished papers in all fields of medicine, so presented as to be of value and interest to primary care physicians. Articles must not be under consideration for publication elsewhere.

Manuscript format
Papers should be typewritten double-spaced, and the original and a copy should be submitted. The text should comprise a maximum of about 2,000 words. In addition, a prefatory abstract of about 45 words, a brief closing summary, and selected references should be provided. Illustrative material is welcome. A cover page should indicate the title, and the full names, affiliations (primary first), and current addresses of all of the authors, and in the case of multiple authorship, should designate which author is handling the correspondence and where reprint requests should be sent.

Manuscripts are acknowledged upon receipt, and the author is notified within 60 days of acceptance or rejection.

Manuscripts and all correspondence regarding them should be addressed to the Editorial Department, POSTGRADUATE MEDICINE, 4530 W 77th St, Minneapolis, MN 55435.

Manuscript review
All papers received are submitted to referees in the field or fields of medicine represented for review prior to acceptance or rejection. Material accepted for publication is subject to editing. A typescript of the edited manuscript is sent to the designated author for review and approval. Galley proofs or page proofs are not routinely submitted. Authors are responsible for all changes in the manuscript, including those made by the manuscript editor.

Title
The title should be short and meaningful for purposes of indexing.

Author names and affiliations
The full name and highest pertinent academic degrees should be given for each author. An affiliation giving professional appointments and interests is used with the author photograph on an inside page of the article. The journal regularly publishes photographs of authors of major articles. If there are more than three authors, a picture of the senior author only is used. Photographs are requested at the time the paper is accepted and are returned to the author when they have been processed.

References
References should be limited to about 20 and should be cited in the text in numerically consecutive order. Personal communications and unpublished data should not be included, but may be designated as such in the text. References to journals must include the surname and initials of all authors, complete title, name of the journal abbreviated according to *Index Medicus*, volume number, first and last page numbers, and year of publication. References to books or other publications must include the surname and initials of all authors or editors, title, number of edition after the first, place of publication, name of publisher, year of publication, volume number if there is more than one, and page numbers. Specific page numbers must be given for all quoted material.

Tables
Tables should be titled and should be numbered consecutively according to their citation in the text. If the data have been published previously, an appropriate reference should be included.

Illustrations
The journal welcomes illustrations to accompany articles. The illustrations should be cited consecutively in the text in numerical order, and short descriptive legends should be provided. Illustrations should be submitted in duplicate and should have on the back the author's name and figure number, and the top should be indicated. Glossy prints are preferred to original artwork, and x-ray films are preferred to glossy prints. X-ray films and photomicrographs should have crop marks indicated at the edge, and the legends for photomicrographs should give the stain and magnification. If illustrations have been published previously, a complete reference to the original publication and copies of the publisher's and author's permission to use the figure must be included. Illustrations are returned after publication.

Reprints
Reprints are available, and an order form and price list are sent to the designated author shortly before publication.

Fig. A4-6. Information for authors for *Postgraduate Medicine*. Reproduced by permission.

A5 □ Uniform requirements for manuscripts submitted to biomedical journals

PREFACE

The editors of the journals listed at the end of this document have agreed to receive manuscripts prepared and submitted in accordance with the requirements described on the following pages. Authors *must* also consult the instructions printed in the journal to which they plan to submit their manuscripts for information as to what clinical or scientific material is suitable for that particular journal and the types of papers that may be submitted (for example, original articles, review articles, case reports, and brief reports). In addition, the journal's own instructions contain important information concerning acceptable languages, length of articles, approved abbreviations besides those listed in this document, number of copies of manuscripts to be submitted, and requirements for transfer of copyright.

The material in this document will be revised at intervals. Inquiries and comments originating in North America should be sent to Edward J. Huth, M.D., Annals of Internal Medicine, 4200 Pine Street, Philadelphia, PA 19104; those originating in other regions should be sent to Stephen Lock, M.A., M.B., British Medical Journal, British Medical Association, Tavistock Square, London WC1H 9JR, United Kingdom.

SUMMARY OF REQUIREMENTS

Type manuscript double spaced, including title page, abstract, text, acknowledgments, references, tables, and legends.

Each manuscript component should begin on a new page, in this sequence:

Title page
Abstract and key words
Text
Acknowledgments
References
Tables: each table, complete with title and footnotes, on a separate page
Legends for illustrations

Illustrations must be good quality, unmounted glossy prints usually 12.7 by 17.3 cm (5 by 7 in.) but no larger than 20.3 by 25.4 cm (8 by 10 in.).

Submit the required number of copies of manuscript and figures (*see* journal's instructions) in heavy-paper envelope. Submitted manuscript should be accompanied by covering letter, as described under "Submission of Manuscripts," and permissions to reproduce previously published materials or to use illustrations that may identify subjects.

Follow journal's instructions for transfer of copyright. Authors should keep copies of everything submitted.

PREPARATION OF MANUSCRIPT

Type manuscript on white bond paper, 20.3 by 26.7 cm or 21.6 by 27.9 cm (8 by 10½ in. or 8½ by 11 in.) or ISO A4 (212 by 297 mm) with margins of at least 2.5 cm (1 in.). Use double spacing throughout, including title page, abstract, text, acknowledgments, references, tables, and legends for illustrations. Begin each of the following sections on separate pages: title page, abstract and key words, text, acknowledgments, references, individual tables, and legends. Number pages consecutively, beginning with the title page. Type the page number in the upper right-hand corner of each page.

Manuscripts will be reviewed for possible publication with the understanding that they are being submitted to one journal at a time and have not been published, simultaneously submitted, or already accepted for publication elsewhere. This does not preclude consideration of a manuscript that has been rejected by another journal or of a complete report that follows publication of preliminary findings elsewhere, usually in the form of an abstract. Copies of any possibly duplicative published material should be submitted with the manuscript that is being sent for consideration.

Title page

The title page should contain [1] the title of the article, which should be concise but informative; [2] a short running head or footline of no more than 40 characters (count letters and spaces) placed at the foot of the title page and identified; [3] first name, middle initial, and last name of each author, with highest academic degree(s); [4] name of department(s) and institution(s) to which the work should be attributed; [5] disclaimers, if any; [6] name and address of author responsible for correspondence about the manuscript; [7] name and address of author to whom requests for reprints should be addressed, or statement that reprints will not be available from the author; [8] the source(s) of support in the form of grants, equipment, drugs, or all of these.

Abstract and key words

The second page should carry an abstract of not more than 150 words. The abstract should state the purposes of the study or investigation, basic procedures (study subjects or experimental animals and observational and analytic methods), main findings (give specific data and their statistical significance, if possible), and the principal conclusions. Emphasize new and important aspects of the study of observations. Use only approved abbreviations (*see* list of Commonly Used Approved Abbreviations elsewhere in this document).

Key (indexing) terms: Below the abstract, provide and identify as such, three to 10 key words or short phrases that will assist indexers in cross-indexing your article and that may be published with the abstract. Use terms from the Medical Subject Headings list from *Index Medicus* whenever possible.

Text

The text of observational and experimental articles is usually—but not necessarily—divided into sections with the headings Introduction, Methods, Results, and Discussion. Long articles may need subheadings within some sections to clarify their content, especially the Results and Discussion sections. Other types of articles such as case reports, reviews, and editorials are likely to need other formats, and authors should consult individual journals for further guidance.

Introduction: Clearly state the *purpose* of the article. Summarize the rationale for the study or observation. Give only strictly pertinent references, and do not review the subject extensively.

Methods: Describe your selection of the observational or experimental subjects (patients or experimental animals, including controls) clearly. Identify the methods, apparatus (manufacturer's name and address in parenthesis), and procedures in sufficient detail to allow other workers to reproduce the results. Give references to established methods, including statistical methods; provide references and brief descriptions of methods that have been published but are not well known; describe new or substantially modified methods, give reasons for using them, and evaluate their limitations.

When reporting experiments on human subjects, indicate whether the procedures followed were in accord with the ethical standards of the Committee on Human Experimentation of the institution in which the experiments were done or in accord with the Helsinki Declaration of 1975. When reporting experiments on animal subjects, indicate whether the institution's or the National Research Council's guide for the care and use of laboratory animals was followed. Identify precisely all drugs and chemicals used, including generic name(s), dosage(s), and route(s) of administration. Do not use patients' names, initials, or hospital numbers.

Include numbers of observations and the statistical significance of the findings when appropriate. Detailed statistical analyses, mathematical derivations, and the like may sometimes be suitably presented in the form of one or more appendixes.

Results: Present your results in logical sequence in the text, tables, and illustrations. Do not repeat in the text all the data in the tables and/or illustrations: emphasize or summarize only important observations.

Discussion: Emphasize the new and important aspects of the study and *conclusions* that follow from them. Do not repeat in detail data given in the Results section. Include in the Discussion the implications of the findings and their limitations and relate the observations to other relevant studies. Link the conclusions with the goals of the study but avoid unqualified statements and conclusions not completely supported by your data. Avoid claiming priority and alluding to work that has not been completed. State new hypotheses when warranted, but clearly label them as such. Recommendations, when appropriate, may be included.

Acknowledgments

Acknowledge only persons who have made substantive contributions to the study. Authors are responsible for obtaining written permission from everyone acknowledged by name because readers may infer their endorsement of the data and conclusions.

References

Number references consecutively in the order in which they are first mentioned in the text. Identify references in text, tables, and legends by arabic numerals (in parenthesis). References cited *only* in tables or in legends to figures should be numbered in accordance with a sequence established by the first identification in the text of the particular table or illustration.

Use the form of references adoped by the U.S. National Library of Medicine and used in *Index Medicus*. Use the style of the examples cited at the end of this section, which have been approved by the National Library of Medicine.

The titles of journals should be abbreviated according to the style used in *Index Medicus*. A list of abbreviated names of frequently cited journals is given near the end of this document; for others, consult the "List of Journals Indexed," printed annually in the January issue of *Index Medicus*.

Try to avoid using abstracts as references; "unpublished observations" and "personal communications" may not be used as references, although references to written, not verbal, communications may be inserted (in parenthesis) in the text. Include among the references manuscripts accepted but not yet published; designate the journal followed by "in press" (in parenthesis). Information from manuscripts submitted but not yet accepted should be cited in the text as "unpublished observations" (in parenthesis).

The references must be verified by the author(s) against the original documents.

Examples of correct forms of references are given below.

Journal

1. Standard Journal Article (List all authors when six or less; when seven or more, list only first three and add et al.)

    Soter NA, Wasserman SI, Austen KF. Cold urticaria: release into the circulation of histamine and eosinophil chemotactic factor of anaphylaxis during cold challenge. N Engl J Med 1976; 294:687-90.

2. Corporate Author

    The Committee on Enzymes of the Scandinavian Society for Clinical Chemistry and Clinical Physiology. Recommended method for the determination of gammaglutamyltransferase in blood. Scand J Clin Lab Invest 1976; 36:119-25.

Books and other monographs

3. Personal Author(s)

    Osler AG. Complement: mechanisms and functions. Englewood Cliffs: Prentice-Hall, 1976.

4. Corporate Author

    American Medical Association Department of Drugs. AMA drug evaluations, 3rd ed. Littleton: Publishing Sciences Group, 1977.

5. Editor, Compiler, Chairman as Author

    Rhodes AJ, Van Rooyen CE, comps. Textbook of virology: for students and practitioners of medicine and the other health sciences. 5th ed. Baltimore: Williams & Wilkins, 1968.

6. Chapter in Book

    Weinstein L, Swartz MN. Pathogenic properties of invading microorganisms. In: Sodeman WA Jr, Sodeman WA, eds. Pathologic physiology: mechanisms of disease. Philadelphia: WB Saunders, 1974:457-72.

7. Agency Publication

    National Center for Health Statistics. Acute conditions: incidence and associated disability, United States July 1968-June 1969. Rockville, Md.: National Center for Health Statistics, 1972. (Vital and health statistics. Series 10: Data from the National Health Survey, no. 69) (DHEW publication no. (HSM)72-1036).

Other articles

8. Newspaper Article

    Shaffer RA. Advances in chemistry are starting to unlock mysteries of the brain: discoveries could help cure alcoholism and insomnia, explain mental illness. How the messengers work. Wall Street Journal 1977 Aug 12:1(col. 1), 10(col. 1).

9. Magazine Article

    Roueché B. Annals of medicine: the Santa Claus culture. The New Yorker 1971 Sep 4:66-81.

Tables

Type each table on a separate sheet; remember to double space. Do not submit tables as photographs. Number tables consecutively and supply a brief title for each. Give each column a short or abbreviated heading. Place explanatory matter in footnotes, not in the heading. Explain in footnotes all nonstandard abbreviations that are used in each table. For footnotes, use the following symbols in this sequence: *, †, ‡, §, ‖, ¶, **, ††. . . . Identify statistical measures of variations such as SD and SEM.

Omit internal horizontal and vertical rules.

Cite each table in the text in consecutive order.

If you use data from another published or unpublished source, obtain permission and acknowledge fully.

Having too many tables in relation to the length of the text may produce difficulties in the layout of pages. Examine issues of the journal to which you plan to submit your manuscript to estimate how many tables to use per 1000 words of text.

The editor on accepting a manuscript may recommend that additional tables containing important backup data too extensive to be published may be deposited with the National Auxiliary Publications Service or made available by the author(s). In that event, an appropriate statement will be added to the text. Submit such tables for consideration with the manuscript.

Illustrations

Submit the required number of complete sets of figures. Figures should be professionally drawn and photographed; freehand or typewritten lettering is unacceptable. Instead of *original* drawings, roentgenograms, and other material, send sharp, glossy black-and-white photographic prints, usually 12.7 by 17.3 cm (5 by 7 in.) but no larger than 20.3 by 25.4 cm (8 by 10 in.). Letters, numbers, and symbols should be clear and even throughout, and of sufficient size that when reduced for publication each item will still be legible. Titles and detailed explanations belong in the legends for illustrations, not on the illustrations themselves.

Each figure should have a label pasted on its back indicating the number of the figure, the names of the authors, and the top of the figure. Do not write on the back of the figures or mount them on cardboard, or scratch or mar them using paper clips. Do not bend figures.

Photomicrographs must have internal scale markers. Symbols, arrows, or letters used in the photomicrographs should contrast with the background.

If photographs of persons are used, either the subjects must not be identifiable or their pictures must be accompanied by written permission to use the photograph.

Cite each figure in the text in consecutive order. If a figure has been published, acknowledge the original source and submit written permission from the copyright holder to reproduce the material. Permission is required, *regardless of authorship or publisher,* except for documents in the public domain.

For illustrations in color, supply color negatives or positive transparencies and, when necessary, accompanying drawings marked to indicate the region to be reproduced; in addition, send two positive color prints to assist editors in making recommendations. Some journals publish illustrations in color only if the author pays for the extra cost.

Legends for illustrations

Type legends for illustrations double spaced, starting on a separate page with arabic numerals corresponding to the illustrations. When symbols, arrows, numbers, or letters are used to identify parts of the illustrations, identify and explain each one clearly in the legend. Explain internal scale and identify method of staining in photomicrographs.

ABBREVIATIONS

Use only standard abbreviations (*see* below for lists of commonly used approved abbreviations). Consult the following sources for additional standard abbreviations: [1] CBE Style Manual Committee. Council of Biology Editors style manual: a guide for authors, editors, and publishers in the biological sciences. 4th ed. Arlington: Council of Biology Editors, 1978; and [2] O'Connor M, Woodford FP. Writing scientific papers in English: an ELSE-Ciba Foundation guide for authors. Amsterdam, Oxford, New York: Elsevier-Excerpta Medica, 1975. Avoid abbreviations in the title. The full term for which an abbreviation stands should precede its first use in the text unless it is a standard unit of measurement.

In most countries the International System of Units (SI) is standard or is becoming so. Report measurements in the units in which they were made. Journals may use these units, convert them to another system, or use both.

Commonly used approved abbreviations

Term	Abbreviation or symbol
Standard units of measurement	
ampere	A
ångström	Å
barn	b
candela	cd
coulomb	C
counts per minute	cpm
counts per second	cps
curie	Ci
degree Celsius	°C
disintegration per minute	dpm
disintegration per second	dps
electron Volt	eV
equivalent	Eq
farad	F
gauss	G
gram	g
henry	H
hertz	Hz
hour	h
international unit	IU
joule	J
kelvin	K
kilogram	kg
liter, litre	l or L
meter, metre	m
minute	min
molar	M
mole	mol
newton	N
normal (concentration)	N
ohm	Ω
osmol	osmol
pascal	Pa
revolutions per minute	rpm
second	s
square centimeter	cm^2
volt	V
watt	W
week	wk
year	yr

Combining prefixes		
tera-	(10^{12})	T
giga-	(10^{9})	G
mega-	(10^{6})	M
kilo-	(10^{3})	k
hecto-	(10^{2})	h
deca-	(10^{1})	da
deci-	(10^{-1})	d
centi-	(10^{-2})	e
milli-	(10^{-3})	m
micro-	(10^{-6})	μ
nano-	(10^{-9})	n
pico-	(10^{-12})	p
femto-	(10^{-15})	f
atto-	(10^{-18})	a

Statistical terms

correlation coefficient	r
degrees of freedom	df
mean	$\bar{x}$
not significant	NS
number of observations	n
probability	p
standard deviation	SD
standard error of the mean	SEM
"Student's" t test	*t* test
variance ratio	F

Others

adenosinediphosphatase	ADPase
adenosine 5'-diphosphate (adenosine diphosphate)	ADP
adenosine 5'-monophosphate (adenosine monophosphate, adenylic acid)	AMP
adenosine triphosphatase	ATPase
adenosine 5'-triphosphate (adenosine triphosphate)	ATP
adrenocorticotropic hormone (adrenocorticotropin)	ACTH
bacille Calmette-Guérin	BCG
basal metabolic rate	BMR
body temperature, pressure, and saturated	BTPS
central nervous system	CNS
coenzyme A	coA
deoxyribonucleic acid (deoxyribonucleate)	DNA
dihydroxyphenethylamine	dopamine
electrocardiogram	ECG
electroencephalogram	EEG
enteric cytopathogenic human orphan (virus)	ECHO
ethyl	Et
ethylenediaminetetraacetate	EDTA
gas-liquid chromatography	GLC
guanosine 5'-monophosphate (guanosine monophosphate, guanylic acid)	GMP
hemoglobin	Hb
logarithm (to base 10; common logarithm)	log
logarithm, natural	ln
methyl	Me
Michaelis constant	K_m
negative logarithm of hydrogen ion activity	pH
partial pressure of CO_2	P_{CO_2}
partial pressure of O_2	P_{O_2}
per	/
percent	%
radiation (ionizing, absorbed dose)	rad
respiratory quotient	RQ
specific gravity	sp gr
standard atmosphere	atm
standard temperature and pressure	STP
ultraviolet	uv
volume	vol
volume ratio (volume per volume)	vol/vol
weight	wt
weight per volume	wt/vol
weight ratio (weight per weight)	wt/wt

Abbreviations of names of frequently cited journals

Acta Medica Scandinavica	Acta Med Scand
American Family Physician	Am Fam Physician
American Heart Journal	Am Heart J
American Journal of Cardiology	Am J Cardiol
American Journal of Clinical Nutrition	Am J Clin Nutr
American Journal of Clinical Pathology	Am J Clin Pathol
American Journal of Digestive Diseases	Am J Dig Dis
American Journal of Diseases of Children	Am J Dis Child
American Journal of Human Genetics	Am J Hum Genet
American Journal of Medical Sciences	Am J Med Sci
American Journal of Medicine	Am J Med
American Journal of Obstetrics and Gynecology	Am J Obstet Gynecol
American Journal of Ophthalmology	Am J Ophthalmol
American Journal of Pathology	Am J Pathol
American Journal of Physical Medicine	Am J Phys Med
American Journal of Physiology	Am J Physiol
American Journal of Psychiatry	Am J Psychiatry
American Journal of Public Health	Am J Public Health
AJR; American Journal of Roentgenology	AJR
American Journal of Surgery	Am J Surg
American Journal of Tropical Medicine and Hygiene	Am J Trop Med Hyg
American Review of Respiratory Disease	Am Rev Respir Dis
Anaesthesia	Anaesthesia
Anesthesiology	Anesthesiology
Annals of Allergy	Ann Allergy
Annals of Internal Medicine	Ann Intern Med
Annals of Otology, Rhinology and Laryngology	Ann Otol Rhinol Laryngol
Annals of Surgery	Ann Surg
Annals of Thoracic Surgery	Ann Thorac Surg
Archives of Dermatology	Arch Dermatol
Archives of Environmental Health	Arch Environ Health
Archives of General Psychiatry	Arch Gen Psychiatry
Archives of Internal Medicine	Arch Intern Med
Archives of Neurology	Arch Neurol
Archives of Ophthalmology	Arch Ophthalmol
Archives of Otolaryngology	Arch Otolaryngol
Archives of Pathology and Laboratory Medicine	Arch Pathol Lab Med
Archives of Physical Medicine and Rehabilitation	Arch Phys Med Rehabil
Archives of Surgery	Arch Surg
Arthritis and Rheumatism	Arthritis Rheum

Blood; Journal of Hematology	Blood
Brain; Journal of Neurology	Brain
British Heart Journal	Br Heart J
British Journal of Obstetrics and Gynaecology	Br J Obstet Gynaecol
British Journal of Radiology	Br J Radiol
British Journal of Surgery	Br J Surg
British Medical Journal	Br Med J
Canadian Journal of Public Health	Can J Public Health
Canadian Medical Association Journal	Can Med Assoc J
Cancer	Cancer
Chest	Chest
Circulation; Journal of the American Heart Association	Circulation
Circulation Research	Circ Res
Clinical Pediatrics	Clin Pediatr (Phila)
Clinical Pharmacology and Therapeutics	Clin Pharmacol Ther
Clinical Science and Molecular Medicine	Clin Sci Mol Med
Clinical Toxicology	Clin Toxicol
Diabetes	Diabetes
DM; Disease-a-Month	DM
Endocrinology	Endocrinology
Gastroenterology	Gastroenterology
Geriatrics	Geriatrics
Gut	Gut
Human Pathology	Hum Pathol
Investigative Radiology	Invest Radiol
JAMA; Journal of the American Medical Association	JAMA
Journal of Allergy and Clinical Immunology	J Allergy Clin Immunol
Journal of Applied Physiology	J Appl Physiol
Journal of Biological Chemistry	J Biol Chem
Journal of Bone and Joint Surgery; American Volume	J Bone Joint Surg [Am]
Journal of Bone and Joint Surgery; British Volume	J Bone Joint Surg [Br]
Journal of Clinical Endocrinology and Metabolism	J Clin Endocrinol Metab
Journal of Clinical Investigation	J Clin Invest
Journal of Clinical Pathology	J Clin Pathol
Journal of Experimental Medicine	J Exp Med
Journal of Gerontology	J Gerontol
Journal of Immunology	J Immunol
Journal of Infectious Diseases	J Infect Dis
Journal of Investigative Dermatology	J Invest Dermatol
Journal of Laboratory and Clinical Medicine	J Lab Clin Med
Journal of Laryngology and Otology	J Laryngol Otol
Journal of Medical Education	J Med Educ
Journal of Nervous and Mental Disease	J Nerv Ment Dis
Journal of Neurosurgery	J Neurosurg
Journal of Pathology	J Pathol
Journal of Pediatrics	J Pediatr
Journal of Physiology	J Physiol
Journal of Thoracic and Cardiovascular Surgery	J Thorac Cardiovasc Surg
Journal of Trauma	J Trauma
Journal of Urology	J Urol
Lancet	Lancet
Medical Clinics of North America	Med Clin North Am
Medical Letter on Drugs and Therapeutics	Med Lett Drugs Ther
Medicine (Baltimore)	Medicine (Baltimore)
New England Journal of Medicine	N Engl J Med
Obstetrics and Gynecology	Obstet Gynecol
Pediatric Clinics of North America	Pediatr Clin North Am
Pediatrics	Pediatrics
Physiological Reviews	Physiol Rev
Plastic and Reconstructive Surgery	Plast Reconstr Surg
Postgraduate Medicine	Postgrad Med
Progress in Cardiovascular Diseases	Progr Cardiovasc Dis
Public Health Reports	Public Health Rep
Radiology	Radiology
Rheumatology and Rehabilitation	Rheumatol Rehabil
Seminars in Roentgenology	Semin Roentgenol
Surgery	Surgery
Surgery, Gynecology and Obstetrics	Surg Gynecol Obstet

SUBMISSION OF MANUSCRIPTS

Mail the required number of manuscript copies in a heavy paper envelope, enclosing the manuscript copies and figures in cardboard, if necessary, to prevent bending of photographs during mail handling. Place photographs and transparencies in a separate heavy paper envelope.

Manuscripts should be accompanied by a covering letter from the author who will be responsible for correspondence regarding the manuscript. The covering letter should contain a statement that the manuscript has been seen and approved by all authors. The letter should give any additional information that may be helpful to the editor, such as the type of article the manuscript represents in the particular journal, information on publication of any part of the manuscript, and whether the author(s) will be willing to meet the cost of reproducing color illustrations. Include copies of any permissions needed to reproduce published material or to use illustrations of identifiable subjects.

PARTICIPATING JOURNALS (TENTATIVE LIST)

American Journal of Diseases of Children
American Review of Respiratory Disease
Annals of Internal Medicine
Archives of Dermatology
Archives of General Psychiatry
Archives of Internal Medicine
Archives of Neurology
Archives of Ophthalmology
Archives of Otolaryngology
Archives of Pathology and Laboratory Medicine
Archives of Surgery
British Medical Journal
Canadian Journal of Public Health (Revue Canadienne de Santé Publique)
Canadian Medical Association Journal
Clinical and Investigative Medicine
Circulation
Journal of the American Medical Association
The Lancet
The New England Journal of Medicine

A6 □ Journal flow sheet: copyediting and production procedures

A. *Incoming manuscript:* Manuscript accepted for publication arrives from editor accompanied by two copies of transmittal slip. Duplicate slip returned to editor's office to acknowledge receipt.
   1. Transmittal slip gives cataloguing data used in editor's office, authors' names and affiliations, address of corresponding author to whom galley proof is to be sent, title of article, dates of submission and acceptance, section of journal in which article will appear, and number of figures and tables. Accompanying permission letters, if any, receipt of copyright transfer from authors by editor (to be retained in editor's file), and special comments pertaining to article are noted.
   2. Information on transmittal slip is used to type central file record, which will be pulled by reprint department after contents are prepared.
   3. Manuscript is sent to production department for sizing of illustrations.
   4. If color illustration is included, author is asked to verify that he is willing to pay estimated cost of production. If so, color is processed and proof is sent to author for ok in advance of galley proofs.

B. *Manuscript to copy editor:* Copy editor prepares manuscript for typesetter. This includes editing for grammatical construction, consistency of usage, conformity to journal style, querying author as necessary for clarity and discrepancies in content, checking reference citations in text against reference list, and checking legend copy against figures to see that designations on figure match explanations in legend. Copy editor also checks that permissions of publisher and author for quotes and previously published figures and tables are included as well as patient consent form if full face views are used. If not, he or she contacts editor's office to have author supply. Copy editor would also bring to editor's attention illustrations submitted that are not reproducible. After seeing that the type is marked adequately for typesetter, manuscript with tables, figures, and legends is sent down for typesetting.

C. *Galley proof from typesetter:* Galley proof, proofs of figures, and original manuscript are returned by typesetter. Production department logs in, checks galley proof against manuscript to see that typesetter followed instructions, checks proof of figures against originals for quality of reproduction, and turns over to copy editor. Copy editor checks master set of galley proof to see that all queries have been carried, answers any queries from typesetter and production department, and measures copy to see how many journal pages the article will make. Corrections and questions are transferred to author's and editor's set. Copy editor retains master set, original copy, and paste-up set in file and mails out author's and editor's sets. If for some reason author does not return proof and cannot be located before text ok date, editor is contacted by copy editor and asked to read and approve for author. When proofs are returned, corrections are transferred to master set and changes affecting make-up are noted on the paste-up set.

D. *List to editor:* Copy editor sends list of articles set in type to editor approximately 2 weeks before articles are scheduled for paste-up, designating number of journal pages each article will make. Editor selects articles for current issue, keeping within the established number of pages, and returns the list to the copy editor with the order of publication numbered to the side. Obviously, the schedule is too tight at this point to accommodate articles that are not already set in type or in the process of being set.

E. *Assembling for paste-up:* Copy editor pulls articles (hopefully with all author corrections back and transferred) that editor has selected and gives to paste-up in proper sequence of publication within each section of the journal.

F. *Paste-up:* In laying out the journal, production:
   1. Checks style file for specific information concerning journal style.
   2. Pastes journal using template and referring to style folder and most recent issue of journal. Checks master galleys for each article and calculates gains and losses due to author corrections.
   3. Gives paste-up to copy editor with a list of anything that needs the copy editor's attention.

G. *Paste-up checked and sent to printer:*
   1. Copy editor:
      a. Writes in running heads on dummy.
      b. Checks list of queries from production, gaining and losing lines as necessary for make-up.
      c. Checks consecutive order of figures and tables and that legends accompany correct figure.
      d. Double-checks that footnotes are on same page with mentions and symbols have been altered as necessary.
      e. Checks folios and looks at dummy page for general appearance and esthetics.
      f. Transfers authors corrections that have arrived since material turned over to production. Makes list of any author corrections that are still outstanding.

g. Types contents, assembles front matter, and makes up information sheet with production data.

2. Production:
   a. Repastes to allow for author corrections, if any, and for any other changes that copy editor has asked for.
   b. Pulls film of illustrations for each article from file to send with paste-up.

H. *Pages from printer:*
   1. Production:
      a. Checks pages for alignment and proper depth. Checks illustrations against paste-up for proper position and sequence. Checks pages for general spacing and appearance.
      b. Checks page proofs against master galleys line for line, brackets any lines that have been reset and not marked by printer. Checks number of contents as well as first and last page numbers of text and special items such as color plates.
      c. Gives page proof to copy editor.
   2. Copy editor:
      a. Compares pages with master set of galleys, reading reset lines, adding author corrections if still coming in, and checking remade figures.
      b. Makes line adjustments required by production and answers any queries.
      c. Checks consecutive order and positioning of figures, legends, and tables. Checks section heads.
      d. Reads contents against page proof and checks front matter.
      e. Stamps "Showproof" on pages with corrections and "OK" on those pages ready for press. Makes list of showproof pages that must be revised.
      f. At this stage, any articles that have not been approved by author must be pulled, and copy editor must trace author for phone approval or get editor's approval to proceed.
      g. Returns master set of pages to production with list of pages needing further adjustment, articles held for approval, and total number of showproof pages.
   3. Production:
      a. Holds ok'd front matter pages in file until ad layout received so that folios can be changed accordingly.
      b. Checks pages once again for author additions or deletions that may require page adjustments.
      c. Releases to printer for final corrections.

I. After all showproof pages are ok'd, the final production cycle begins. Negatives and ok'd pages are sent to printer for assembly into printing forms. Printer sends Dylux proofs of forms for final check for alignment, positioning, etc. After Dylux ok'd, a set of printed forms are assembled in proper binding sequence and checked by production and copy editor before printer given ok to bind and mail.

A7 □ Journal comparison of specifications for publication

	Page limitation	Accept case reports	Time		Rate acceptance	Assignment of copyright
			Submission → Decision	Decision → Publication		
Am. J. Surg.	No requirement	Yes, but discouraged	1 month	6-9 months	36%	Yes
Am. Surg.	No requirement	2/issue	10 months	7 months	78-80%	Yes
Arch. Surg.		Yes	2-3 months	4-8 months	40-50%	Yes
Ann. Pl. Surg.	8 pages max. recommended	Yes	6 months	5 months	65%	Yes
Br. J. Plast. Surg.	No requirement	Yes	0-2 months	6-12 months	35%	Yes
Cleft Palate Journal	8 page max. recommended	Yes	3-6 months	3-6 months	—	Both hold
Curr. Surg.	13 pages max. recommended	No	1 month	3 months	80%	Yes
J. Hand Surg.	No requirement	No separate section	2 months	7-9 months	78%	Yes
J. Thor. Card. Surg.	No requirement	No separate section	6-8 weeks	7 months	40%	Yes
Plast. Reconstr. Surg.	Max. 4,000 words + 10 ills (accept 6,000 words less 100 words/ill)	Yes	2-3 months	4-5 months	40%	Yes
Surgery	No requirement	No separate section	4-6 weeks	6-8 months	35-40%	Yes
Surg. Gynecol. Obstet.	No requirement	No	1-2 weeks	6 months	40%	Yes

Possible costs to author				Author receives			Changes allowed		
Page	B/W photos	4/C photos	Proof changes	Edited ms	Galley	Page	Edited ms	Galley	Page
—	—	$290/1st $90/2nd $60/others	—		X			X	
—	—	At cost	—						
—	—	$270 up to 6 on 1 page	—	X			X		
$100/page over 8 pages	—	$350 up to 6 on 1 page	—	X	X		X	X	
—	—	$500/photo	—	X		X	X		X
$40/page over 8 pages	—	$950/photo if excessive		X	X		Errors only	Errors only	
—	—		—		X	X			
		At cost			X			X	
		At cost			X			X	
$75/page over 10 pages	—	$350/page			X			Mini- mal	
		At cost			X			X	
—	—	At cost	None unless ms is reset		X			X	

A8 □ **The rejection**

Rare is the writer who maintains sweetness of disposition in the face of a rejected manuscript. Too old to cry, he rereads in disbelief the cruel judgment of a distant editor. Enraged, he indulges in several moments or more of paranoid thinking to which he is understandably entitled. Soon, hopefully, he will realize that the decision of the Editorial Board was not a vendetta. He may console himself with the thought that the reviewers were too muddled to appreciate the merits of the manuscript; and that accusation, in fact, is sometimes valid. Many a classic has bounced from journal to journal and publisher to publisher before its merit was recognized.

As an editor who still has papers rejected, I empathize with those whose written offerings have been refused.

In a writer's Utopia (but not a reader's), every paper would be accepted. In an editor's Shangrila, every manuscript would be brilliantly crafted and would contain a momentous message. The editor, moreover, would be able to publish unstintingly since cost and space would not be limiting factors. Alas, the reality is that papers vary greatly in their quality and importance; and editors must heed financial exigencies. Moreover, editors must protect their readers from trivia and mediocrity by properly screening, actively soliciting, and continually upgrading literary inflow and output. A good editor must be a reader's ombudsman as well as a writer's servant and sometimes his teacher. If those challenges were not difficult enough, a medical editor also has the obligation to promote learning, with a vision toward improving the human condition. Nevertheless, these idealistic desiderata do not course through the mind of a turned-down author. Like the thwarted lover, he feels the slap and remembers it.

All this is prologue to my confessing that the most unpleasant aspect of my position is to preside over the process of rejecting a manuscript. I am the one whose signature appears in the doomsday letter. Realizing that into every paper goes part of the soul and viscera of the author, I spend considerable time, as do the Associate Editors, before judging a manuscript unacceptable.

I should like to think that any author who receives a negative notice will not become one less friend, or worse, one more enemy. For protection, however, an editor soon grows a carapace to go with his red pencil. He will endure the slings and arrows to get something of quality. My criteria of a good paper are that it advances our field, provides worthwhile information, or both. In most areas of human activity, great leaps are rare. The writings of a Pasteur, Darwin, Freud, or Einstein are singular events; we must settle for smaller accomplishments. Yet an apparently trivial observation may lead someone else to a significant discovery. I would rather have a poorly written paper with an original idea than a wondrously wrought rehash. The former gains majesty through rewriting; the latter can never be transformed by even the cleverest alchemist.

Plastic and Reconstructive Surgery receives approximately 1,000 manuscripts a year and can accept only about 350. That so many papers come from meetings of the American Society of Plastic and Reconstructive Surgeons, the American Association of Plastic Surgeons, the American Society of Maxillofacial Surgeons, and the American Society for Aesthetic Plastic Surgery has advantages and disadvantages. The obvious advantage is the flow of material, since *Plastic and Reconstructive Surgery* has the right of first acceptance. The disadvantage is that not every paper presented at a meeting will make a good journal article. All too familiar is the sequence of "another meeting, another paper."

As editor, my primary objective and that of the Board is excellence, with balance, so the Journal can meet the many needs and interests of its diverse readership. We would prefer to publish fewer articles and maintain the Journal's superior quality rather than succumb to spiraling mediocrity. Few would argue against high standards unless he or she is negatively affected.

Unlike what is inscribed on the Statue of Liberty, the Editors do not wish to receive "your tired . . . wretched refuse." We want your brilliant best.

Reprinted from Goldwyn, R.M.: The rejection (editorial), Plast. Reconstr. Surg. **65**:346, March 1980.

Book writing

B1 □ New book proposals specification form

This form provides guidelines for the type of information necessary for a publisher to evaluate a proposed book for possible publication.

1. Names, titles, addresses, and telephone numbers of authors/editors
2. Number of contributors to book
3. Tentative book title
4. Present stage of manuscript: idea( ), 50% ( ), more than 50% ( )
5. Probable date for manuscript completion
6. Mechanical dimensions of manuscript:
   _____ Estimate of printed pages (approximately two double-spaced, typewritten pages to one printed page; two tables or illustrations to one page)
   _____ Number of tables
   _____ Number of line drawings
   _____ Number of halftones (photos)
   _____ Number of color illustrations (explain)
7. Description of purpose and scope of the book
8. Listing of primary and secondary professional and/or student markets for which the book is intended with emphasis on the level of readership at which it is aimed
9. Estimate of approximate price range for the book
10. Listing of competing titles (include author, title, pulisher, date of publication, and price)
11. Comparison of proposed book to competing titles, highlighting unique features offered by proposed book

When providing this information, the author should also include:

Curriculum vitae
Introductory or prefatory statement
Table of contents (detailed outline of project)
Contributor list (if applicable)
Sample chapter(s)

B2 □ Editorial instructions for author

TEXT

1. Manuscript should be typed, *double-spaced*, with 1 inch margins, on 8½ × 11 inch bond paper. Please prepare tabular material, references, and footnotes in this way also. We suggest you make a carbon copy for your records.
2. Number manuscript pages consecutively in the upper right-hand corner.
3. Number tables consecutively within each chapter. If chapter numbers have been assigned, use the chapter number as a prefix. For example, the second table in Chapter 6 would be numbered Table 6-2.
4. Outline each chapter including all headings; indent to indicate subordinate headings. The outlines will be used as a guide in the selection of type to indicate the relative importance of headings within each chapter.
5. Enclose all directly quoted material in quotation marks and include the complete source of original publication in a footnote. The following information should be in the footnote:
   a. If quote is from a *book:* author or editor, title of book, year, and publisher.
   b. If quote is from a *journal:* author, title of article, volume, page, year.
   Check to make sure the quotation is verbatim. See Section III for details on obtaining permissions to reproduce quotations more than 100 words in length.
6. Include the following front matter with the manuscript:
   a. Title page—listing name, degrees, and affiliations *exactly* as you want them listed in the book.
   b. Preface.
   c. Table of contents—check to make sure chapter titles are consistent with those used in the manuscript.
   You may also want to include:
   a. Contributor listing—with names, degrees, and affiliations of all persons who contributed chapters to the manuscript.
   b. Dedication.
   c. Acknowledgements—these can usually be included with the preface but can be separate if necessary.
   d. Foreword—written by someone other than author or editor of the book.

ILLUSTRATIONS
Photographs

1. Photographs should be prepared for a ⅓ off reduction, for example: 7½ inches reduced to 5½ inches. This does not pertain to photomicrographs and elec-
tronmicrographs, which are not reduced unless specified.
2. Photographs should be original glossy prints, 5 × 7 or 8 × 10 inches in size.
3. If you do not wish all of the photograph to appear in the finished illustration, indicate crop marks in the margins with a china marking pencil.
4. Photographs should not be mounted and the surface should not be marred by the use of pins or paper clips.
5. If it is necessary to block the eyes on a photograph, note this on the back of the illustration. Please refer to Section III for information on obtaining permission from persons whose full faces appear in photographs.
6. Submit original glossy prints for borrowed photographs.
7. Indicate "top" and the figure number on the back of each photograph writing *lightly with pencil* to avoid embossing the photo.

Line and tone drawings

1. Drawings should be prepared with India ink on white quality artboard. Prepare for ⅓ off reduction.
2. Labels should be positioned on a tissue overlay as this material will be edited and set in type. Lead lines should be positioned on the overlay also.

Legends (Each figure must have a legend.)

1. Legends should be typed on 8½ × 11 inch paper, *double-spaced*, with 1 inch margins. We suggest you keep a copy for your records.
2. Legends should not be attached to illustrations or typed in the manuscript.
3. Legend numbers should correspond with the figure numbers in the text.
4. Please refer to Section III for information on credit lines to be included with legends.

PERMISSIONS
Illustrations

Obtain written permission from the original publisher and author(s) for the use of previously published illustrations. This includes the publisher of your own works. (See Appendix B-5). The credit line following the legend should contain the following information.

1. For a *book:* author or editor, title, edition, city in which publisher is located, year, publisher.
2. For a *journal:* authors, journal abbreviation, volume, page, and year. If appropriate, include month of publication or supplement number.

Tables

Obtain written permission of the original publisher and author(s) for the use of directly reproduced tabular material. This includes the publisher of your own works. Include the complete source of publication in a footnote accompanying the table. The footnote should include the following information:

1. For a *book:* author or editor, title of book, edition, city in which publisher is located, year, and publisher.
2. For a *journal:* authors, title of article, journal abbreviation, volume, page, and year.

Full faces

Obtain written permission of all patients and personnel shown in illustrations (parent or guardian of minors). If permission is not obtained the eyes will be blocked except where they are the primary reason for the illustration (see Appendix B-5).

General

1. Include permissions with the pertinent chapter. It is important to indicate in the margin of each letter the manuscript page number on which the quotation appears or the table or illustration number to which it refers.
2. If you are borrowing from Mosby publications, it will *not* be necessary to obtain Mosby permission. It will, however, be necessary to obtain the author's permission.
3. In the case of illustrations that are redrawn or modified from another illustration, it is necessary to obtain permission to redraw from whomever owns the copyright of the original illustration.

REFERENCES

1. Type references *double-spaced* on 8½ × 11 inch paper with 1 inch margins, just as other manuscript copy.
2. Use references of recent origin and latest editions of books, unless of historical value.
3. Check spelling of authors' names in the text against spelling in the references.
4. Do not underline journal and book titles and volume numbers for italics or boldface.
5. In citing medical, nursing, and dental journals, use the style of abbreviations recommended in the latest *Cumulated Index Medicus.*
6. Include the lists of references with the manuscript, numbered as manuscript pages, at the end of a chapter, section, part, unit, or at the end of the book. The principal consideration in determining their placement should be convenience for the reader.
7. References should include the full facts of publication:
   a. *Book:* author or editor, title, edition, city in which publisher is located, year of publication, publisher (the exact corporate name should be used, not a short form except to abbreviate Company, Incorporated, and Limited), volume number and page number (when essential).
   b. *Journal:* authors' names, title of article, name of journal (abbreviated without periods), volume number, initial page number, year of publication. (In some instances it is desirable to include month of publication, supplement number, and other information.)
8. A reference is a citation that is actually referred to in the text. If specific citations are not included in the text, the following listings can be used:
   a. Additional readings: not actually cited in the text but contain information that you believe will be of aid or interest.
   b. Bibliography: an extensive list of readings that should appear in the back of the book as an alphabetized unnumbered listing.

B3 □ Reference styles

Two styles of references that are preferred in our medical and dental publications are:

ALPHABETICAL-NUMERICAL

References are *listed alphabetically and numbered according to that sequence.* These numbers are used each time the reference is cited in the text. They should be *typed as superscript numbers,* not in parentheses. Text citations then are not in numerical order. Any additional readings not cited in text but which contain information of interest to the reader are alphabetized but unnumbered.

Example: This subject has been covered thoroughly by Clark.[2] Management of heart disease is discussed in Brams[1] while Cook[3] has covered the subject of quackery in medicine.

1. Brams, W. A.: Managing your coronary, ed. 2, Philadelphia, 1956, J. B. Lippincott Co.

AUTHOR-DATE

In the text, *dates of publication are placed in parentheses after the author's name* to refer to a citation. References are *alphabetized, but not numbered,* at the end of the chosen unit. (This system has the advantage of making it relatively easy to add or delete references at any stage of preparation and early stages of production, since no renumbering is required and additional readings need not be listed separately from cited references.)

Example: This subject has been covered thoroughly by Clark (1962). Management of heart disease is discussed in Brams (1956), while the subject of quackery in medicine has been covered elsewhere (Cook, 1958a).

Brams, W. A. 1956. Managing your coronary, ed. 2, Philadelphia, J. B. Lippincott Co.

SAMPLE REFERENCES
Alphabetical-numerical style

BOOKS
Two authors

6. Folta, J. R., and Deck, E. S.: A sociological framework for patient care, New York, 1966, John Wiley & Sons, Inc.

With volume number

12. Bourne, H. G., editor: World review of nutrition and diet therapy, Vol. 5, New York, 1965, Hafner Publishing Co., Inc., pp. 79-131.

Part of edited book

9. Kahan, B. M., and Goodhart, R. S.: The vitamins. In Wohl, M. G., and Goodhart, R. S., editors: Modern nutrition in health and disease, Philadelphia, 1964, Lea & Febiger.

JOURNALS

2. Barboriak, J. J., and others: Breakfast menu and blood lipids, J. Am. Diet. Assoc. **49:**204, 1966.
5. Editorial, J. Am. Dent. Assoc. **61:**247, 1960.

THESES

10. Kerkhove, B. C., Jr.: A clinical and television densitometric evaluation of the indirect pulp capping technique (thesis), Indiana University, 1964.

UNPUBLISHED MATERIAL

7. Gass, J. D. M., and Norton, E. W. D.: Follow-up study of cystoid macular edema following cataract extractions, Trans. Am. Acad. Ophthal. Otolaryng., 1968. (In press.)
24. Tanzer, P. C.: Personal communication, 1968.

Author-date style
BOOKS
With more than 4 authors

White, A., et al. 1964. Principles of biochemistry, ed. 3, New York, McGraw-Hill Book Co.

Part of edited book

Kahan, B. M., and Goodhart, R. S. 1964. The vitamins. In Wohl, M. G., and Goodhart, R. S., editors: Modern nutrition in health and disease. Philadelphia, Lea & Febiger.

Edited volume

Landsberg, H., and Van Mieghem, J., editors: 1962. Advances in geophysics. New York, Academic Press.

JOURNALS

Sweatman, T. W., Selzer, A., and Cohn, K. 1970. Echocardiographic diagnosis of ruptured chordae tendineae, Am. J. Cardiol. **26:**661.

TRANSLATION

Kretschmer, E. 1925. Physique and character, ed. 2, translated by W. J. H. Spratt, New York, Harcourt, Brace & World, Inc.

SERIAL PUBLICATION

Heinstein, M. 1963. Behavioral correlate of breast-bottle regimes under varying parent-infant relationships, Monograph, Society for Research in Child Development, No. 88, Vol. 28.

ABSTRACT

Cohen, M. M. 1955. Gingiva at puberty, J. Dent. Res. **34:**679 (abst).

B4 □ Copyright information

PERMISSIONS AND FAIR USE

The following sections are guidelines for use by Mosby authors in interpreting the fair use section of the copyright law. Although guidelines have no legal standing, Mosby considers these policies to be prudent.

General guidelines

Responsibility. Obtaining permission to borrow is the author's responsibility. You, as the author, have primary control over the substance of your book and thus a large share of the legal responsibility as well. Getting your own permissions has some advantages:

1. Permission is more easily obtained. An author or publisher is more willing to give permission to you as a fellow scholar and prospective book buyer than to Mosby, a prospective rival.
2. If permission is refused, you can more easily decide how to replace or omit the material in the manuscript.
3. You may receive permission letters that correct or update the original; you can then incorporate this new information in your manuscript.

Get permissions early. As soon as you know what sources you will use, begin sending permission requests. You should have all permissions ready when you submit the manuscript to Mosby. *Failure to do so may delay or prevent publication of your book.*

Having applied for permission, you are responsible for following the stipulations of the grantor. Usually these are requests for fees, free copies of the book, and particular phrasing in credit lines. If you believe the stipulations to be too stringent—for example, that fees charged are excessive—contact your Mosby acquisition editor and discuss alternatives. You may pay fees personally or Mosby may in some instances pay them as an advance against royalties.

Be sure to obtain permission to borrow from your own work, unless you own the copyright, if it has been published by someone other than Mosby.

If material is to be borrowed from a Mosby copyrighted book for use in another Mosby book, *publisher* permission is generally automatic if you secure permission from the senior author of the original book and if the borrowing is not excessive. If the source is a collective work, such as a symposium, request permission from the author of the original paper or chapter instead.

Requesting permissions. A good procedure to follow in securing permissions is the following:

1. Send your request to the permissions department of the publisher of the work in question. If the publisher does not own or control the rights involved, he will pass your request on or notify you. If the publisher tells you that you must obtain the author's approval, please do so. Publishers' addresses are listed in the *Literary Market Place* and *International Literary Market Place*.
2. Use a permission request letter similar to that shown in Appendix B5.
3. Try to obtain all the rights mentioned in the sample request letter.
4. If you want to adapt material, be sure to specify in your request exactly how you plan to do so.
5. Follow up on your request by letter or telephone if you have not heard from the publisher within a few weeks; confer with your acquisition editor if problems arise.

Handling permission letters. When you receive permission, mark on the permission letter the page, figure, or table number in your manuscript that it pertains to. If the source is not clearly given in the letter (with complete publication data: author, title, date, publisher, and pages), add that, too. Make copies and place the originals in your permissions file. When that file is complete, send it to Mosby with your completed manuscript.

Is permission ever unnecessary? Permission is not legally necessary for some types of borrowed material. These include the following:

1. Works in the public domain
   a. "A work prepared by an officer or employee of the United States Government as part of that person's official duties."* Most government works are in the public domain, although the government can own copyrights bequeathed or assigned to it and governmental works can include privately generated copyrighted material. The originals of such works should show a copyright note, although lack of such a note does not always mean that the work is in the public domain. If you are in doubt about a specific work, contact the Copyright Office or the agency that distributed the work.
2. Noncopyrightable material
   a. "Computing and measuring devices such as slide rules, wheel dials, and nomograms."† However, if such a device appears in a copyrighted work, it is best to seek permission.

From Mosby author's guide, St. Louis, 1981, The C. V. Mosby Co., pp. 32-41.

*From 17 USC 101, 105.

†From U.S. Copyright Office: Computing and measuring devices, Circular 33, Washington, D.C., 1978, U.S. Government Printing Office.

b. "Ideas or procedures for doing, making, or building things; scientific or technical methods or discoveries; business operations or procedures; mathematical principles; formulas; or any other sort of concept, process, method of operation, or plan of action."* You may not, however, use the literary, graphic, artistic, or other form in which information or ideas are expressed. That form is protected by copyright, as are the selection, organization, and arrangement of otherwise noncopyrightable materials, such as the selection and arrangement of facts.

c. "Blank forms and similar works designed to record rather than to convey information," even though they may contain "names, titles, and phrases or clauses such as column headings, simple checklists, and the like. The format, arrangement, or typography of a blank form or similar work is not a copyrightable element."† However, if such a form contains within it an original literary or pictorial expression, *that portion* is copyrightable.

d. "Works consisting entirely of information that is common property containing no original authorship; such as, for example: standard calendars, height and weight charts, tape measures and rulers, schedules of sporting events, and lists or tables taken from public documents or other common sources."‡

Giving credit. Include all credit lines in your manuscript before sending it to Mosby. Always acknowledge borrowed material, whether or not you have obtained permission.

In granting permission many publishers stipulate that a credit line be given on the page on which the borrowed material appears. For this reason, Mosby normally does so for all lengthy borrowed material. If an entire chapter or article is used, put the credit line in a footnote at the bottom of the first page. For tables, place the credit line immediately under the borrowed table; for illustrations, at the end of the legend. For long quotations that are set off in a block, give credit in a marked footnote at the bottom of the page; very short quotations may merely be marked by a reference number.

If the copyright holder stipulates particular wording or placement, use it exactly. Otherwise, use the following format:

---

*From U.S. Copyright Office: Ideas, plans, methods, or systems, Circular 31, Washington, D.C., 1978, U.S. Government Printing Office.
†From U.S. Copyright Office: Blank forms and other uncopyrightable works, Circular 32, Washington, D.C., 1978, U.S. Government Printing Office.
‡Ibid.

Book

From Author, J. A.: Title of book, City of publication, 1900 (date of publication), Publisher's full name, p. 000.

Journal

From Author, J. A.: Abbreviated journal title, volume number: page number, date of publication. (For tables and illustrations; for footnotes, add title of article after author's name.)

Secondary quotations. If you quote a passage for which you must obtain permission and it contains a quotation from a second source, you may also need to obtain permission from the second source.

Paraphrase. Organization and specific word combinations (style) are copyrightable, whereas facts and ideas are not. Therefore a paraphrase is probably fair use if you convey the key ideas or facts of the original but in an organization and style that are clearly your own. Paraphrasing in lieu of obtaining permission can be dangerous; similarity of wording or sequence of thought may constitute an infringement.

Specific guidelines
Discrete textual material

1. Always secure permission to use textual material that is complete in itself, such as tables, separate outlines, abstracts, summaries, chapters of books, complete pamphlets, and journal, magazine, or newspaper articles.
2. If material is to be used in a book of readings or an anthology, get permission for each copyrighted selection, no matter how short. *In such a work, no portion of the manuscript will be set in type until Mosby has all permissions for the book.*

Quotations

1. Whenever possible, quote directly from the original source rather than a derivative one, such as an anthology or collection of readings. Doing so leads to more accurate quotation, and it is usually easier to get more precise copyright information from the original source.
2. All quotations must be clearly identifiable as such in the manuscript. A quotation of not more than four or five typewritten lines should be enclosed in quotation marks. A longer quotation should be inset at least five spaces from the rest of the text at each margin, typed double-spaced and without quotation marks. If necessary to distinguish such quotes from other special material in your text, note "quotation" in the margin. Use ellipses (. . .) to indicate points where material has been omitted from the quotation. If the omission occurs at the end of a sentence, use four dots, the first being the period. Material that *you* have italicized for emphasis within the quotation should be indicated as

such by a footnote: "Italics mine." Any additions of your own must be placed within brackets, [ ], not parentheses, ( ). Parentheses should appear *only* as used by the original author. Check each quotation to be sure it is absolutely verbatim.

3. Obtain permission from the copyright holder for any quotation that may not be fair use. In general, longer quotations are more likely to be considered fair use if the source is a published textbook or other scholarly book; if the quote is clearly used for criticism, comment, scholarship, or support or refutation of research; and if proper credit is given in a footnote. Consider both the length of individual quotes and the cumulative length of scattered short quotations from the same work.

4. Even shorter quotations may necessitate permission. If the source itself is relatively brief, such as a scholarly journal article, encyclopedia article, or essay, less can be borrowed without overstepping the bounds of fair use.

If the quote is from a trade publication, obtain permission if you quote more than a sentence or two even though more extensive borrowing may appear to be fair use. Examples are fiction, popularized nonfiction, or popular magazines.

If the quote is from unpublished material, get permission regardless of the length even though copyright law provides for fair use of material either published or unpublished. Such matter includes letters or other private documents, theses, dissertations, and lectures. *Note:* In each instance, obtain permission from the *author*, not the owner or holder of the material (such as a library or university).

If the quotation is from a copyrighted poem, secure permission to quote any portion, regardless of length. *Note:* A poem published in the United States before the turn of the century is in the public domain. But if it appears in a later anthology or edited work, it may have been edited, and such editing is subject to copyright; therefore use the original published version if at all possible.

If any quotation is used for ornamental purposes or to "set a tone" for your work (for example, a quote used as display at the beginning of a chapter), obtain permission whatever the length unless the material is in the public domain.

If you are in doubt, ask for permission; however, if you are certain that your use is fair, *do not* apply for permission. You may wish to consult your acquisition editor about borderline cases.

Illustrations

1. For *any* map, chart, photograph, or illustration that is copyrighted or is from a copyrighted source

(book, journal, etc.), get permission from the copyright owner. Use a request letter similar to that shown in Appendix B5.

2. If the illustration is to be borrowed from a Mosby book for use in another Mosby copyrighted book, the same guidelines that appeared on p. 251 may be followed. *Note:* If you contemplate using more than three illustrations from any one Mosby book, check with your acquisition editor in advance.

3. If you are using the services of a professional illustrator, be sure you have a clear, written understanding of what you are buying. Preferably you should own the illustrations *and* the unlimited right to their use. You may wish to discuss this with your acquisition editor.

4. To make an adaptation of a line drawing from a copyrighted source, it is generally best to get permission. However, it is the *style* of a drawing that is copyrightable, not the object being presented. Simple outline drawings of everyday objects (such as a light bulb) have few stylistic characteristics that are copyrightable. But do not use the unique stylistic features of another person's original drawing (for example, its particular perspective, shading, or use of complex line, any of which may be copyrightable) without permission.

PHOTOGRAPHIC SUBJECT PERMISSIONS

The preceding parts of this appendix have dealt with the copyright law and fair use. Although the topic of permission by the subjects of photographs does not involve copyright questions, it does involve laws concerning rights of privacy.

If you acquire photographs from a commercial photographer or an archival source, explain in writing that you want to use them in a book and ask whether any release or permission is needed in addition to the one the source is supplying you.

The best procedure is to obtain a signed release from the subject of *any* photograph. Although photographs of normal persons in common public activities might not seem to need permission, invasion of privacy can be alleged even in these circumstances. It is safest to have permission even if the subject is a friend of yours.

If you are dealing with the photograph of a minor, obtain from the minor and from the parent or guardian written permission that includes an agreement that the parent or guardian will indemnify you against any claim that the minor might make involving disaffirmance of written permission.

Photographs of patients, retarded or handicapped persons, mentally ill persons, prisoners, or accident victims should be accompanied by permission except as noted hereafter. Any photograph showing an identifiable person nude or in an embarrassing pose or circumstance must be accompanied by permission. If the subject is not mentally competent, obtain permission from a parent or guardian. Photographs of public personalities such as politicians, well-known athletes, or movie celebrities may be used for, among other things, their news or historical value without subject permission.

If a photograph of *any* person is to be used for a book cover or in advertising, get permission.

Books that must use photographs of patients' faces for teaching or case verification present special problems. If it is not possible to obtain the patient's permission, consult your acquisition editor about alternative measures such as cropping the illustration or blocking the patient's eyes. If such measures cannot be used, as when the patient's condition affects both the face and the eyes, Mosby may be willing to waive the requirement for permission if you have attempted unsuccessfully to obtain permission or cannot trace the patient *and* agree to assume responsibility for the use.

FAIR CRITICISM AND LIBEL

Libel may be defined as a written statement that accuses another person of immoral, unlawful, or ridiculous conduct and holds that person up to public contempt or injures his or her standing in the community, in business, or in personal relations. All parties to the dissemination of libelous material are held to be responsible and may be sued. The truth of the libelous material is an important defense, but truth may be hard to prove. Regardless of whether the defendant in a libel suit wins or loses, fighting a court case costs time and money.

The most important measure in avoiding libel is to verify your sources of information. Be certain that your statements are accurate. It may, of course, not be necessary to use real names. Be as objective as possible when you are criticizing an act or a condition that could result in libel charges. When in doubt, consult your acquisition editor. Mosby retains a legal counsel who can help in questions involving libel.

B5 □ Permission form letters

This form letter to be used when requesting permission to reproduce illustrations, graphs, or charts

To: Publisher (Author)

Dear Sir or Madam:

I would like to have your permission to reproduce the following figure(s):

Fig. No.   *Page*

____________________   _________

____________________   _________

from (if a *book*, insert Title, Edition and Year)
     (if a *journal*, insert Name of Journal and Article, Vol. No., page and year)

by _____________________, in a book I am writing under the title of ___________________, to be published by The C. V. Mosby Company, 11830 Westline Industrial Drive, St. Louis, MO 63141, for international distribution. This request shall include all future editions in all languages thereof.

Credit to the original source will be included in the legend(s).

(To publisher only) If permission from the author is also necessary, kindly provide me with his/her address so that I may request his/her permission, as well as the use of the original illustration copy.

Sincerely,

____

PLEASE USE RELEASE FORM BELOW
____

Permission is granted on the terms stated in this letter.

Date _________________________________   Name _________________________________

                                                 Address _________________________________

This form letter to be used when requesting permission to quote from books or journal articles (for quotes over 100 words)

To: Publisher (Author)

Dear Sir or Madam:

I would like to have permission to quote the following material:

"____

____

____"

from (if a *book*, insert Title, Edition, and year)
     (if a *journal*, insert name of journal and article, vol. no., page, and year)

by ________________________, in a book I am writing under the title of ________________________, to be published by The C. V. Mosby Company, 11830 Westline Industrial Drive, St. Louis, MO 63141, for international distribution. This request shall include all future editions in all languages thereof.

Credit to the original source of publication will be properly given in a footnote following the quotation.

(To publisher only) If permission of the author is also necessary, kindly provide me with his/her address.

                            Sincerely,

               ____

PLEASE USE RELEASE FORM BELOW

Permission to quote is granted on the terms stated in this letter.

Date ________________________   Name ________________________

                                  Address ________________________

Consent to use name or picture

                               Date: ________________________

I hereby irrevocably consent that my name and/or any picture or portrait of me, or of any part of me, and reproductions thereof, may be used by ________________________ for such purposes as he/she may desire in connection with his/her research, writing and professional activities, may be used, exhibited, and published through any medium whatsoever as part of or in connection with research, writing and professional activities, even though such use may be for advertising purposes or purposes of trade.

I hereby certify and represent that I am (am not) over 21 years of age.

                              ____
                                       (Name)

                              ____
                                    (Address)

Consent of parent or guardian (to be obtained when person signing above is under 21 years of age)

Date: ____

I, ___________________________, am the parent/guardian of ___________________________, and I hereby irrevocably consent that his/her name and/or any picture or portrait of him/her or any parts of him/her and reproductions

thereof, may be used by ___________________________ for such purposes as he may desire in connection with his/her
research, writing, and professional activities, and may be used, exhibited, and published through any medium whatsoever as part of or in connection with his/her research, writing, and professional activities, even though such use may be
for advertising purposes or purposes of trade.

____
(Name)

____
(Address)

B6 □ Corrected galley proof

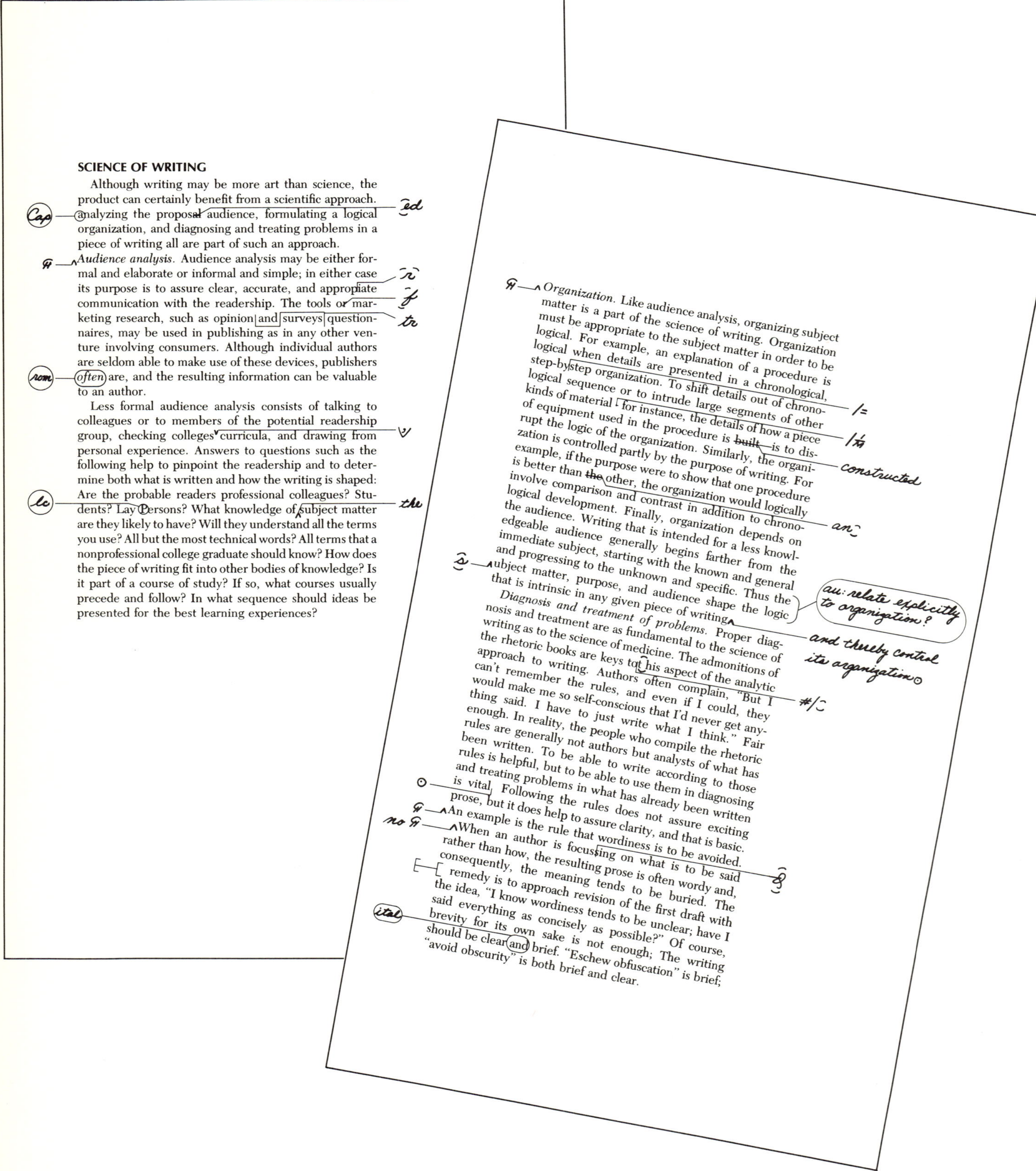

Fig. B6-1. Galley proofs with an exaggerated number of corrections to illustrate proofreading symbols in use. The corrections caused by these marks are shown in Appendix B7.

SCIENCE OF WRITING

Although writing may be more art than science, the product can certainly benefit from a scientific approach. Analyzing the proposed audience, formulating a logical organization, and diagnosing and treating problems in a piece of writing all are part of such an approach.

Audience analysis. Audience analysis may be either formal and elaborate or informal and simple; in either case its purpose is to assure clear, accurate, and appropriate communication with the readership. The tools of marketing research, such as opinion surveys and questionnaires, may be used in publishing as in any other venture involving consumers. Although individual authors are seldom able to make use of these devices, publishers often are, and the resulting information can be valuable to an author.

Less formal audience analysis consists of talking to colleagues or to members of the potential readership group, checking colleges' curricula, and drawing from personal experience. Answers to questions such as the following help to pinpoint the readership and to determine both what is written and how the writing is shaped: Are the probable readers professional colleagues? Students? Lay persons? What knowledge of the subject matter are they likely to have? Will they understand all the terms you use? All but the most technical words? All terms that a nonprofessional college graduate should know? How does the piece of writing fit into other bodies of knowledge? Is it part of a course of study? If so, what courses usually precede and follow? In what sequence should ideas be presented for the best learning experiences?

Organization. Like audience analysis, organizing subject matter is a part of the science of writing. Organization must be appropriate to the subject matter in order to be logical. For example, an explanation of a procedure is logical when details are presented in a chronological, step-by-step organization. To shift details out of chronological sequence or to intrude large segments of other kinds of material—for instance, the details of how a piece of equipment used in the procedure is constructed—is to disrupt the logic of the organization. Similarly, the organization is controlled partly by the purpose of writing. For example, if the purpose were to show that one procedure is better than another, the organization would logically involve comparison and contrast in addition to chronological development. Finally, organization depends on the audience. Writing that is intended for a less knowledgeable audience generally begins farther from the immediate subject, starting with the known and general and progressing to the unknown and specific. Thus the subject matter, purpose, and audience shape the logic that is intrinsic in any given piece of writing and thereby control its organization.

Diagnosis and treatment of problems. Proper diagnosis and treatment are as fundamental to the science of writing as to the science of medicine. The admonitions of the rhetoric books are keys to this aspect of the analytic approach to writing. Authors often complain, "But I can't remember the rules, and even if I could, they would make me so self-conscious that I'd never get anything said. I have to just write what I think." Fair enough. In reality, the people who compile the rhetoric rules are generally not authors but analysts of what has been written. To be able to write according to those rules is helpful, but to be able to use them in diagnosing and treating problems in what has already been written is vital. Following the rules does not assure exciting prose, but it does help to assure clarity, and that is basic.

An example is the rule that wordiness is to be avoided. When an author is focusing on what is to be said rather than how, the resulting prose is often wordy and, consequently, the meaning tends to be buried. The remedy is to approach revision of the first draft with the idea, "I know wordiness tends to be unclear; have I said everything as concisely as possible?" Of course, brevity for its own sake is not enough; The writing should be clear *and* brief. "Eschew obfuscation" is brief; "avoid obscurity" is both brief and clear.

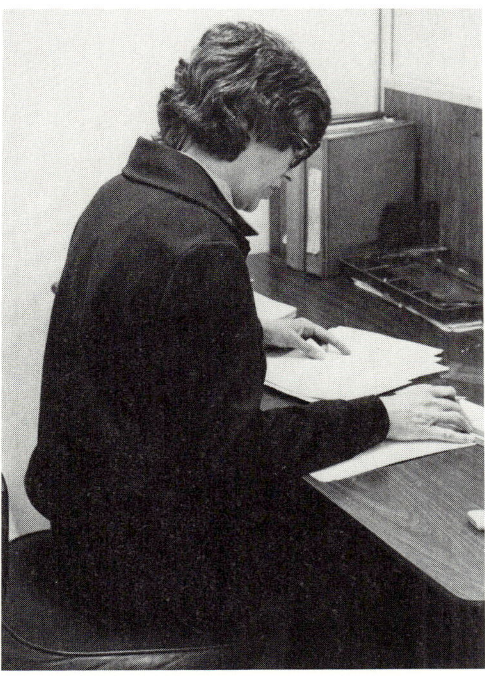

Fig. B7-1. Page proofs with the corrections marked in Appendix B6 made. Note the amount of resetting caused by the addition of "the" in the second paragraph. This is the reason that alterations charges accumulate so rapidly.

B8 □ **Proofreading marks**

PROOFREADING MARKS

Instruction	Mark	Example
Dele, or delete, take out		We are crafts/men printers.
Insert space	#	We arecraftsmen printers.
Turn over	9	We are craftsmen printers.
Close up, no space	⌒	We are craftsmen print⌒ers.
Insert apostrophe where indicated	⋁	We are printers craftsmen.
Character of wrong size or style, wrong font	wf	We are crafts**m**en printers.
Put in lower case	lc	We are craftsmen PRINTERS.
Reset in bold face	bf	We are craftsmen printers.
Put in italic type	ital	We are craftsmen printers.
Let it stand; ignore marks above dots	stet	We are craftsmen printers.
Defective letter	X	We are craftsmen printers.
Make paragraph	¶	printers. ⌐We are craftsmen
No paragraph	no ¶	printers. ⌐We are craftsmen printers.
Insert period	⊙	We are craftsmen printers
Carry to the left	L	We are craftsmen printers.
Carry to the right	⌐	We are craftsmen printers.
Lower to place indicated	⊔	We are craftsmen printers.
Raise to place indicated	⊓	We are craftsmen printers.
Transpose	tr	We are craftsmen printer.
Insert hyphen	/=/	We are craftsmen printers.
Put in small capitals	sc	We are craftsmen printers.
Insert comma	⋏	Yes we are craftsmen printers.
Query to author	are	We craftsmen printers.
Spell out words marked with a circle	spellout	We are 2nd to none.
Push down space	⊥	We are craftsmen printers.
Space more evenly	eq #	We are craftsmen printers.
Indent 1 em	□	We are craftsmen printers.
Indent 2 ems	□□	We are craftsmen printers.
1-em dash	/em/	We are craftsmen printers
2-em dash	/em/	We are craftsmen printers
En dash	/n/	We are craftsmen printers.
Straighten alignment	=	We are craftsmen printers.
Enclose in quotation marks	⌣ ⌣	We are craftsmen printers.
Put in roman type	rom	We are craftsmen printers.
Words are omitted from, or in, copy	out see copy	We printers.
Put in capitals as indicated	caps	We are craftsmen printers.

B9 □ **Preparation of illustrations**

PLANNING FOR ILLUSTRATIONS

Deciding how and when to use illustrations is an important part of planning your book. Good illustrations can make a valuable contribution to the text while bad illustrations may serve only to distract the reader.

Because you know your book better than anyone else, you are the logical one to decide whether or not illustrations are appropriate to your subject. If you are in doubt, confer with your acquisition editor, seek advice from your colleagues, and consult other books in the field to see what other authors have thought suitable for the subject.

As you write your first draft, note places where you think illustrations would be appropriate, and keep a list of those places and the kind of illustrations that would seem best suited. Each time you consider using an illustration, ask yourself these questions: How much will the illustration contribute to the book? Will an illustration *show* readers something far more clearly, effectively, and concisely than the text can *tell* them? What kind of illustration is best suited to the subject being discussed?

The subject matter of illustrations can be either informative or decorative. Informative illustrations contribute to the understanding of the text and can be charts, graphs, diagrams, drawings, and photographs. Decorative illustrations, intended to set a mood or establish an atmosphere, are usually drawings or photographs, may be of an abstract nature, and are sometimes used as part- or chapter-opening illustrations.

SOURCES OF ILLUSTRATIONS

Illustrations can be obtained in several ways: by commissioning a professional illustrator, by acquiring permission to use previously published illustrations, by using illustrations in the public domain, or by providing them yourself. Remember, you want your book to appear as professional as possible, so seek the assistance of professionals when preparing the illustrations. If you are affiliated with an institution, there may well be a department or an individual on staff who can assist you or refer you to someone who does the kind of work you need. Your colleagues or your acquisition editor can also be a valuable resource for suggestions.

Literary Market Place lists many artists, art services, and suppliers of photographs. Other books in your field will show sources of photographs and art in the picture credits.

United States government departments and agencies often can supply material related to their particular prov-

inces. If you need illustrative material related to a particular industry, write to companies in that industry. Their public relations departments often supply photographs without charge. Museums, libraries, and historical societies are good sources of illustrations in such fields as art, history, anthropology, and archeology.

Many commercial photo services and press syndicates can supply stock photographs. *Literary Market Place* lists these as well as professional photographers who will take pictures to your specifications.

TYPES OF ILLUSTRATIONS

Illustrations can be broken into two categories: line and continuous tone. Line illustrations are black and white with no intermediate tones and are exemplified by charts, graphs, diagrams, maps, and simple drawings. Continuous tone illustrations range from black through intermediate shades of gray to white. Examples include photographs, ink wash or water color, and pencil drawings.

Line illustrations

Line illustrations should be prepared with sharp, well-defined edges and maximum contrast. Although it is possible to reproduce faint lines and to drop out gray or colored backgrounds, a loss of quality will result. Your artist should be providing you will illustrations characterized by clean, even lines with clearly defined edges. It is usually a good idea to submit samples of the illustrations you intend to use to your acquisition editor for evaluation. This can save time and money in the long run and avoid the disappointment of a book with mechanically substandard illustrations.

Most artists prefer to prepare illustrations larger than they will appear in the book. To allow your artist to properly proportion the work and provide you with illustrations that will fit the format of your book, you should ask your acquisition editor to furnish you with the dimensions proposed for your book. Original line illustrations are always preferred. Line illustrations clipped from books or magazines or quality photographic copies are acceptable if originals are not available. However, remember that permission must be obtained for the use of illustrations borrowed from other publications.

Continuous tone illustrations

Photographs should be glossy black-and-white prints with a wide range of tones from highlights to deep shadows. In printing, shades of gray are achieved by using dots of various sizes to create the illusion of tone. This is called the halftone process. In this process the interme-

From Mosby authors guide, St. Louis, 1981, The C. V. Mosby Co., pp. 46-52.

diate tones tend to flatten out. Therefore it is usually best to submit photographs with slightly more contrast than is wanted in the finished book. A 5 by 7 inch print is a convenient size to handle; however, larger or smaller prints are acceptable as long as they are not smaller than they will appear in the book. It is important to handle photographs with care. Smudges, cracks, and indentations will all show up when the photograph is reproduced. Take special precautions not to write heavily and emboss the face of photographs or to use rubber stamps that will cause ink to bleed through or offset onto the next photograph. Never use a paper clip without adequate padding between the clip and the photograph.

If a group of photographs is to appear as a single figure in the book, indicate the grouping by letter designation or by a rough sketch accompanying the illustrations. Do not mount the photographs on paper or cardboard.

When you mail photographs, to prevent them from curling or being otherwise damaged, place them between two stiff pieces of cardboard somewhat larger than the photographs and hold them together firmly with tape or rubber bands.

LABELING

Protecting illustrations with a tissue overlay is a good idea. Labels should always be indicated on a tissue rather than directly on the illustration. Lead lines may be included on the tissue, or to ensure pinpoint accuracy they can be applied directly to the illustration by the illustrator. Be sure to check the tissue overlay to assure accuracy and completeness so that expensive changes will not be made after production has begun. It is a good idea to use marks to register the illustration to the tissue to ensure accuracy. Your illustrator can assist with this. A manuscript editor will review your labels, legend, and text to be sure they are in agreement. Labels will then be set in a typeface that is consistent in style and size with the typography in your book. For reasons of time, expense, consistency, and duplication of effort your illustrator should not spend time hand lettering or setting type for labels.

CROPPING

Proper cropping can greatly improve the value of an illustration. Your illustration can be larger and more effective if only the area of primary interest is reproduced. Proper cropping will emphasize the important part of your illustration and eliminate unimportant parts. Cropping should be indicated in the border of the illustration with a china marking pencil or on the tissue overlay with a soft lead pencil. The reduction of the illustration will depend on the format of the book; however, if you have specific suggestions for the sizing of your illustrations, indicate the reduction on the back of the illustration.

X-RAY REPRODUCTION

If you wish to have x-ray films reproduced in your book, furnish black and white glossy prints. Some loss of detail is always experienced when x-ray negatives are reduced and converted to photographic prints. By making prints you can control the detail and properly crop your illustrations before they are submitted for publication. The subtle shadings of gray showing the internal soft tissues are especially difficult to reproduce. If there is an area of particular importance in your x-ray film, attach a tissue overlay and circle the area of interest with a note, "Shoot for this."

COLOR ILLUSTRATIONS

The use of color adds considerably to the cost of producing a book. Arrangements must be made with your acquisition editor if you wish to include color illustrations. Before considering color be sure it is absolutely necessary to the subject of the illustration and will enhance the readers' understanding. Color photographs and color transparencies can be reproduced in black and white with good results in most cases. Full-color photographs will usually be handled as plates and placed into the bound book by hand. Two-color illustrations may be printed and numbered with the rest of the illustrations. If you and your acquisition editor have determined that your book is to be two-color throughout, then your illustrator should incorporate the second color into illustrations in a meaningful way.

LEGENDS

Legends, or captions, should be submitted separately from the manuscript and typed double-spaced on 8½ by 11 inch paper. The legends for each chapter should begin on a new sheet of paper.

Illustrations are sent to a photolithographer, whereas legends are sent to a typesetter (but not necessarily at the same time as the manuscript). For these reasons do not type legends on the manuscript, on pieces of paper fastened to the illustrations, or on the back or front of the illustrations themselves. Keep legends separate, making sure that the numbers correspond.

Legends should be as short as possible. Articles, such as *the*, *a*, and *an*, can usually be omitted without affecting the sense of the legend. Any extensive explanation of an illustration should appear in the text.

When typing legends, make two carbon or xerographic copies. Send one with the original copy and keep one for your files. When the legends have been typed, check each one against the illustration to make sure that everything mentioned in the legend actually appears on the illustration. Be sure that any coined abbreviations, identifying letters, or symbols are explained; but if labels are explained on the illustrations, do not repeat the explanations in the legends.

Courtesy lines

A courtesy line for an illustration from a noncopyrighted source should be included in parenthesis at the end of the legend. Such acknowledgements usually read "Courtesy Amalgamated Widget Co., Anytown, Ohio," or "Courtesy Jane Q. Public, New York, N.Y." Occasionally the courtesy line is reduced and placed directly below the photograph, separate from the legend.

Credit lines

A credit line acknowledges the source of a previously published, copyrighted illustration. Credit lines generally carry the full facts of publication: "From Shane, P. G.: Police and people: a comparison of five countries, St. Louis, 1980, The C.V. Mosby Co." Credit lines may be shortened by omitting the title of a journal article or using a shortened book credit line (omitting place of publication and publisher) when the credit line is repeated often and is given both in the text and in the list of references.

Credit lines can become exceedingly complicated when they refer to an illustration that has been borrowed from one source that has, in turn, modified it from another source. The best course to follow in such instances is to give as much information as you can in the credit line and leave it to the manuscript editor to decide how to include; be sure that the sequence is clearly indicated.

Courtesy and credit lines should appear beneath the illustrations to which they refer, not in the front matter of the book. The exception of this is a book in which all illustrations are from one source, in which case blanket acknowledgement is made in the preface.

BORROWED ILLUSTRATIONS

The number of illustrations borrowed from other publications should be held to a minimum. Borrowed illustrations may present problems in obtaining permission from copyright holders, payment of fees, and difficulty of securing a satisfactory copy for reproduction.

Although a figure from another source is sometimes the best way to make a point, several factors should be taken into account if such illustrations are to be effective.

Will the borrowed illustration be more effective than one of your own? Using many borrowed illustrations may distract from the originality of your manuscript.

Will the borrowed illustration be compatible with your own? Such variations as alternate spellings or different terminology in labels, differences in lettering styles, and differences in complexity of drawings may conflict with your own illustrations. This will give your book an inconsistent appearance.

Will the borrowed illustration fit the size planned for your book? An illustration from an 8½ by 11 inch atlas may be too large to fit well on the page of an average-sized textbook, or an illustration may fit on the page but

be much larger or smaller than your other illustrations. Unless originals of borrowed illustrations are obtained, they cannot be enlarged, reduced, or relabeled.

Will the borrowed illustration be appropriate to your intended audience? Illustrations that are much simpler or more advanced than your text or your other illustrations will seem out of place and may confuse the reader.

When requesting permission it is appropriate to ask if the original is available or if a contact negative of the publisher's negative can be purchased.

GENERAL CONSIDERATIONS

When you send your manuscript to Mosby, send illustrations and legends in envelops or folders, separated by chapters. Illustrations should not be interleaved with manuscript pages.

In numbering your illustrations, write lightly (particularly on a photograph) on the back with a soft pencil and with the illustration on a hard surface to avoid embossing the face. Use the double-numbering system, in which the chapter numbers are used as prefixes to the figure numbers. For example, figures in Chapter 7 are numbered 7-1, 7-2, and so on. In case a figure is deleted or added, you need change only the figure numbers in a single chapter rather than throughout the book. If a figure has several parts, give each part a letter designation, for example, 7-1, *A*; 7-1, *B*; 7-1, *C*. If you are in doubt about the final chapter sequence, omit the chapter prefix and leave space in front of the figure number so that you can easily add the prefix when chapter sequence is finally determined. If it is difficult to distinguish the top from the bottom of an illustration, write "top" on the top of the back.

Reader attention should be directed to illustrations by mentions in the text: "as shown in Fig. 7-1," "(see Fig. 7-2)," and so on. If an illustration is worth including in the book, it is worth mentioning. (However, this suggestion may not apply to books designed to appeal to a wide audience, in which illustrations are frequently more decorative than informative.)

Preferred placement of figures should be noted in the right-hand page margins. "Fig. 7-1 here." Bear in mind, however, that pagination considerations, especially in books with many illustrations, may prevent placing illustrations exactly where they are mentioned.

Avoid "dated" material. When selecting illustrations, be sure that hair and dress styles and other items in the pictures do not date the book. Of course, if the illustrations are being used for their historical value, dating is no problem.

When you send in your manuscript, indicate approximately 10 illustrations that you think would be suitable for advertising purposes. If possible, send duplicate illustrations. Do not recommend illustrations borrowed from other publications.

B10 □ **Preparation of tables**

Tables are often the best and sometimes the only way of presenting essential information. They do, however, have disadvantages. Tables are expensive to typeset, and if they refer to data by years they may date the book. Some readers skip rather than study tables, regarding them as interruptions rather than as essential to their knowledge of the subject they are studying.

If you are contemplating the use of tables in your book, ask yourself two questions.

1. Can I summarize the content of the proposed table in the text? If you can, and if it can be done briefly and completely, by all means do so. It will not force readers to change their pace, and they will be more likely to absorb the information. If a table contains little material, it is best to omit the table and incorporate the material into the text. Extensive statistical material, of course, is much better presented in tabular form.

2. Can I present the material in the table in the form of a graph or chart? Readers are more likely to pay attention to material presented in an attractive graph or chart than to that presented as columns or rows of figures.

If you do decide that a table is the only answer, then confine the material in the table to the table. Do not repeat tabulated material in the text exactly as it is listed in the table. Of course, the text can and should comment on significant points brought out by material in the table.

Plan your table with the thought in mind that it must fit into the planned page size of the book. Long tables can be run over from one page to the next, but wide tables must be set broadside, and the reader must turn the book to study them.

Keep the presentation as simple as you can. Tables with many subheads, sub-subheads, center heads, brackets, and boxes frequently mystify rather than enlighten. Arrange vertical and horizontal entries so that they are not duplicated and so that entries in columns or rows are presented in comparable form. Tables are generally constructed for reading across the columns. If yours are not, perhaps they need restructuring. Columns should be aligned for easy reading. The University of Chicago's *Manual of Style* shows various forms of tabular material and gives complete information on the elements of tables and typographic considerations.

Saving space is important in tables. Use abbreviations or symbols (but easily understood ones) for space-saving reasons. If these are likely to be unfamiliar to the reader, they must be explained in footnotes to the table. Use symbols (*, †, ‡, §, ‖, ¶) or superior letters for reference marks in a table, and position the footnotes directly below the table.

Type tables on separate pages of manuscript, but number them in with the text. They should be typed double-spaced with plenty of space between columns and around heads to allow the manuscript editor to mark type for the typesetter. Do not insert rules; the designer and the editor will decide if vertical and horizontal rules are needed.

Tables should be double numbered in the same manner as the illustrations, with the chapter number and an Arabic numeral, although if there are only a few tables in the book, they can be numbered consecutively throughout the book. Table titles should be as concise as possible, and every numbered table should have a title. Occasionally short, simple listings that will cause no problems in page makeup need not be numbered or carry a title.

Numbered tables should always be cited in the text. References to these tables should be by table numbers. Do not refer to "the table that follows" or "the table above." Problems in page makeup may make it necessary to change the location of the table.

Check column totals to make certain that they are correct. If discrepancies must occur, explain why in a footnote to the table.

Tables borrowed from copyrighted sources must carry a credit line as a footnote; a courtesy line is desirable if the table is from a noncopyrighted source. If the source has been cited at the end of the chapter or book in a reference list and in the text, an abbreviated form can be used for the credit line.

Some books contain tabular material that is of significance to the book as a whole, tables that contain conversions, logarithms, square and cube roots, and similar materials. Such tables, which contain data not related to a particular chapter or section, are best placed in an appendix at the end of the book.

From Mosby author's guide, St. Louis, 1981, The C. V. Mosby Co., pp. 53-54.

Audiovisual preparation

C1 □ Type styles

STANDARD RANGE PAGE INDEX

These four pages list all 358 type-styles in the catalog. They've been grouped into Serif, Sans Serif, Decorative & Letragraphica and its page number indicated.

SANS SERIF

Pg.
13 Alternate Gothic 2
15 Antique Olive MEDIUM
15 Antique Olive SEMI BOLD
15 Antique Olive BOLD
16 Antique Olive BOLD CONDENSED
16 Antique Olive COMPACT
16 Antique OLIVE NORD
17 Avant Garde GOTHIC EXTRA LIGHT
18 Avant Garde GOTHIC MEDIUM
18 Avant Garde GOTHIC BOLD
24 Cable LIGHT
25 Cable HEAVY
33 Compacta LIGHT
33 Compacta
34 Compacta ITALIC
34 Compacta BOLD
36 Compacta BLACK
35 COMPACTA OUTLINE
35 COMPACTA BOLD OUTLINE

Pg.
39 Din 16 mi
39 Din 17 mi
41 ENGINEERING STANDARD
42 Eurostile MEDIUM EXTENDED
42 Eurostile BOLD EXTENDED
43 Folio LIGHT
44 Folio MEDIUM
45 Folio BOLD CONDENSED
44 Folio MEDIUM EXTENDED
44 Folio BOLD
45 Folio EXTRA BOLD
47 Franklin Gothic EXTRA CONDENSED
46 Franklin Gothic CONDENSED
46 Franklin Gothic
48 Franklin Gothic ITALIC
48 Franklin Gothic BOLD
49 Franklin Gothic CONDENSED REVERSED
49 Futura LIGHT
50 Futura MEDIUM

Pg.
50 Futura MEDIUM ITALIC
51 Futura BOLD CONDENSED
52 Futura DEMI BOLD
53 Futura EXTRA BOLD CONDENSED
54 Futura DISPLAY
51 Futura BOLD
52 Futura BOLD ITALIC
53 Futura EXTRA BOLD
53 Futura BLACK
55 Gill Sans LIGHT
56 Gill Sans
56 Gill Sans BOLD CONDENSED
56 Gill Sans BOLD
54 Gill EXTRA BOLD CONDENSED
54 Gill EXTRA BOLD
55 Gill EXTRA BOLD OUTLINE
55 Gill Kayo
58 Grotesque 7
58 Grotesque 9
58 Grotesque 9 ITALIC

Pg.
59 Grotesque 215
59 Grotesque 216
60 Helvetica EXTRA LIGHT
62 Helvetica LIGHT CONDENSED
61 Helvetica LIGHT
62 Helvetica LIGHT ITALIC
64 Helvetica MEDIUM CONDENSED
63 Helvetica MEDIUM
64 Helvetica MEDIUM ITALIC
65 Helvetica BOLD CONDENSED
65 Helvetica BOLD
66 Helvetica BOLD ITALIC
66 Helvetica EXTRA BOLD
66 Helvetica MEDIUM OUTLINE
67 Horatio LIGHT
67 Horatio MEDIUM
67 Horatio BOLD
73 Microgramma MEDIUM EXTENDED
73 Microgramma BOLD EXTENDED
75 News Gothic CONDENSED

Pg.
75 News Gothic
75 News Gothic BOLD
81 Pump LIGHT
81 Pump MEDIUM
81 Pump
82 Pump TRILINE
86 Simplex BOLD
89 Standard EXTRA BOLD CONDENSED
88 Standard MEDIUM
93 Univers 45
94 Univers 59
94 Univers 57
93 Univers 55
93 Univers 53
95 Univers 67
94 Univers 65
95 Univers 75
96 Venus BOLD EXTENDED

SERIF

13 Aachen MEDIUM
13 Aachen BOLD
14 Annlie EXTRA BOLD
14 Annlie EXTRA BOLD ITALIC
18 Baskerville OLD FACE

Pg.

19 Belwe LIGHT
19 **Belwe** MEDIUM
19 **Belwe** BOLD
20 Berling
20 *Berling* ITALIC
20 **Berling** BOLD
21 Beton MEDIUM
21 **Beton** BOLD
21 **Beton** EXTRA BOLD
22 **Bookman** BOLD
22 *Bookman* BOLD ITALIC
26 **Carousel**
26 Caslon 540
26 **Caslon Black**
27 Century SCHOOLBOOK BOLD
28 Cheltenham OLD STYLE
28 Cheltenham MEDIUM
28 **Cheltenham** BOLD
30 Clarendon MEDIUM
31 **Clarendon** BOLD
32 **Clearface** GOTHIC EXTRA BOLD
32 **Clearface** HEAVY
32 Cloister BOLD
37 COPPERPLATE GOTHIC HEAVY
41 **Egyptienne** BOLD CONDENSED

Pg.

54 EGYPTIAN OUTLINE
57 **Goudy** EXTRA BOLD
57 **Goudy** HEAVYFACE CONDENSED
60 **Hawthorn**
68 I.T.C. Caslon REGULAR 223
68 *I.T.C. Caslon* REGULAR ITALIC 223
68 **I.T.C. Caslon** BOLD 223
69 **I.T.C. Caslon** EXTRA BOLD 223
69 Jenson MEDIUM
69 **Jenson** EXTRA BOLD
71 Lectura
71 Lectura BOLD
73 Melior
74 Modern No. 20
76 Optima
76 Optima MEDIUM
77 **Optima** BOLD
77 **Palatino** SEMI BOLD
79 **Plantin** BOLD
79 **Plantin** BOLD CONDENSED
85 **Salisbury** BOLD
86 Serifa
86 Souvenir LIGHT
87 **Souvenir** MEDIUM
87 **Souvenir** DEMI BOLD

Pg.

87 **Souvenir** BOLD
91 Times NEW ROMAN
90 **Times** BOLD
91 *Times* BOLD ITALIC
91 **Times** EXTRA BOLD
92 **Trooper Roman**
97 **Windsor** BOLD
97 Windsor ELONGATED

DECORATIVE

14 AMERICAN UNCIAL
17 Arnold Bocklin
22 **Blanchard** SOLID
23 **Bottleneck**
23 **Broadway**
23 Brody
24 *Brush Script*
24 Bulletin TYPEWRITER
25 **Candice**
25 **Candice** INLINE
27 CHARRETTE
29 City LIGHT
29 City MEDIUM
29 **City** BOLD
36 **Cooper Black**
36 *Cooper Black* ITALIC

Pg.

37 Countdown
38 Data 70
38 DAVIDA
38 De Vinne ORNAMENTED
39 Dom Casual
40 Dynamo MEDIUM
40 **Dynamo**
43 *Flash* LIGHT
43 *Flash*
45 Fraktur BOLD
46 Eckmann Schrift
57 **Goudy Fancy**
60 Hobo
70 *Juliet*
70 Kalligraphia
70 **Lazybones**
71 *Le Griffe*
72 LETTRES ORNÉES
72 **Loose New Roman**
72 Manuscript CAPS
74 *Murray Hill Bold*
76 Old English
77 *Palace Script*
78 Peignot LIGHT
78 Peignot MEDIUM

Pg.

78 **Peignot** BOLD
79 Playbill
80 **Pretorian**
80 PRISMA
80 PROFIL
82 QUENTIN
82 **Revue**
83 Ringlet
83 Rockwell LIGHT 390
83 Rockwell 371
84 **Rockwell** BOLD 391
84 **Rockwell** EXTRA BOLD
84 ROMANTIQUES
85 SANS SERIF SHADED
85 SAPPHIRE
89 STENCIL BOLD
89 Tabasco MEDIUM
90 **Tabasco** BOLD
92 Tiptopetto
92 **Tip Top**
95 University Roman
96 University ROMAN BOLD
96 Vivaldi
97 Zipper

Helvetica Medium Haas

Ea E1a E1a E1a

47-192-C (707) 3 N C	47-192-L (708) 3 C	47-144-CN (709) 2 C	47-144-L (710) 2 C	47-120-CN (711) 2 C	47-120-L (712) C

E1a E1a E1a E1a E1a E1a E1a

47-96-CN (713) C	47-96-L (714) C	47-84-CN (715) C	47-84-L (716) C	47-72-L (717) N C	47-72-L (718) C	47-60-CN (719) N C	47-60-L (720) C
47-48-CN (721) N C	47-48-L (722) C						

Ea1 Ea1 Ea1 Ea1 Ea1 Ea1 Ea1 Ea1 Ea1 Ea1

47-42-CLN (724) N C	47-36-CLN (2120) C	47-30-CLN (725) N C	47-24-CLN (727) C	47-18-CLN (728) C	47-14-CLN (1568) C	47-12-CLN (2121) C	47-10-CLN (1569) C	47-8-CLN (1570) C	47-6-CLN (1571) C

ABCDEFGHI abcdefghijkl
JKLMNOPQ mnopqrstuv
RSTUVWXY wxyz12345
Z&?!ß£$ 67890;—

HELVETICA MEDIUM

C2 □ Photographic film guide (Kodak)

KODAK BLACK-AND-WHITE FILMS

KODAK Film (Code)	Properties and Purpose	Speeds	
Roll Films		**Daylight**	**Tungsten**
VERICHROME Pan (VP)—rolls and for Cirkut cameras	All-round use.	125	125
PLUS-X Pan (PX)—135①	General-purpose film.	125	125
TRI-X Pan (TX)①	Very fast. For limited light action.	400	400
PANATOMIC-X (FX)—135① PANATOMIC-X Professional (FXP)—120	Extremely fine grain, very high resolving power.	32	32
PLUS-X Pan Professional (PXP)— 120 and 220 in 5-roll pro-pack	General-purpose film, retouching surface on emulsion side.	125	125
TRI-X Pan Professional (TXP)— 120 and 220 in 5-roll pro-pack; film packs	Superior highlight brilliance, good contrast control, retouching surface on both sides.	320	320
ROYAL-X Pan (RX)—120 only	Ultra-fast. For existing light.	1250③	1250③
Recording 2475 (ESTAR-AH Base) (RE)—135-36①	Ultra-fast panchromatic. For adverse light conditions.	—	1000-3200③
High Speed Infrared (HIE)—135-20 only	Haze penetration, special effects and purposes.	—③	—③
Technical Pan 2415①	High to normal contrast, depending on development.	25③	20
Sheet Films	**Properties and Purpose**	**Daylight**	**Tungsten**
EKTAPAN 4162 (ESTAR Thick Base)②	For portraits by electronic flash and general use.	100	100
PLUS-X Pan Professional 4147 (ESTAR Thick Base)②	Excellent definition. For portrait and commercial work.	125	125
SUPER-XX Pan 4142 (ESTAR Thick Base)	Long tonal gradation. Color-separation negatives.	200	200
TRI-X Pan Professional 4164 (ESTAR Thick Base)②	Superior highlight brilliance, good contrast control.	320	320
TRI-X Ortho 4163 (ESTAR Thick Base)	Superior body highlight brilliance. For portraits and commercial subjects.	320	200
ROYAL Pan 4141 (ESTAR Thick Base)②	High Speed. General purpose.	400	400
ROYAL-X Pan 4166 (ESTAR Thick Base)	Ultra-fast. For available-light exposure.	1250③	1250③
Commercial 6127 and 4127 (ESTAR Thick Base)	Blue-sensitive. For continuous-tone copying, transparencies.	50 (20④)	8
Contrast Process Ortho 4154 (ESTAR Thick Base)	Extremely high contrast. For line copies.	100④	50
Contrast Process Pan 4155 (ESTAR Thick Base)	Extremely high contrast. For copies of colored line originals.	100④	80
Professional Copy 4125 (ESTAR Thick Base)	Retains highlight gradation in copies.	25④	12
High-Speed Infrared 4143 (ESTAR Thick Base)	Haze penetration, special effects. Document copying.	—③	—④
Long Rolls **(Wider than 16 mm)**	**Properties and Purpose**	**Daylight**	**Tungsten**
PLUS-X Pan Professional 2147 (ESTAR Base)	Good definition and excellent latitude.	125	125
PLUS-X Portrait 5068	For portrait and school work. Retouching surface.	125	125
Direct Positive Panchromatic 5246	For reversal processing to slides.	80	64

NOTES: ① Also available in long rolls, 35 mm perforated.
② Also available in long rolls, 3½ in. wide.
③ See film instructions.
④ Speed to white-flame arc.

Copyright by the Eastman Kodak Company. Reprinted with permission.

KODAK COLOR FILMS

KODAK Color Film (Code) — Roll Films	Balanced for	Daylight Speed	Daylight Filter	Flash Bulb	Flash Filter	Photolamps (3400 K) Speed	Photolamps (3400 K) Filter	Tungsten (3200 K) Speed	Tungsten (3200 K) Filter	Electronic Flash Filter	Processing ◆ KODAK Chemicals®
KODACHROME 25 (Daylight) (KM) For color slides[1]	Daylight, Electronic Flash, Blue Flash	25	None	Blue	None	8	80B	6	80A	None	Not for user processing — By Kodak labs and by photofinishers. Sent to Kodak by dealers or direct by users with KODAK Mailers.
KODACHROME 40, 5070 (Type A) (KPA) For color slides[1] 135-36 only	Photolamps (3400 K)	25	85	Blue	85	40	None	32	82A	85	
KODACHROME 64 (Daylight) (KR) For color slides[1]	Daylight, Electronic Flash, Blue Flash	64	None	Blue	None	20	80B	16	80A	None	
KODACOLOR II (C) For color prints[2]	Daylight, Electronic Flash, Blue Flash	100	None	Blue	None	32	80B[6]	25	80A[6]	None	FLEXICOLOR® Process C-41 — By Kodak, other labs, or users. Sent to Kodak by dealers or direct by users with KODAK Mailers.
KODACOLOR 400 (CG) For color prints[2]	Daylight, Electronic Flash, Blue Flash	400	None	Blue	None	125	80B[6]	100	80A[6]	None	
EKTACHROME 64 (Daylight) (ER) For color slides[1]	Daylight, Electronic Flash, Blue Flash	64	None	Blue	None	20	80B	16	80A	None[7]	Process E-6 — By Kodak, other labs, or users. Sent to Kodak by dealers or direct by users with KODAK Mailers.
EKTACHROME 200 (Daylight) (ED) For color slides[1]	Daylight, Electronic Flash, Blue Flash	200	None	Blue	None	64	80B	50	80A	None[7]	
EKTACHROME 160 (Tungsten) (ET) For color slides[1]	Tungsten	100	85B	—	—	125	81A	160	None	—	
EKTACHROME 64 Professional (Daylight) (EPR)[1] 120, 135-36,[3] long rolls (5017)	Daylight, Electronic Flash, Blue Flash	64[4]	None	Blue	None	20	80B	16	80A	None[7]	
EKTACHROME 50 Professional (Tungsten) (EPY)[1] 120, 135-36,[3] long rolls (5018)	3200 K Tungsten	32 at 1/60 sec	85B	—	—	40 at 1/10 sec	81A	50[4] at 1/10 sec	None	—	
EKTACHROME 200 Professional (Daylight) (EPD)[1] 120, 135-36,[3] long rolls (5036)	Daylight, Electronic Flash, Blue Flash	200[4]	None	Blue	None	64	80B	50	80A	None[7]	
EKTACHROME 160 Professional (Tungsten) (EPT)[1] 120, 135-36,[3] long rolls (5037)	Tungsten	100	85B	—	—	125	81A	160[4]	None	—	
VERICOLOR II Professional, Type S (VPS)[2] 120, 135-20, 135-36, 220 Expose 1/10 sec or less	Electronic Flash, Daylight, or Blue Flash	125	None	Blue[5]	None	40	80B	32	80A	None	FLEXICOLOR Process C-41 — By Kodak, user labs, or professional finishers. Sent to Kodak by dealers or direct by users with KODAK Mailers. Type L film is not printed by Kodak.
VERICOLOR II Professional, Type L (VPL)[2] 120 only Expose 1/50 to 60 sec	3200 K Tungsten	64 at 1/50 sec	85B	Not recom.		64 at 1 sec	81A	80 at 1 sec[4]	None	Not recom.	

C3 □ List of materials and equipment necessary for preparing visual aids

Minimum equipment

Drawing board
T-square
Triangle
Tackle box for storage of materials
Metal rule
Compass
Scissors
X-Acto knife or #11 scalpel
Drawing pen with variety of nibs
Light source
Burnisher for transfer letters

Advanced equipment

Drafting table and stool
Tabouret for storage of supplies
Lettering guides
Mat knife
Paper cutter
Light box
Technical pens

Basic materials

Pencils with hard and soft lead
Erasers
Illustration board
Tracing paper
Transfer letters
Drafting (or masking) tape
Colored pencils
Spray fixative
Rubber cement and rubber cement thinner
India ink
White paint for touch-up

Advanced materials

Inks or paints for adding color
Self-adhesive color films
Adhesive shading mediums
Colored adhesive tapes
Colored papers or illustration board
Graphite tracing paper
Acetate sheets

C4 □ List of suppliers and equipment for graphic materials

This by no means represents all materials available. It is, rather, a list of those that are commonly available in art supply or stationery stores.

Pens and pencils

Drawing and colored pencils, color markers

Koh-I-Noor mechanical pencil
    Koh-I-Noor Rapidograph, Inc.
    100 North Street
    Bloomsbury, NJ 08804
Mongol Pencils
    Eberhard Faber, Inc.
    Crestwood, Wilkes-Barre, PA 18773
Prismacolor Pencils
    Eagle Pencil Co.
    Eagle Road
    Danbury, CN 06810
Pantone Markers
    Letraset USA, Inc.
    40 Eisenhower Drive
    Paramus, NJ 07652

Lettering pens

Osmiroid Pens
    Hunt Manufacturing Co.
    Statesville, NC 28677
Pelikan Pens
    Koh-I-Noor Rapidograph Co.
    100 North Street
    Bloomsbury, NJ 08804
Speedball Pens and Nibs
    Hunt Manufacturing Co.
    Statesville, NC 28677

Technical pens

Faber Castell
    Faber Castell Co.
    41-47 Dickerson St.
    Newark, NJ 07103
Koh-I-Noor Rapidograph
    Koh-I-Noor Rapidograph, Inc.
    100 North Street
    Bloomsbury, NJ 08804

Mars Technical Pen
J. S. Staedtler, Inc.
Boonton Ave.
Montville, NJ 07045

Transfer letters and symbols

Chartpak
Chartpak
1 River Road
Leeds, MA 01053
Formatt
Graphic Products Corporation
Rolling Meadows, IL 60008
Letraset
Letraset USA, Inc.
40 Eisenhower Drive
Paramus, NJ 07652
Tachtype
Tachtype
127 W. 26th Street
New York, NY 10001

Charting and graphic arts tape

Chartpak
Chartpak
1 River Road
Leeds, MA 01053
Formaline
Graphic Products Corporation
Rolling Meadows, IL 60008
Letraline
Letraset USA, Inc.
40 Eisenhower Drive
Paramus, NJ 07652

Color adhesive overlays

Letrafilm
Pantone Color Film
Letraset USA, Inc.
40 Eisenhower Drive
Paramus, NJ 07652
Zipatone
Zipatone, Inc.
150 Fencl Lane
Hillside, IL 60162

Lettering guides

Leroy Lettering Set
Keuffel & Esser Co.
40 East 43rd Street
New York, NY 10017
Varigraph
Varigraph, Inc.
1480 Martin Street
Madison, WI 53701
Wrico Lettering Set
The Wood-Regan Instrument Company
184 Franklin Avenue
Nutley, NJ 07110

Illustration board and art papers

Crescent
Crescent Cardboard Company
P.O. Box XD
100 West Willow Road
Wheeling, IL 60090
Pantone Color Paper
Letraset USA, Inc.
40 Eisenhower Drive
Paramus, NJ 07652
Strathmore
Strathmore Paper Company
Westfield, MA 01085

Planning boards and cards

Medro Educational Products
P.O. Box 8463
Rochester, NY 14618

Light boxes

Companion
Technology Products Company
Irvine, CA 92714

Transparent watercolors (Also useful for coloring Kodalith slides)

Martin's Water Colors
Salis International
Hollywood FL 33020

C5 □ List of suppliers for photographic equipment

This list includes the most widely available and popular photographic equipment. The omission of any equipment does not mean that it is not acceptable for clinical use. Most camera manufacturers supply lenses and flash units that are particularly suited for use on their equipment. Independent suppliers, however, manufacture both lenses and flash equipment that is suitable for use with other manufacturer's cameras. The best source of information about camera equipment is from a local photo supplier. If, however, you wish additional information, contact the manufacturer.

35 mm single lens reflex cameras

Canon
    Canon USA, Inc.
    10 Nevada Drive
    Lake Success, NY 11042
Chinon
    Chinon Corporation of America, Inc.
    43 Fadem Road
    Springfield, NJ 07081
Contax
    Yashica, Inc.–Contax Division
    411 Sette Drive
    Paramus, NJ 07652
Fujica
    Fuji Photo Film, USA
    350 Fifth Ave.
    New York, NY 10001
Konica
    Konica Camera Division Berkey Marketing Companies
    25-20 Brooklyn-Queens Expressway W.
    Woodside, NY 11377
Leica
    Ernst Leitz, Inc.
    Link Drive
    Rockleigh, NJ 07647
Mamiya
    Bell & Howell/Mamiya Company
    Box 1128
    Highland Park, IL 60035
Minolta
    Minolta Corporation
    101 Williams Drive
    Ramsey, NJ 07446
Nikon
    Nikon, Inc.
    623 Stewart Ave.
    Garden City, NY 11530

Olympus
    Olympus Camera Corporation
    Crossways Park
    Woodside, NY 11377
Pentax
    Pentax Corporation
    35 Inverness Drive East
    Englewood, CO 80112
Ricoh
    Braun North America
    55 Cambridge Parkway
    Cambridge, MA 02142
Rolleiflex
    Rollei of America
    Box 1010
    Littleton, CO 80160
Topcon
    Photo America Corporation
    7491 N.W. 8th Street
    Miami, FL 33126
Yashica
    Yashica, Inc.
    411 Sette Drive
    Paramus, NJ 07652

Lenses

Asanuma
    Asanuma Corporation
    1639 E. Del Amo Boulevard
    Carson, CA 90746
Osawa
    Osawa & Co., Ltd.
    521 Fifth Ave.
    New York, NY 10017
Quantaray
    Ritz Camera
    11710 Baltimore Avenue
    Beltsville, MD 20705
Sigma
    Unitron Instruments, Inc., Photo Division
    101 Crossways Park W.
    Woodbury, NY 11797
Soligor
    AIC Photo, Inc.
    168 Glen Cove Road
    Carle Place, NY 11514
Tamron
    Tamron Division Berkey Marketing Companies, Inc.
    25-20 Brooklyn-Queens Expressway W.
    Woodside, NY 11377

Vivitar
Vivitar Corporation
1630 Stewart Street
Santa Monica, CA 11797

Electronic flash units
Ascorlight
Berkey Marketing Companies, Inc.
25-20 Brooklyn-Queens Expressway W.
Woodside, NY 11377
Bogen-Bowens
Bogen Photo Corporation
100 South Van Brunt Street
Englewood, NJ 07631
Braun
Braun North America
55 Cambridge Parkway
Cambridge, MA 02142
Hanimex
Hanimex, Inc.
1801 W. Touhy Avenue
Elk Grove Village, IL 60007
Metz
Unitron Instruments, Inc. Photo Division
101 Crossways Park W.
Woodbury, NY 11797
Spiralite
Spiratone
135-06 Northern Boulevard
Flushing, NY 11354
Sunpak
Sunpak Division Berkey Marketing Companies, Inc.
25-20 Brooklyn-Queens Expressway W.
Woodside, NY 11377

Vivitar
Vivitar Corporation
1630 Stewart Street
Santa Monica, CA 90406

Ringlights
Ascorlight
Berkey Marketing Companies, Inc.
25-20 Brooklyn-Queens Expressway W.
Woodside, NY 11377
Spiratone ringlite
Spiratone
135-06 Northern Boulevard
Flushing, NY 11354

Special equipment
Combination ring and point light
Lester A. Dine, Inc.
2080 Jericho Turnpike
New Hyde Park, NY 11041
K-ring flash bracket
Klinger Precision Fine Mechanics and Optics
439 S. LaCienega Boulevard
Los Angeles, CA 90048

Incandescent studio lighting
Smith-Victor Corporation
301 N. Colfax St.
Griffith, IN 46319

Spiratone
135-06 Northern Boulevard
Flushing, NY 11354

C6 □ List of suppliers of materials and equipment for preparing scientific exhibits

Rear screen modules for slide projectors or movies

Rappaport Exhibits
3608 Payne Avenue
Cleveland, OH 44114

Prefabricated folding panel exhibits

Downing Displays, Inc.
115 W. McMicken Ave.
Cincinnati, OH 45210

Rear screen, synchronized slide projectors and video equipment

Fairchild Industrial Products
75 Mall Drive
Commack, NY 11725

LaBelle Industries
657 S. Worthington St.
Oconomowoc, WI 53066

Buhl, Inc.
Dept. 50
5 Paul Kohner Place
Elmwood Park, NJ 07407

Bell & Howell
Audio-Visual Products Division
7100 N. McCormack Rd.
Dept. 8876
Chicago, IL 60645

Electrosonic Systems Inc.
4575 W. 77th St.
Minneapolis, MN 55435

Video equipment

Sony Video Information Center
Department 1076
P.O. Box 1594
Trenton, NJ 08607

Videodetics Corporation
2121 South Manchester Ave.
Anaheim, CA 92802

Projectors

Eastman Kodak Company
Department A 5 017
Rochester, NY 14650

C7 □ Setting up an office photographic system

Equipment and facilities

Equipment. First make a decision about the type system you will use. This can vary from a simple camera with an attached electronic flash to a more complex system, using a sophisticated camera and studio lighting. If you are just getting started or if you plan to have your office personnel take most of the photographs, a relatively simple system will be better.

The minimum equipment for a simple system is:

> 35 mm single lens reflex camera
> 100 mm macro lens
> Electronic flash

If most of your photographs will be of extremities or the trunk, you may want to add a 50 mm macro lens.

Set aside a photographic area in the office. There are several option for this. You can designate a specific location and use it for photography only, or each treatment room can be designed with an area for photography. Regardless of your choice, certain criteria must be considered if the area is to be satisfactory for good clinical photographs.

First, the background must be suitable. Second, the room should be large enough that the patient can be positioned at least two, preferably three, feet from the background to eliminate shadows. The room must also be long enough to allow the necessary camera-to-subject distance, particularly when photographing the trunk or extremities with a 100 mm lens.

Background. The background should be plain and unobtrusive. Use a neutral color, preferably blue or medium gray. Avoid either black or white. Above all, avoid any distracting features such as doors, windows, figured wallpaper, or equipment in the background.

A portion of a wall may be painted a suitable color or you may use a large movable panel. A continuous roll of colored paper may be hung from a bracket and pulled down for a background. Try to have the surface smooth; curtains or drapes may wrinkle or fold and be distracting.

The junction between the wall and floor can be distracting when photographing the lower extremity. A good way to eliminate this is to use a continuous background such as a roll of paper or a flap of material attached to a mobile cart. If this is not feasible, provide a small stool for the patient to stand on that will elevate the feet above the level of the wall-floor junction.

Adapted from suggestions by Louis Charles Hacker, M.D.

Establish standards

Set standards for each area to be photographed. In order to have uniform photographs of any given anatomic area, you must establish standards for each. For example, photographs of the head or face should be taken with the lens set at 1:10 magnification. Similar decisions should be made about all other areas to be photographed. A suggested guide is given in Chapter 19.

Make test exposures. After you have determined the standards for each region, make test exposures to determine the best combination of lens settings and lighting. First determine what is calculated to be the best exposure, then "bracket" this by making exposures one-half to one stop over and under this. Keep careful records of these test exposures, then examine each to see which best and most accurately depicts the subject.

Make a guidebook. After all standards have been established, a good way to maintain uniformity is to make a guidebook for your personnel. Each page in this book should include:

A. Area to be photographed
B. Examples of standard views
C. Examples of any special views
D. Center of viewpoint
E. Camera and lens settings
F. Position of lighting
G. Background
H. Frequency of photographs (preop, postop intervals)

Train personnel

After you have obtained your equipment, established standards, and developed a guidebook, spend some time training your personnel. Many of them not only may be unfamiliar with photographic equipment, but also may be overawed by its complexity and afraid to use it. A few hours of instruction and reassurance should overcome this and give them confidence. Plan to invest in several rolls of film and processing, give each of them an opportunity to use the equipment, then go over the results with each person until each is familiar with and comfortable with the equipment.

The training sessions should include:

A. Operation of camera
 1. General description
 2. Loading film
 3. Selection of proper lens
 4. Adjustment of settings
 5. Operation of flash or other lighting
B. Preparation of the patient
 1. Explanation of what is going to be done
 2. Removal of clothing or draping

3. Removal of jewelry
4. Pull back hair, if necessary
C. Positioning and photographing the patient
   1. Refer to guidebook for standard views
   2. Be sure background is suitable
   3. Assure
      a. Proper focal length lens
      b. Sharp focus
      c. Camera centered on subject
      d. Correct angle of view
      e. Light source proper and in correct position
      f. Background plain and uncluttered
D. Practice session

Monitor quality

Even after the training sessions are completed, it is still desirable to continuously monitor the quality of the photographs taken by your personnel. A good way to do this is to review each batch of slides after they have been labeled and identified but before they have been filed. At this time any problems can be identified and recommendations for their correction made. Projecting a group of slides occasionally may help even more to point out problems.

Common faults to be looked for during these sessions are:

A. Selection of wrong lens
B. Improper focusing
C. Improper exposure
D. Wrong, or no, film in camera
E. Failure to remove jewelry, clothing, or cosmetics
F. Distracting background
G. Failure to follow standard views
   1. Improper magnification
   2. Photographs not centered
   3. Nonstandard lighting
   4. Wrong angle of view
   5. Failure to take full complement of views

Filing

Slides may be filed in the patient's chart or they may be put in a separate file, identified by name and chart number. Regardless of the method of filing, set up a cross-reference file so that slides that are useful for teaching or illustration of talks or papers may be retrieved easily.

The cross-reference system should be tailored to your needs. You may want to identify slides by anatomic regions, by diagnosis, by operation, or by a combination of all of these. Regardless of which system you choose, cross-reference the slides at the time they are returned from the processor and before they are filed. Otherwise, you will be faced with the almost insurmountable job of cross-referencing several thousand slides, which is so discouraging that the task will probably never be done and retrieval of slides becomes almost impossible.

C8 □ Using tape to make graphs

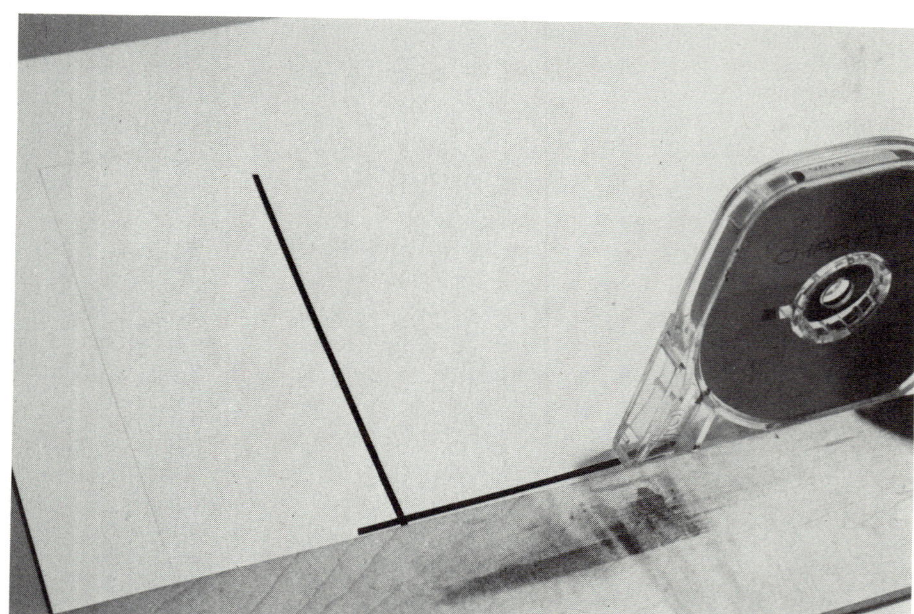

Fig. 1. First make the axis lines. This can be done by using a straightedge as a guide or by placing the tape over lightly penciled guidelines. The axis lines should be easily visible, but not as bold as the information lines.

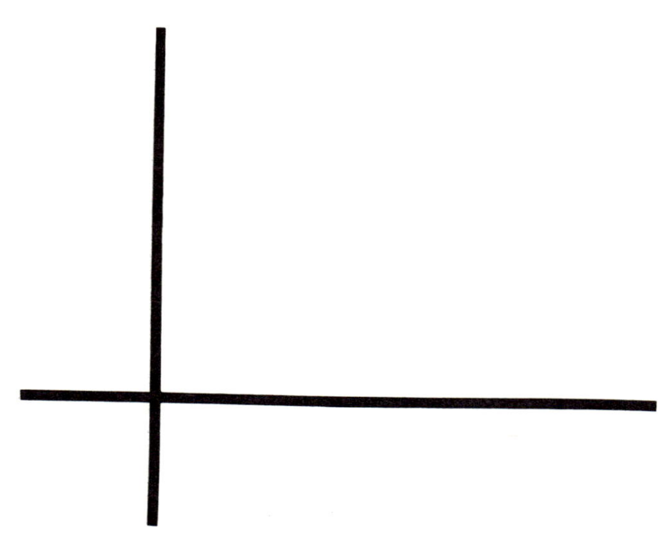

Fig. 2. Allow the tape to overlap at the corners.

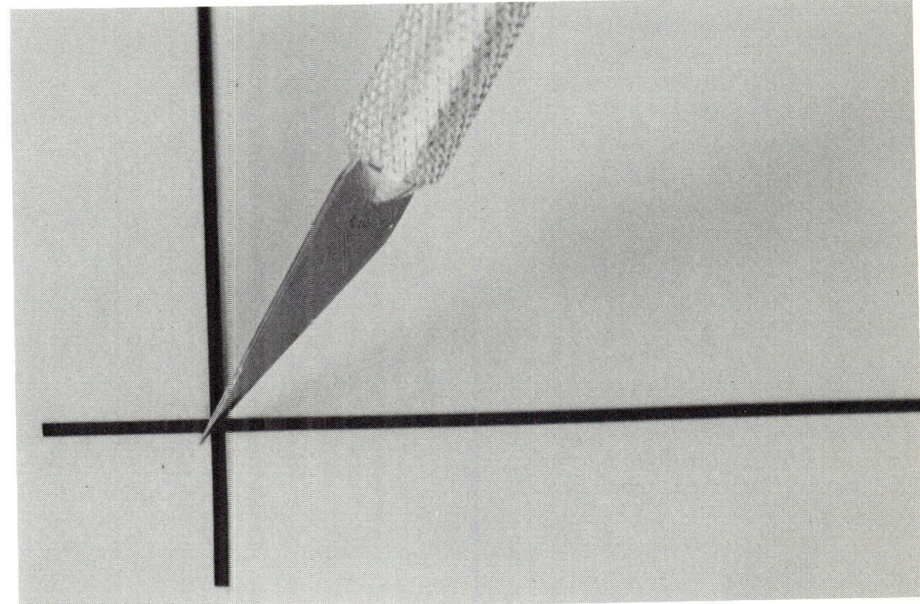

Fig. 3. Cut through both tapes at the corner at a 45-degree angle, using a sharp knife.

Fig. 4. This will result in a perfectly mitered corner.

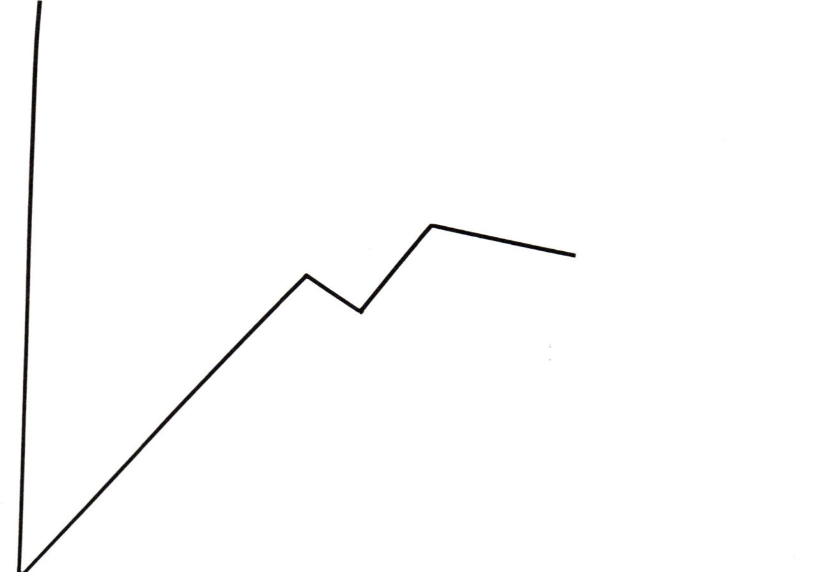

Fig. 5. Information lines can be placed on the graph following guidelines and the junctions cut as described for the corners of the axis lines.

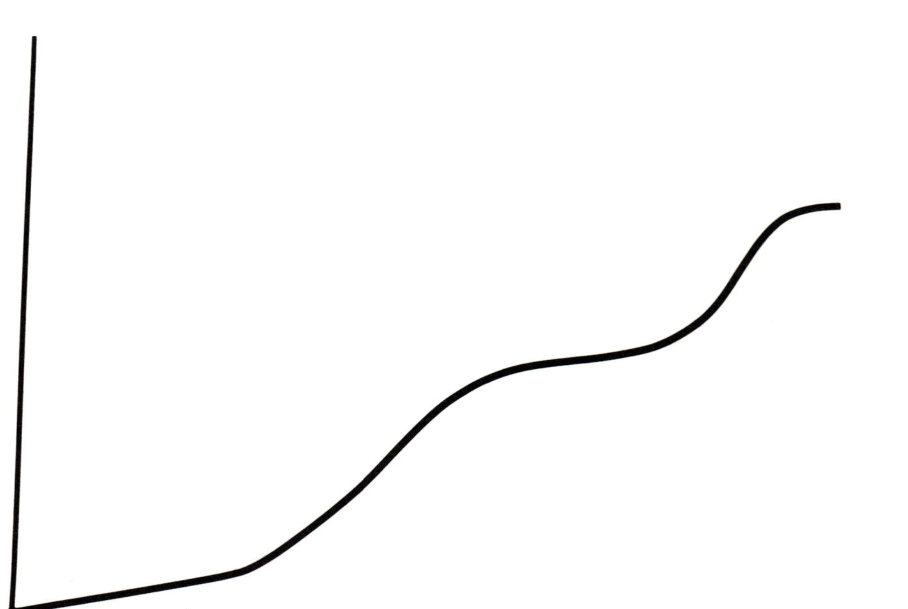

Fig. 6. Flexible tapes may be used to make curved information lines.

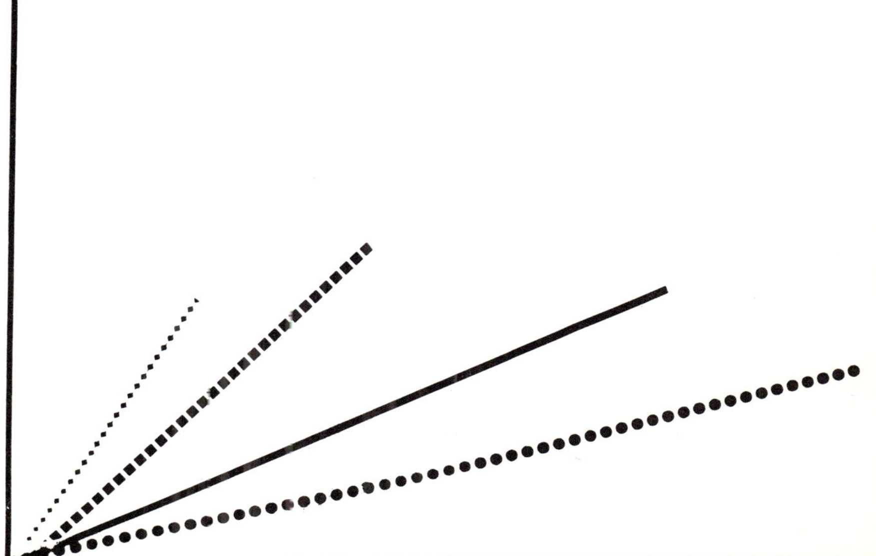

Fig. 7. If multiple information lines are used, select tapes with enough contrast in design to clearly delineate each.

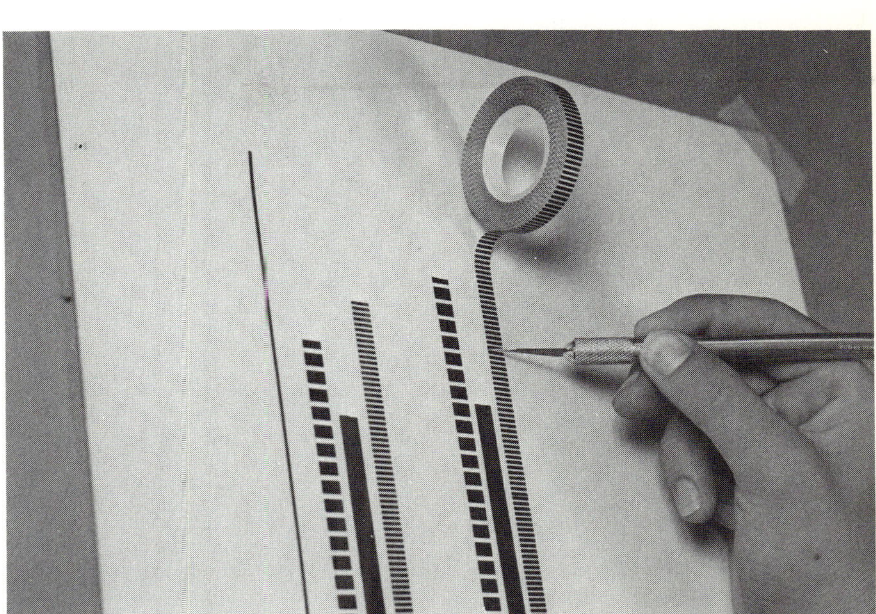

Fig. 8. Wider tapes can be used to make bar graphs.

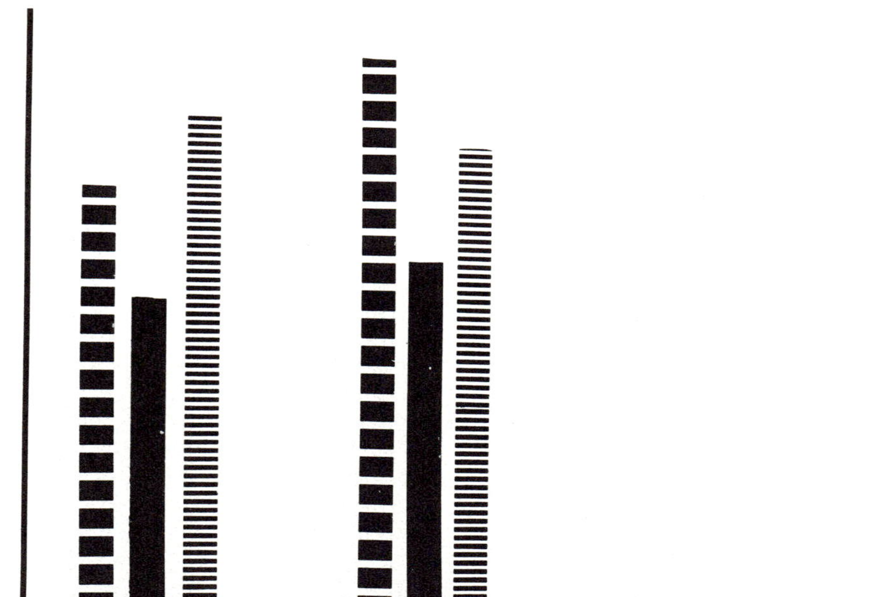

Fig. 9. As with other graphs, select tape designs that will be distinctive enough to prevent confusion with other bars.

C9 □ Using transfer letters

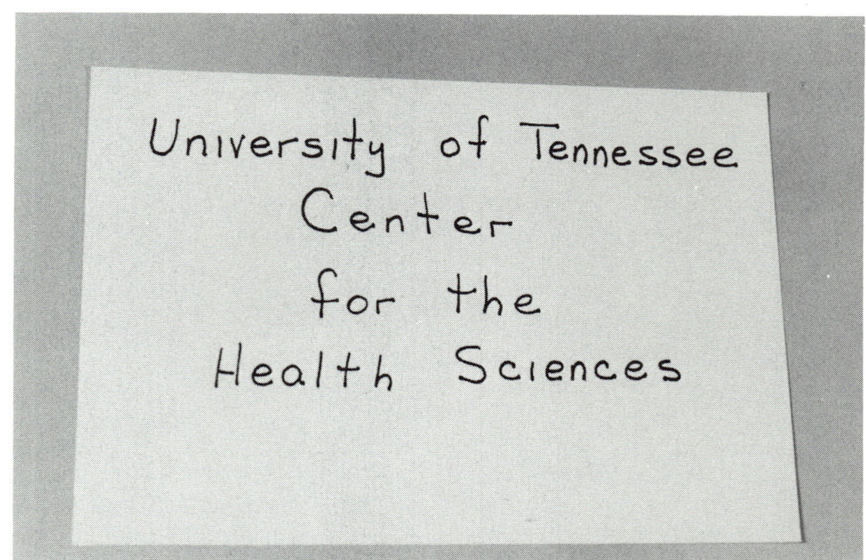

Fig. 1. Make a rough sketch or "thumbnail" arranged as you want the finished graphic to appear.

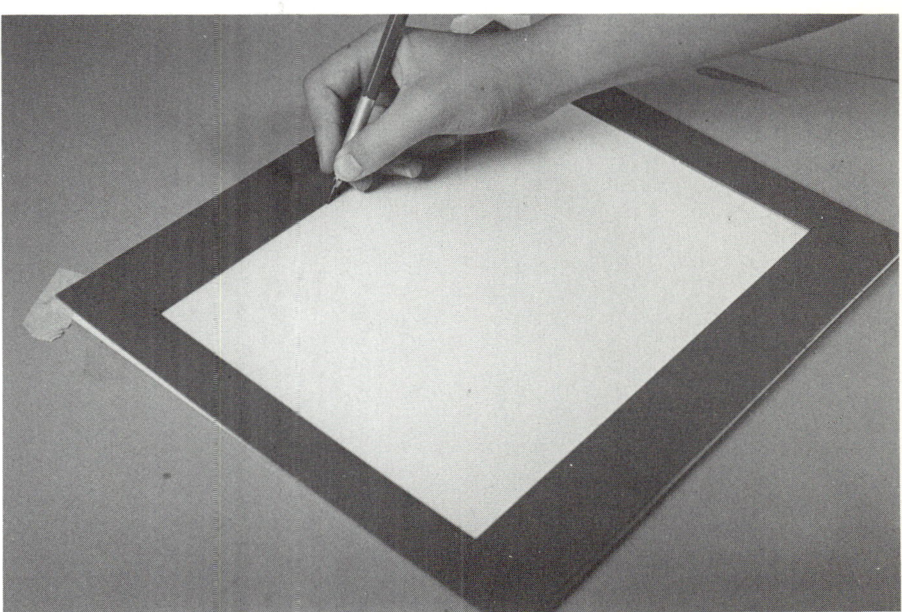

Fig. 2. Using a template, outline the working area on the artboard.

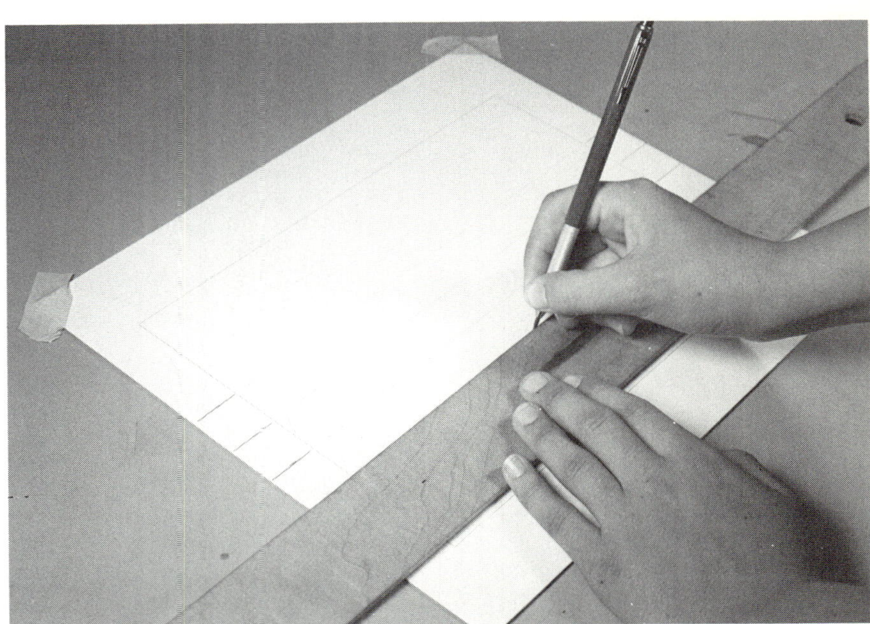

Fig. 3. Draw guidelines lightly on the artboard, following the arrangement on the rough sketch.

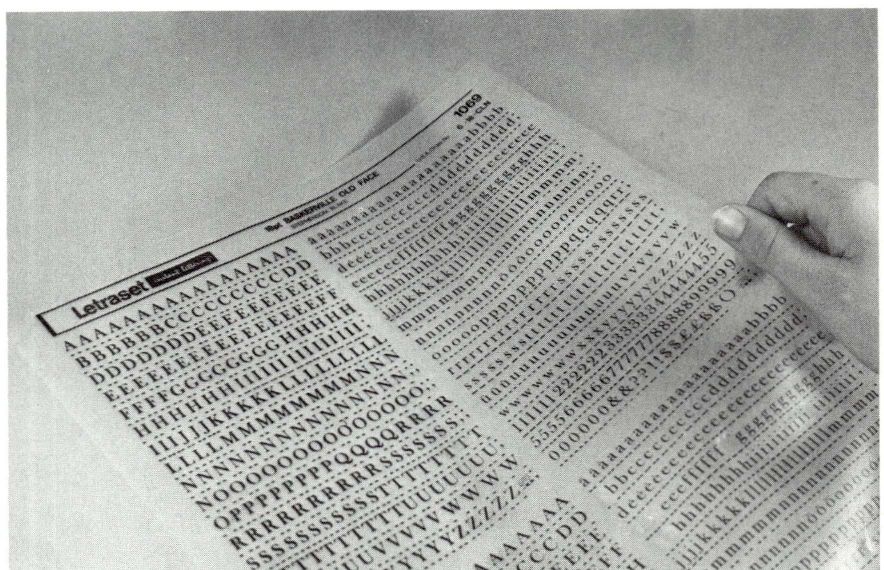

Fig. 4. Select the appropriate sheet of transfer letters.

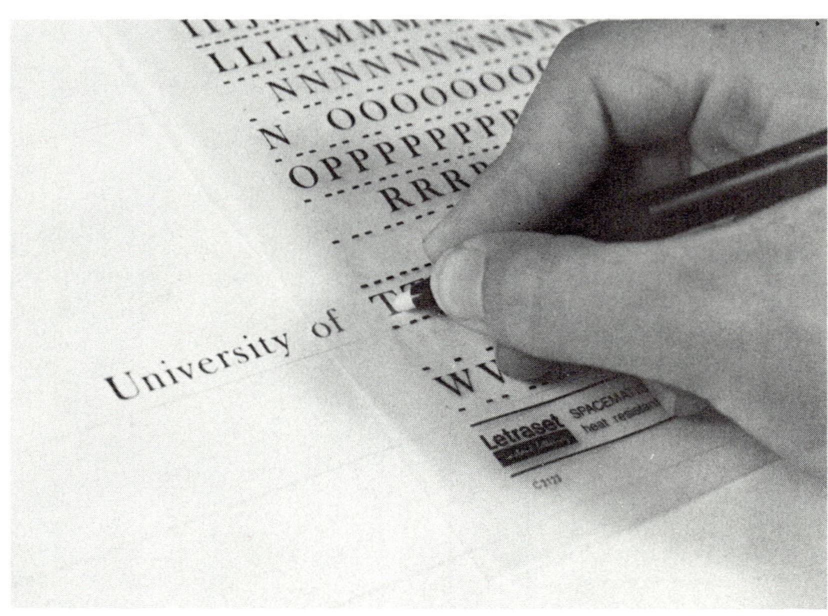

Fig. 5. Position the carrier sheet in position and transfer the letter by lightly burnishing over it.

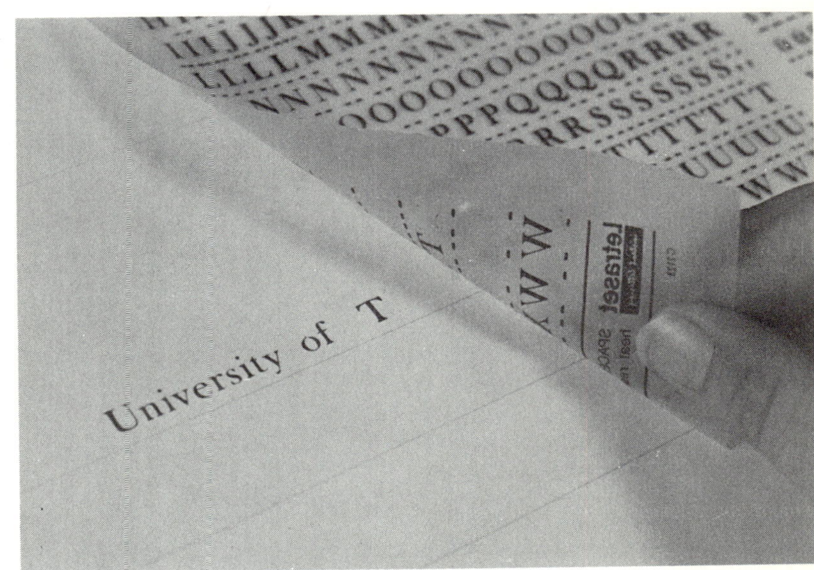

Fig. 6. When you lift the carrier sheet away, the letter will adhere to the art-board.

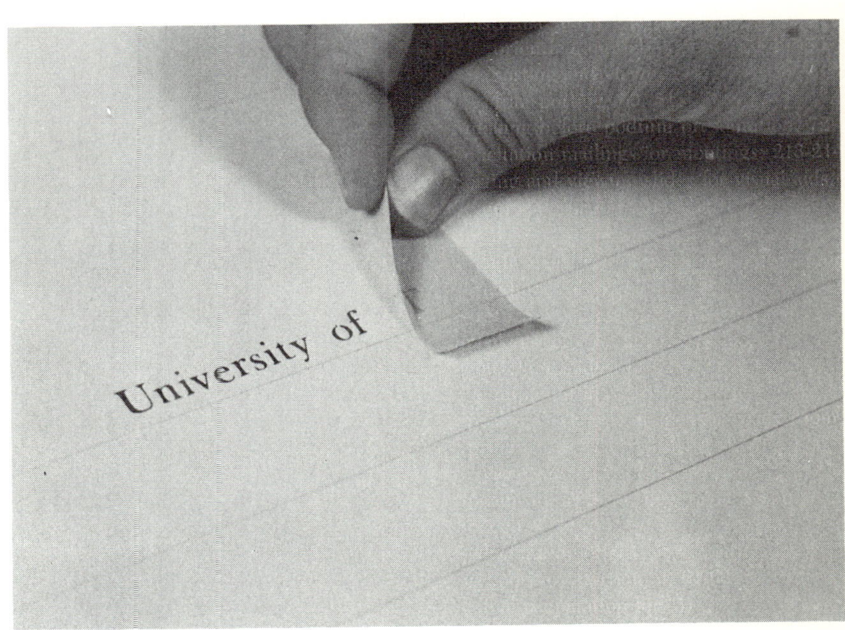

Fig. 7. If you make a mistake, the letter or letters can be lifted from the art-board with Scotch or drafting tape.

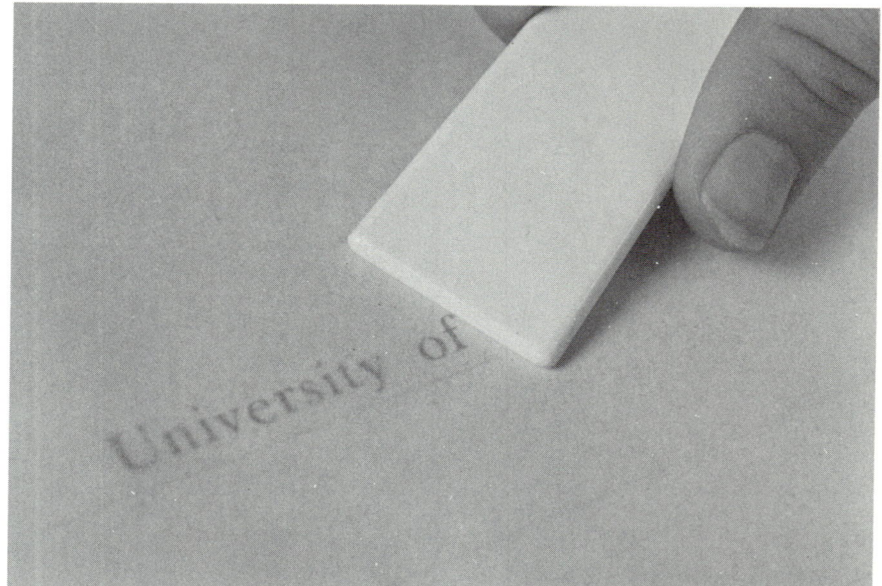

Fig. 8. After the correct lettering is applied to the artboard, cover it with the transfer letter backing sheet and burnish firmly. This will cause the letters to adhere permanently.

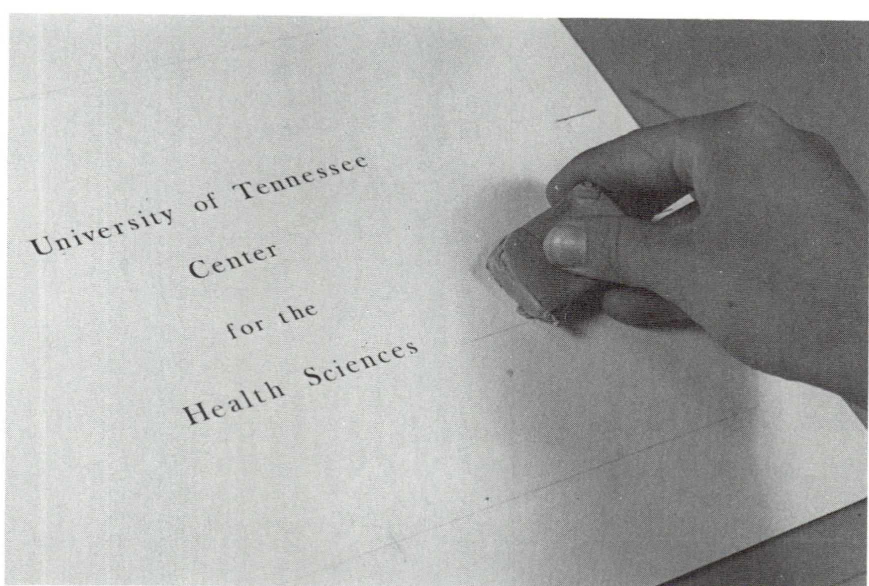

Fig. 9. When all lettering is complete and has been burnished onto the artboard, erase the guidelines.

C10 □ Adding color to artwork with adhesive color film

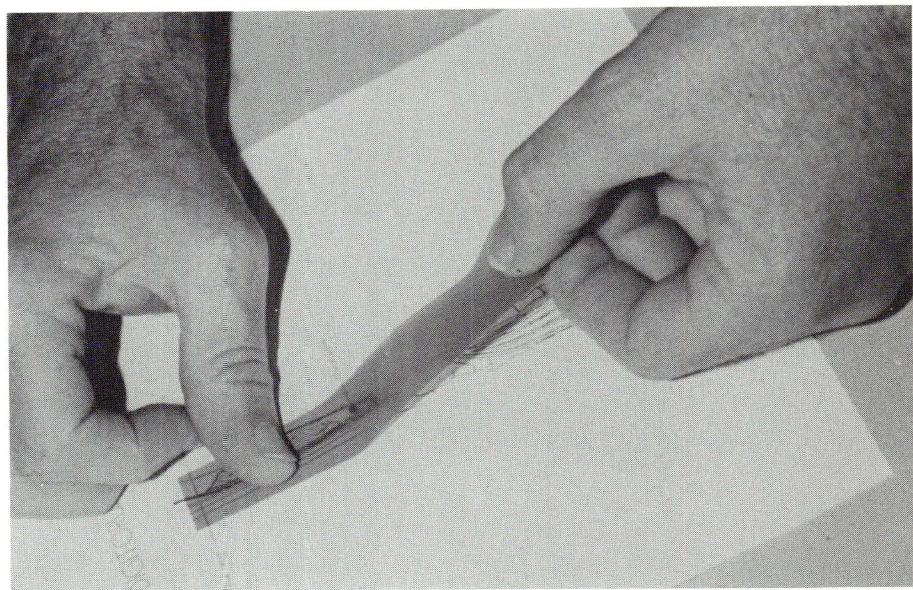

Fig. 1. Cover the area to be colored with adhesive-backed color film. This should be larger than the area to be colored.

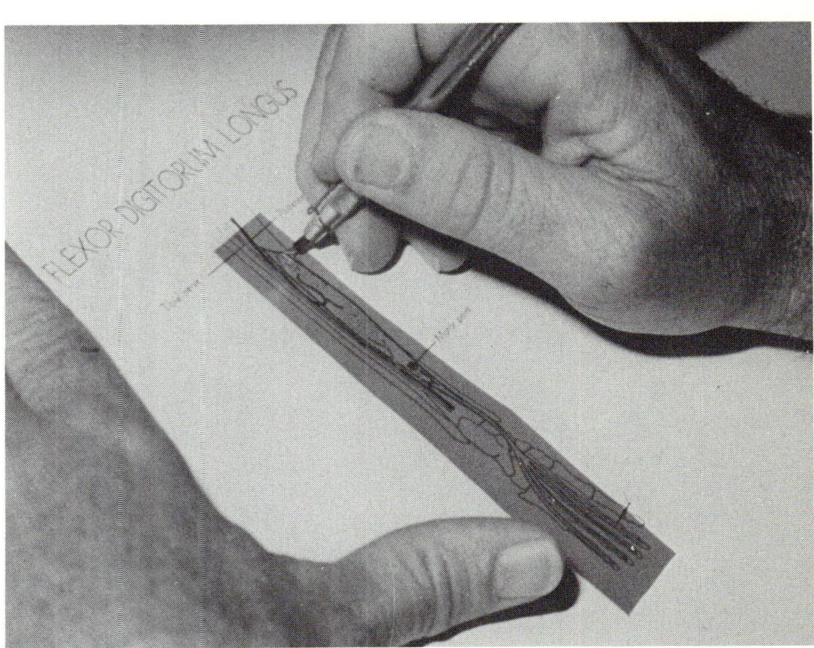

Fig. 2. Cut through the film, following the outline of the area to be emphasized.

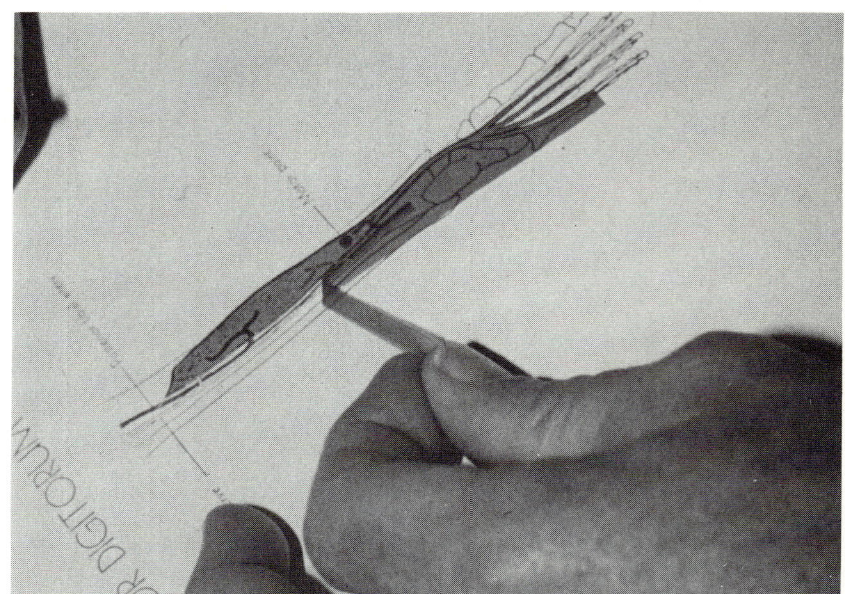

Fig. 3. Peel away the unwanted materi-al. Burnish the remaining film to make it adhere firmly.

C11 □ Effective slide preparation

ARTWORK LETTERING SIZES

Assuming you are using 10 × 12 inch artwork and your screen size will be 10 × 10 feet, the following is a guide to the minimal letter size that will be necessary for greatest legibility.

Distance of farthest viewer (feet)	Minimal letter height (inches)
32	3/32
64	3/16
96	1/4
128	5/16
160	7/16
192	1/2

BEST COLOR COMBINATIONS

1. Black on yellow
2. Black on orange
3. Orange on blue
4. Green on white
5. Red on white
6. Black on white
7. Blue on white
8. White on blue*
9. Orange on black
10. White on black

*Refers to white lettering on blue paper, not diazo slides.

C12 □ Effective slide lectures

Rehearse your slide presentation several times so that you will be familiar with the sequence and timing of the slides.

Several days in advance, let the program chairman know the size and mounting (glass, metal, Kodak Ready-Mount, etc.) of your slides and the kind of tray you will use, so that you will be provided with the right projector. Be sure you use a widely accepted mount.

On your trip, carry your slides with you—in the tray, if possible. Do not check them with your luggage.

Check with the projectionist early concerning the required projector. If necessary, plan for the time it will take to load a projector tray.

Request a projector with remote control that you can operate from the lectern. Otherwise, have a signal light for the projectionist or arrange some other means of signaling; for instance, provide a copy of the commentary marked to show the slide changes.

Give your slides to the projectionist before the meeting when you will have time to discuss any special instructions. If you wait until just before your talk, the projectionist may be busy with the previous speaker's slides.

Use the slides to supplement and support your oral presentation, not simply to repeat what you are saying.

Request a pointer, if needed.

Consider your audience size in terms of screen size and projector output. As an example, an audience of 400 needs a screen image 8 feet (2.4 m) high.

Meeting planning

D1 □ Meeting planning worksheet

Name or subject of meeting ____

Length of meeting ____

Proposed date ____

Alternate date(s) ____

Expected attendance ____

   Members ____

   Guests ____

   Faculty ____

   Total ____

Number of sleeping rooms ____

Meeting rooms:

	Number	Attendance
General sessions		
Breakout or workshops		

Food functions:

	Number	Attendance
Breakfast		
Luncheon		
Dinner		
Reception		
Coffee break		

Number of exhibits   Scientific ______________________ Commercial ______________________

Proposed location ____

Hotel (first choice) ____

Hotel (alternate) ____

Airport ____

Adequacy of air service ____

Limousine to hotel? ____

Other public transportation ____

D2 □ **Hotel checklist**

Lobby	Yes	No
Attractive	____	____
Clean	____	____
Long lines at check-in counter	____	____
Long lines at cashier	____	____
Furnishings and carpet in good repair	____	____

Elevators	Yes	No
Sufficient number	____	____
In good working order	____	____

Hotel staff	Yes	No
Courteous	____	____
Neatly groomed	____	____
Attentive to customers	____	____
Helpful	____	____

Sleeping rooms	Satis.	Unsatis.
Cleanliness	____	____
Furnishings and drapes	____	____
Size of closets	____	____
Storage space	____	____
Size of vanity	____	____

Coffee shop	Yes	No
Menu standard	____	____
Any interesting or different entrees	____	____
Service pleasant and competent	____	____
Tables cleared promptly	____	____
Long lines for seating	____	____
Order taken promptly	____	____
Food served promptly	____	____
Food attractively served	____	____
Quality of food good	____	____
Prices reasonable	____	____

	Satis.	Unsatis.
Number of towels	____	____
Soundproofing	____	____
Everything in good repair	____	____
Convenience to ice, soft drinks	____	____

Meeting rooms

Name	Size	Ceiling height	Blackout drapes	Projection obstructions

	Yes	No
Sound system available	____	____
Adequate soundproofing	____	____
Convenient control of lights	____	____

	Yes	No
In-house audiovisual staff	____	____
Pad, pencils, and water provided	____	____

D3 □ **Meeting planning checklist**

Function	Time prior to meeting	Function	Time prior to meeting
1. *Determine schedule and requirements for the meeting*	8 months	i. Housing information j. Transportation information	

2. *Contact the hotel sales office*
  a. Determine style of meeting room setup necessary
  b. Figure room capacity desired for projected attendance
	8 months	5. *Plan the miscellaneous*
		  a. Order signs
		  b. Arranging badges
		  c. Ordering badgeholders
		  d. Ordering a bulletin typewriter
			2 months

3. *Budgeting, programming, selection of suppliers*
  a. Brochure printing and mailing
  b. Honoraria and faculty expense
  c. Program printing
  d. Food function expense (breakfast, luncheons, dinners, receptions, coffee breaks—including tax and gratuity)
  e. Ticket printing
  f. Gratuities to outstanding hotel personnel
  g. Bulletin typewriters
  h. Badges and badgeholders
  i. Audiovisual equipment and projectionists
  j. Sound equipment and sound personnel
  k. Telephone
  l. Busing
  m. Signs
  n. Security
  o. Office expenses (postage, photocopying, etc.)
	6-7 months	e. Ordering registration personnel
		  f. Printing a final program
		  g. Handling the faculty or VIP housing
		  h. Determining final room setups for the meeting rooms to be used
		  i. Ordering security
		  j. Obtaining necessary supplies
		  k. Finalizing audiovisual requirements
		  l. Printing tickets
		  m Ordering handouts and brochures from convention bureau	

		6. *Submit final requirements to the hotel*
		  a. Schedule of events
		  b. Room setup requirements and floor plans
		  c. Menu selections
		  d. Coffee breaks
		  e. Hotel posting instructions
		  f. Billing instructions
			1 month

4. *Solicitation mailings and registration*
  a. Dates of meeting
  b. Name of meeting
  c. Location of meeting
  d. Registration fees
  e. Schedule of events
  f. List of speakers
  g. Refund policies
  h. Where to send registration
	3-6 months	7. *Submit final audiovisual requirements to supplier*
		  a. Carousel projectors (35 mm)
		  b. Film projectors (16 mm)
		  c. Screens
		  d. Overhead projectors
		  e. Electric pointer
		  f. Marking pens
		  g. Speaker timer and warning light
		  h. Tape recorders and tapes
		  i. Professional projectionist
		  j. Microphone and sound requirements
			1 month

D4 □ Seating capacity for meeting

Schoolroom style

Room 700 square feet or larger:

$$\frac{\text{Total square feet}}{14} = \text{Occupancy}$$

Room 700 square feet or less:

$$\frac{\text{Total square feet}}{17} = \text{Occupancy}$$

Theater

$$\frac{\text{Total square feet}}{10} = \text{Occupancy}$$

Luncheon or banquet

$$\frac{\text{Total square feet}}{10} = \text{Occupancy}$$

Reception

$$\frac{\text{Total square feet}}{7.5} = \text{Occupancy}$$

D5 □ Function sheet

**American Society of Plastic and Reconstructive Surgeons/
Its Educational Foundation/American Society of Maxillofacial Surgeons**
29 East Madison — Suite 800
Chicago, Illinois 60602
(312) 641-0593

FUNCTION SHEET

HOTEL _______________________________________

Group _______________________________	Date of Function _______________________
_______________________________________	Day of Function ________________________
Contact ______________________________	Room Assigned __________________________
Address ______________________________	Function Begins ______________ Ends __________
_______________________________________	ALL ROOMS SET AND OPEN 1/2 HOUR PRIOR TO START
Telephone (______) __________________	Maximum Count ____________ GUARANTEE ____________

ROOM SETUP PREFERRED
□ Theater   □ Conference
□ Schoolroom   □ U-Shape
□ T-Shape   □ Rounds
□ Stand-up Reception *(Cocktail seating)*
□ Speaker table to seat _______________
□ Table Lectern   □ Floor Lectern
Indicate Number of Mikes Below:
(   ) table   (   ) neck   (   ) lectern   (   ) floor

AUDIOVISUAL EQUIPMENT:
□ ASPRS to order   □ Hotel to order
□ 35mm Projector   □ 16mm Projector
□ Overhead Projector   □ Screen
□ Projectionist — Hours _______________
□ Other _______________________________
____
____

SPECIAL EQUIPMENT:
□ Chalkboard, Chalk and Eraser
□ Pencils   □ Easel   □ Pens
□ 6' tables — number _________________
□ Other _______________________________
____
____
____
____
____
____

BAR SETUP: Bartender □ Hours: _______________
Cash Bar □   Sponsored Bar □
Premium Brands □   House Brands □

MENU SELECTION: Serving time _______________
Tickets collected □ Yes   □ No

Wine Selection _______________________________

COFFEE BREAKS:

TIME	COFFEE	TEA	BANKA	SOFT DRINKS	JUICE	DANISH
______ A.M.						
______ A.M.						
______ P.M.						
______ P.M.						

BILLING INSTRUCTIONS:
□ ASPRS Master Account   □ EF Master Account
□ ASMS Master Account   □ Bill to Above
□ As indicated below:

D6 □ How to select a room for audiovisual program

Room size

Attendance times 7 square feet per person equals square feet for audience times 150% for screen, stage, aisles, etc., equals minimal size of room in square feet.

For example, expected attendance of 300:

$$300 \times 7 = 2100 \times 150\% = 3150 \text{ feet (room size needed)}$$

An exception to this is for groups of 25 to 150, where 70% extra is needed for the stage, aisles, etc.

The chart below gives good guidelines for most meetings:

Audience size	Total square feet
25	400
50	675
75	975
100	1,200
150	1,700
200	2,100
300	3,150
400	4,200
500	5,250
750	7,875
1000	10,500

Screen size

Room length divided by 6 equals suggested screen height plus 5 feet from floor to bottom of screen equals minimum ceiling height.

For example, a room 60 feet long:

$$60 \div 6 = 10 + 5 = 15 \text{ feet (minimum ceiling height)}$$

For lower ceilings divide by 8 instead of 6 and lower the bottom of the screen to 4 feet above the floor.

D7 □ Guidelines for ordering audiovisual equipment for a meeting

2 × 2 inch slide projector: Kodak AF-2 with ELH lamp
Screen: DaLite Picture King Matt White
16 mm projector: Kodak 126TR with DFD 1000 watt lamp
3¼ × 4 inch projector: Beseler Slide King with DDB lamp
Electric pointer: Ednalite 120A
Overhead projector: Beseler VGC 614 with DYS lamp
Screen for above: DaLite with Keystoner Mat White
Video cassette playback: Sony Model VP-1200 or Panasonic Model NV-2110M

Video monitor: Sharp Model XR-2194 or Panasonic Model CT-911V
Video receiver: Sharp Model C-1950 or Sony Trinitron Model KV-1711
Lavalier microphone: Shure 570
Projection stand: Welt Safelock Model 56

This list is far from complete, but it does cover most of the items needed for a meeting. It is important to specify not only the manufacturer but also the model number and especially the projection lamp.

Bibliography

WRITING

American Medical Association: Advice to authors, Chicago, 1964, Scientific Publications Division, American Medical Association.

Albutt, T. C.: Notes on the composition of scientific papers, London, 1923, The Macmillan Co.

Alverez, W. C.: The art of holding the reader's interest, New Physician **10**:66, 1961.

Asher, R.: Six honest serving men for medical writers, J.A.M.A. **208:** 83, 1969.

Baker, S.: The practical stylist, ed. 4, New York, 1977, Thomas Y. Crowwell Co., Inc.

Bean, W. B.: Tower of Babel 1961, Archives of Internal Medicine **108:**4, 1961.

Beatty, W. K.: Searching the literature comes before writing the literature. How clinicians can use the printed bibliographies, tapes and computers, Annals of Internal Medicine **79**(6):917, 1973.

Borgman, D. A.: Language on vacation, New York, 1965, Charles Scribner's Sons.

Brodman, E.: The development of medical bibliography, Baltimore, 1954, Waverly Press, Inc.

Buhler, C. F., McManaway, J. G., and Wroth, L. C.: Standards of bibliographical description, Philadelphia, 1949, University of Pennsylvania Press.

Celnik, M.: Physician's book compendium, New York, 1970, Physician's Book Compendium, Inc.

Chalmers, T. C.: Peer review of manuscripts, New England Journal of Medicine **293**:285, 1977.

Cousins, N.: March's thesaurus dictionary, New York, 1958, Hanover House.

Crow, E. L., Davis, F. A., and Maxfield, M. W.: Statistics manual, New York, 1960, Dover Publications, Inc.

Crichton, M.: Medical obfuscation: structure and function, New England Journal of Medicine **293**:1257, 1975.

Croxton, F. E.: Elementary statistics with applications in medicine and the biological sciences, New York, 1953, Dover Publications, Inc.

Cross, L. M.: The preparation of medical literature, Philadelphia, 1959, J. B. Lippincott Co.

Day, R. L.: Criteria for publication, New England Journal of Medicine **296**:107, 1977.

DeBakey, L.: Rewriting and the by-line: is the author the writer? Surgery **75**:38, 1974.

DeBakey, L., editor: The scientific journal: editorial policies and practices; guidelines for editors, reviewers and authors, St. Louis, 1976, The C. V. Mosby Co.

DeBakey, L.: Up with excellence, J.A.M.A. **228**:1521, 1974.

DeBakey, S.: *Cacoethes scribendi*, The New Physician **10**:75, 1961.

DeBakey, S.: Common types of medical papers, Southern Medical Bulletin **53**:5, 1965.

DeBakey, S.: Some types of medical papers, Southern Medical Journal **52**:1530, 1959.

Devlin, J. M. A.: Dictionary of synonyms and antonyms, Cleveland, 1938, The World Publishing Co.

Dorland's illustrated medical dictionary, ed. 25, Philadelphia, 1974, W. B. Saunders Co.

Douglas, W. I.: Editorial review—peerless pronouncements, New England Journal of Medicine **296**:285, 1977.

Ede, C.: The art of the book, New York, 1951, The Studio Publications.

Evans, B.: Dictionary of quotations, New York, 1968, Delacorte Press.

Fadiman, C.: Reading I've liked, New York, 1941, Simon & Schuster, Inc.

Fishbein, M.: Medical writing, Springfield, Ill., 1972, Charles C Thomas, Publisher.

Fishbein, M.: Medical writing: the technique and art, New York, 1957, McGraw-Hill Book Co.

Fishbein, M.: My greatest teacher—experience, New Physician **10**:66, 1961.

Flesh, R.: The art of readable writing, New York, 1962, Collier Books.

Fowler, W. H.: A dictionary of modern English usage, New York, 1965, Oxford University Press, Inc.

Garland, J.: A fourth estate, New Physician **10**:71, 1961.

Garland, J.: The printed word, Journal of Medical Education **38**:292, 1963.

Gather, E. M., and Cordasco, F.: Research and report writing, New York, 1959, Barnes & Noble Books.

Gibson, W.: Tough, sweet and stuffy, Bloomington, Ind., 1966, Indiana University Press.

Gill, R. S.: Author, publisher, printer complex, Baltimore, 1949, The Williams & Wilkins Co.

Gordon, C.: Writing, revising and editing, New York, 1969, Doubleday & Co., Inc.

Gorn, J.: Style guide, New York, 1973, Simon & Schuster, Inc.

Greenfield, H.: Books—from writer to reader, New York, 1976, Crown Publishers, Inc.

Gregg, A.: For future doctors, Chicago, 1957, University of Chicago Press.

Gross, G.: Editors and editing, New York, 1962, Grosset & Dunlap, Inc.

Guth, H. P.: Words and ideas, Belmont, Texas, 1972, Wadsworth Publishing Co., Inc.

Hamalian, L., and Karl, F. R.: Everything you need to know about grammar, New York, 1978, Fawcett Books Group.

Healy, J. B.: Why Do You Write? Lancet **1**:204, 1976.

Hendin, D.: Medical writing, J.A.M.A. **228**:290, 1974.

Hewitt, R. M.: The physician-writer's book: tricks of the trade of medical writing, Philadelphia, 1957, W. B. Saunders Co.

Hewitt, R. M.: Opinions and convictions, some crochety, ingrained or abandoned, New Physician **10**:79, 1961.

Hirschman, J. V.: Sounding board, Medical References, Vol. 299, No. 5, 1978.

Hubbell, G. S.: Writing term papers and reports, New York, 1959, Barnes & Noble Books.

Hull, H.: The writer's book, New York, 1960, Barnes & Noble Books.

Hussey, H.: Medical jargon, J.A.M.A. **235**:1149, 1976.

Hussey, H.: Medical writings: Faults, J.A.M.A. **235**:2327, 1976.

Huth, E. J.: How to judge reliability, Medical Communications **3**:18, 1974.

Inglefinger, F. J.: Criteria for publication, New England Journal of Medicine **292**:107, 1977.

Inglefinger, F. J.: Obfuscation in medical writing, New England Journal of Medicine **293**:1257, 1975.

Inglefinger, F. J.: Peer review in biomedical publication, American Journal of Medicine **56**:686, 1974.

Inglefinger, F. J.: Why the first report is unacceptable, New England Journal of Medicine **290**:740, 1974.

Inglefinger, F. J.: Writing scientific papers in English, New England Journal of Medicine **293**:95, 1975.

Jung, F. T.: What to do about clinical jargon, New Physician **12**:97, 1963.

Kampmeier, R. H.: Instructions to the author, Southern Medical Bulletin **53**:43, 1965.

Kampmeier, R. H.: A word about bibliographic references, Southern Medical Bulletin **53**:53, 1965.

Kelly, A. D.: *Verbum sapiendibus*. Canadian Medical Association Journal **111**:650, 1974.

King, L. S.: Why not say it clearly? A guide to scientific writing, Boston, 1978, Little, Brown & Co.

King, L. S., and Roland, C. G.: Scientific writing, Chicago, 1968, American Medical Association.

Kuehn, H. R.: Resuscitating the medical paper, J.A.M.A. **226**:452, 1973.

Legett, G., Mead, C. D., and Charvat, W.: Prentice-Hall handbook for writers, Englewood Cliffs, N.J., 1965, Prentice-Hall, Inc.

Locke, S.: Thorne's better medical writing, New York, 1977, John Wiley & Sons, Inc.

Manual of style, ed. 12, Chicago, 1969, University of Chicago Press.

Medical writing (a group of four papers), New York, 1955, M.D. Publications, Inc.

Mellis-Wilson, M.: The writing of medical papers, Philadelphia, 1929, W. B. Saunders Co.

Menszel, D. H., Jones, H. M., and Boyd, L. G.: Writing a technical paper, New York, 1961, McGraw-Hill Book Co.

Morehead, P. D.: Roget's thesaurus in dictionary form, New York, 1978, New American Library, Inc.

Murphy, R.: How and where to look it up, New York, 1958, McGraw-Hill Book Co.

Nelms, H.: Thinking with a pencil, New York, 1964, Barnes & Noble Books.

Newman, E.: A civil tongue, Indianapolis, 1975, The Bobbs-Merrill Co., Inc.

Notable medical books, Indianapolis, 1976, Ely Lilly Research Laboratories.

O'Connor, M., and Woodford, E. P.: Writing scientific papers in English, Amsterdam, 1975, Associated Scientific Publishers.

Odessky, M. D.: Scotch with figures, New England Journal of Medicine **290**:636, 1974.

Pei, M.: Weasel words, the art of saying what you don't mean, New York, 1978, Harper & Row Publishers, Inc.

Peterson, M. S.: Scientific thinking and scientific writing, New York, 1959, Barnes & Noble, Books.

Reveno, W. S.: 711 medical maxims, Springfield, Ill., 1951, Charles C Thomas, Publisher.

Roland, C. G.: Pruning your hedges, Anesthesia and Analgesia **53**:200, 1974.

Roland, C. G.: The fallible referee, Medical Communications **3**:11, 1974.

Roland, C. G.: Thoughts about medical writing—crooked thinking, Anesthesia and Analgesia **54**:540, 1975.

Roland, C. G.: Thoughts about medical writing—learning from the ads, Anesthesia and Analgesia **53**:592, 1974.

Roland, C. G.: Thoughts about medical writing—the numbers game, Anesthesia and Analgesia **52**:1015, 1973.

Rondthaler, E.: Alphabet thesarus, New York, 1965, Reinhold Publishing Co.

Roth, A. J., and Altschuler, T. C.: Writing step by step, Boston, 1969, Houghton Mifflin Co.

Sallamder, H.: Bibliotheca Walleriana, Stockholm, 1955, Almquist and Wiksell.

Schullian, D. M., and Sommer, F. E.: A catalogue of incunabula and manuscripts in the Army Medical Library, New York, Henry Schuman, Inc.

Shepard, D. A. E.: The parts of a scientific paper, Medical Communications **3**:22, 1975.

Shindell, S.: Statistics, science and sense, J.A.M.A. **186**:449; **186**:570; **186**:637; **186**:780; **186**:849, 1963.

Shipley, J. T.: Dictionary of word origins, Ames, Iowa, 1959, Littlefield, Adams Co.

Shurter, R. L.: Handy grammar reference, New York, 1959, McGraw-Hill Book Co.

Shuster, J. J.: Statistical review process, J.A.M.A. **235**:534, 1976.

Siegel, I. M.: Games authors play, Lancet **2**:733, 1977.

Silverman, G.: Why do you write? Lancet **1**:364, 1973.

Simmons, G. H., and Fishbein, M.: The art and practice of medical writing, Chicago, 1925, American Medical Association.

Skeat, W. W.: A concise etymological dictionary of the English language, Oxford, 1958, Oxford University Press.

Snively, W. D., Jr.: Prolixity: Its nature and treatment, New Physician **10**:77, 1961.

Snively, W. D., Jr.: With the pen of an angel, Southern Medical Bulletin **53**:11, 1965.

Soffer, A., and Weinberg, S.: Clinician, teacher, investigator—can a specialty journal serve all? Chest **67**:507, 1975.

Soffer, A., and Weinberg, S.: Editorials, review and case reports, Chest **67**:254, 1975.

Soffer, A., and Weinberg, S.: Flexibility in medical writing, Chest **67**:5, 1975.

Soffer, A., and Weinberg, S.: On the content and purpose of a journal, Heart and Lung **3**:889, 1974.

Stedman's medical dictionary, ed. 22, Baltimore, 1972, Williams & Wilkins Co.

Strauss, M. B.: Familiar medical quotations, Boston, 1968, Little, Brown & Co.

Strunk, W., Jr., and White, E. B.: The elements of style, New York, 1972, Macmillan Publishing Co., Inc.

Sturtevant, E. H.: The linguistic change, Chicago, 1962, University of Chicago Press.

Stylebook/Editorial Manual of the AMA, Scientific Publications Division, American Medical Association, Littleton, Mass., 1976, Publishing Sciences Group, Inc.

Swinscow, T. D. V.: Numerical results: some hints on presentation, British Medical Journal **2**:1120, 1976.

Thomas, P. E. L.: A guide for authors, Springfield, Ill., 1951, Charles C Thomas, Publisher.

Thorne, C.: Better medical writing, London, 1970, Pitman Medical.

Thurber, J.: The psychosemanticist will see you now, Mr. Thurber, Science 123:705, 1968.

Urmson, J. O.: How to do things with words, Boston, 1962, Harvard University Press.

Wain, H.: The story behind the word (some interesting origins of medical words), Springfield, Ill., 1958, Charles C Thomas, Publisher.

Warren, R.: The abstract, Archives of Surgery 111:635, 1976.

Warriner, J. E., Whitten, M. E., and Griffith, F.: English grammar and composition, New York, 1977, Harcourt Brace Jovanovich, Inc.

Watanakunakom, C.: How to stop duplicate publication, New England Journal of Medicine 14:726, 1975.

Webster's new collegiate dictionary, Springfield, Mass., 1979, G. & C. Merriam Co.

Webster's new dictionary of synonyms, Springfield, Mass., 1978, G. & C. Merriam Co.

Wilson, P. L.: Medical publishing: an editor's viewpoint, Medical Communications 6:9, 1978.

Zollinger, R. M., Pace, W. C., and Kiensel, G. J.: Practical outline for preparing medical papers and talks, New York, 1961, The Macmillan Co.

SPEAKING

Flesch, R.: The art of plain talk, New York, 1951, Collier Books.

Fluharty, G. W., and Ross, H. R.: Public speaking, New York, 1966, Barnes & Noble Books.

Hayes, H. L.: Physicians can speak with impact: impressiveness in delivery at the medical convention, Southern Medical Bulletin 53:38, 1965.

Hofer, W.: How to give a dull speech, Association Management, Sept., 1975, p. 71.

Kern, R.: Editorial: how to present a scientific paper before a large audience, Annals of Internal Medicine 37:618, 1952.

Lam, C. R.: Speaking before medical groups, Review of Surgery, Vol. 21, No. 6, Nov.-Dec. 1964. Reprinted in Bulletin of the American College of Surgeons 62:20, 1977.

Ott, J.: How to write and deliver a speech, New York, 1976, Cornerstone Library, Inc.

Prochnow, H. V.: The successful speaker's handbook, Englewood Cliffs, N.J., 1951, Prentice-Hall, Inc.

Roper, R.: Improve your speeches by listening to yourself, Association Management, July 1974, p. 100.

Shefter, H.: How to prepare talks and oral reports, New York, 1977, Pocket Books.

Write better, speak better, Pleasantville, N.Y., 1972, Reader's Digest Association.

Zenker, A.: Plain speaking, Boston, 1976, Arnold Zenker Associates.

Zenker, A.: Television—the spectacular machine, Boston, 1976, Arnold Zenker Associates.

Zenker, A.: Toward a better sound, Boston, 1976, Arnold Zenker Associates.

VISUAL AIDS
Correlation of visuals with the manuscript

Audiovisual planning equipment; Kodak Publication S-11, Rochester, N.Y., 1979, Eastman Kodak Co.

Bauer, E., Effective lecture slides, Successful Meetings, Jan. 1976.

Bauer, E.: Improve image quality, Successful Meetings, Feb. 1976.

Bauer, E.: My slides looked terrible, Successful Meetings, Sept. 1974.

Effective lecture slides, Kodak Publication S-22, Rochester, N.Y., 1977, Eastman Kodak Co.

Materials for visual planning and preparation, Kodak Publication S-13, Rochester, N.Y., 1978, Eastman Kodak C.

Planning and producing slide programs, Kodak Publication S-30, Rochester, N.Y., 1975, Eastman Kodak Co.

Ross, D. G.: Selection of visuals to accompany scientific papers, Southern Medical Bulletin 53:22, 1965.

Sheppard, R.: Tips for better slide shows, Petersen's Photographic 7:34, 1978.

Graphics

Basic printing methods, Rochester, N.Y., 1976, Eastman Kodak Co.

Bauer, E.: Effective lecture slides, Successful Meetings, Jan. 1976.

Bauer, E.: Improve image quality, Successful Meetings, Feb. 1976.

Cardamone, T.: Advertising agency and studio skills, New York, 1970, Watson-Guptill Publications.

Copy Preparation, Rochester, N.Y., 1979, Eastman Kodak Co.

Craig, J.: Designing with type, a basic course in typography, New York, 1971, Watson-Guptill Publications.

Cogoli, J. E.: Photo offset fundamentals, Bloomington, Ill., 1973, McKnight Publishing Co.

Effective lecture slides, Kodak Publication S-22, Rochester, N.Y., 1900, Eastman Kodak Co.

Graphic design, Rochester, N.Y., 1976, Eastman Kodak Co.

Gray, B.: Studio tips for artists and graphic designers, New York, 1976, Van Nostrand Reinhold Co.

Hofmann, A.: Graphic design manual, New York, 1965, Van Nostrand Reinhold Co.

Hurley, G. D., and McDougal, A.: Visual impact in print, Chicago, 1971, American Publishers Press.

Legibility—artwork to screen, Kodak Publication S-24, Rochester, N.Y., 1977, Eastman Kodak Co.

Material for visual presentation, Kodak Publication S-13, Rochester, N.Y., 1978, Eastman Kodak Co.

Mayer, R.: The artist's handbook of materials and techniques, New York, 1970, Viking Press.

Reverse text slides, Kodak Publication S-26, Rochester, N.Y., 1977, Eastman Kodak Co.

Snyder, J.: The commercial artist's handbook, New York, 1973, Watson-Guptill Publications.

Stone, B., and Eckstein, A.: Preparing art for printing, New York, 1965, Van Nostrand Reinhold Co.

vanUchelen, R.: Paste-up, New York, 1976, Van Nostrand Reinhold Co.

Zollinger, R.: Next slide please—a good one, American Journal of Surgery 138:398, 1979.

Illustration

Cullen, T. S.: Max Brodel, 1870-1941, Director of the First Department of Art as Applied to Medicine in the World, Bulletin of the Medical Library Association 33:27, 1945.

Demarest, R. J.: Publishers comment, Journal of Biocommunications, vol. 5, 1978.

Diner, J.: Medical art in the courtroom, Journal of the Association of Medical Illustrators 15:21, 1964.

Diner, J.: Medical illustration in the court of law, Journal of the Association of Medical Illustrators 14:21, 1963.

Dusseau, J. L.: The publisher's responsibility to author and artist, Journal of the Association of Medical Illustrators 17:11, 1966.

Holden, C. G.: Visually speaking, Journal of the Association of Medical Illustrators 13:9, 1961.

Holt, C.: Teamwork of medical illustrator and physician, Journal of the Association of Medical Illustrators 19:13, 1970.

Lieberman, J.: A.V. Communication, the constant renewal, Journal of the Association of Medical Illustrators 18:5, 1967.

Loomis, A.: Drawing the head and hands, New York, 1956, Viking Press.

Markowitz, J., Archibald, J., and Downie, H. G.: Experimental surgery (preface), Baltimore, 1964, The Williams & Wilkins Co.

Netter, F.: Cited in Melloni, B.: Frank Netter, Dean of American Medical Illustrators, Visual Medicine 1:38, 1966.

Osburn, W. A.: Editorial, Journal of the Association of Medical Illustrators 16:17, 1965.

Ross, D. G.: Psychology of color preference in projection slides, Journal of the Association of Medical Illustrators 16:13, 1965.

Photography

Bailey, A., and Holloway, A.: The book of color photograpy, New York, 1979, Alfred A. Knopf, Inc.

Beginning creative photography for graphic communication, Kodak Publication GA 11-3, Rochester, N.Y., 1978, Eastman Kodak Co.

Boas, K.: Techniques for innovative slide copying, Kodak Publication AE-111, the eleventh Here's How, Rochester, N.Y., 1979, Eastman Kodak Co.

Chapple, J. G., and Stephenson, K. L.: Photographic misrepresentation, Plastic and Reconstructive Surgery 45:135, 1970.

Clinical photography, Kodak Publication N-3, Rochester, N.Y., 1972, Eastman Kodak Co.

Cornfield, J.: Electronic flash photograpy, Los Angeles, 1976, Petersen Publishing Co.

Dickason, W., and Hann, D. D.: Pitfalls in comparative photography in plastic and reconstructive surgery, Plastic and Reconstructive Surgery 58:166, 1976.

Edgerton, M. T., McKnelly, L. O., and Wolfort, F. G.: Operating room photography for the plastic surgeon, Plastic and Reconstructive Surgery 46:93, 1970.

Filters and lens attachments, Kodak Photo Book AB-1, Rochester, N.Y., 1975, Eastman Kodak Co.

Hedgcoe, J.: Pocket guide to practical photography, New York, 1979, Simon & Schuster, Inc.

Hedgcoe, J.: The art of color photography, New York, 1978, Simon & Schuster, Inc.

Hedgcoe, J.: The book of photography, New York, 1976, Alfred A. Knopf, Inc.

Hedgcoe, J.: The photographer's handbook, New York, 1978, Alfred A. Knopf, Inc.

Helprin, B.: Photolighting techniques, Los Angeles, 1973, Petersen Publishing Co.

Karlan, M. S.: Photographic documentation techniques, Ear, Nose and Throat Journal 58:21, 1979.

Kenny, M. F., and Schmitt, R. F.: Images, images, images,—the book of programmed multi-image production, Kodak Publication S-12, Rochester, N.Y., 1979, Eastman Kodak Co.

Kodak color films, Kodak Data Book E-77, Rochester, N.Y., 1977, Eastman Kodak Co.

Kodak filters for scientific and technical uses, Kodak Publication B-3, Rochester, N.Y., 1973, Eastman Kodak Co.

Lahue, K. C.: Telephoto photography, Los Angeles, 1977, Petersen Publishing Co.

Langford, M.: The step-by-step guide to photography, New York, 1978, Alfred A.Knopf, Inc.

London, B.: A short course in Canon photography, Somerville, Mass., 1979, Curtin and London, Inc.

McComb, S. J.: The preparation of photographic prints for publication, Springfield, Ill., 1950, Charles C Thomas, Publisher.

Morell, D. C., Converse, J. M., and Allen, D.: Making uniform photographic records in plastic surgery, Plastic and Reconstructive Surgery 59:366, 1977.

Owens, W. J.: Close-up photograpy, Los Angeles, 1975, Petersen Publishing Co.

Photography and layout for publication, Kodak Publication Q-74, Rochester, N.Y., 1978, Eastman Kodak Co.

Reverse text slides, Kodak Publication S-26, Rochester, N.Y., 1978, Eastman Kodak Co.

Rothchild, N.: Macro teleconverters, Popular Photography 86:112, 1980.

Sealfon, P.: All about automation, Petersen's Photographic 7:33, 1979.

Shipman, C.: How to select and use Canon SLR cameras, Tucson, Ariz., 1979, Fisher Publishing Co.

Shipman, C.: How to select and use Nikon SLR cameras, Tucson, Ariz., 1979, Fisher Publishing Co.

Shipman, C.: How to select and use Olympus SLR cameras, Tucson, Ariz., 1979, Fisher Publishing Co.

Shipman, C.: How to select and use Pentax SLR cameras, Tucson, Ariz., 1979, Fisher Publishing Co.

Shipman, C.: SLR photographer's handbook, Tucson, Ariz., 1977, Fisher Publishing Co.

Simple copying techniques, Kodak Publication S-40, Rochester, N.Y., 1978, Eastman Kodak Co.

Stensvold, M.: Photo filters, Los Angeles, 1976, Petersen Publishing Co.

Strobel, L., and Todd, H. N.: Dictionary of contemporary photography, Dobbs Ferry, N.Y., 1974, Morgan & Morgan, Inc.

The camera, New York, 1970, Time-Life Books.

The joy of photography, Rochester, N.Y., 1979, Eastman Kodak Co.

Sound-slide presentations

Effective lecture slides, Kodak Publication S-22, Rochester, N.Y., Eastman Kodak Co.

Legibility—artwork to screen, Kodak Publication S-24, Rochester, N.Y., Eastman Kodak Co.

Lord, J., and Pett, D.: Effective presentations, Bloomington, Ind., Indiana University Press.

Planning a slide talk, Kodak Publication P-100-4, Rochester, N.Y., Eastman Kodak Co.

Planning and producing slide programs, Rochester, N.Y., Eastman Kodak Co.

Audio-visual projection

Bauer, E.: How to select a room for A.V., Successful Meetings, Nov., 1974.

Bauer, E.: How to order equipment Successful Meetings, July 1976.

Bauer, E.: Nine factors affect your screen, Successful Meetings, Oct. 1974.

Bauer, E.: Seeing vs interpreting, Part I, Successful Meetings, Sept. 1976.

Bauer, E.: Seeing vs interpreting, Part II, Successful Meetings, Oct. 1976.

Bauer, E.: Speaker A.V. guidelines, Successful Meetings, Oct. 1975.

Bauer, E.: Speakers should be ready to go, Successful Meetings, Sept. 1977.

MEETING PLANNING

Convention liaison manual, ed. 3, by the editors of Successful Meetings Magazine in cooperation with the Convention Liaison Council Editorial Committee. Published by the Convention Liaison Council, 1980.

Making your convention more effective, Washington, D.C., 1972, American Society of Association Executives.

Index